E. JAMES POTCHEN, M.D., *Consulting Editor*

Professor and Chairman
Department of Radiology
Michigan State University
East Lansing, Michigan

Published

GASTROINTESTINAL ANGIOGRAPHY

Stewart R. Reuter, M.D., and Helen C. Redman, M.D.

THE RADIOLOGY OF JOINT DISEASE

D. M. Forrester, M.D., and John W. Nesson, M.D.

RADIOLOGY OF THE PANCREAS AND DUODENUM

S. Boyd Eaton, Jr., M.D., and Joseph T. Ferrucci, Jr., M.D.

THE HAND IN RADIOLOGIC DIAGNOSIS

Andrew K. Poznanski, M.D.

RADIOLOGY OF THE ILEOCECAL AREA

Robert N. Berk, M.D., and Elliot C. Lasser, M.D.

FUNDAMENTALS OF ABDOMINAL AND PELVIC ULTRASONOGRAPHY

George R. Leopold, M.D., and W. Michael Asher, M.D.

RADIOLOGY OF THE ORBIT

G. A. S. Lloyd, B.M., B.Ch.Oxf., F.F.R., D.M.R.D.

Forthcoming Monographs

RADIOLOGIC DIAGNOSIS OF RENAL PARENCHYMAL DISEASE

Alan J. Davidson, M.D.

THE RADIOLOGY OF RENAL FAILURE

Harry J. Griffiths, M.D.

THE RADIOLOGY OF VERTEBRAL TRAUMA

John A. Gehweiler, Jr., M.D., Raymond L. Osborne, Jr., M.D., and R. Frederick Becker, Ph.D.

PEDIATRIC RADIOLOGY OF THE ALIMENTARY TRACT

Edward B. Singleton, M.D., Milton L. Wagner, M.D., and Robert V. Dutton, M.D.

ARTHROGRAPHY: PRINCIPLES AND TECHNIQUES

Tom W. Staple, M.D.

CLINICAL PEDIATRIC AND ADOLESCENT UROGRAPHY

Alfred L. Weber, M.D., and Richard C. Pfister, M.D.

CORONARY ARTERIOGRAPHY

Lewis Wexler, M.D., and Ivo Obrez, M.D.

RADIOLOGY OF THE GALLBLADDER AND BILE DUCTS

Robert N. Berk, M.D., and Arthur R. Clemett, M.D.

RADIOLOGY OF THE LIVER

James McNulty, M.B., F.F.R.

Volume 8 in the Series
SAUNDERS
MONOGRAPHS
IN CLINICAL
RADIOLOGY

SPECIAL PROCEDURES IN CHEST RADIOLOGY

STUART S. SAGEL, M.D.
Associate Professor
Mallinckrodt Institute of Radiology
Washington University School of Medicine
St. Louis, Missouri

1976

W. B. SAUNDERS COMPANY • Philadelphia • London • Toronto

W. B. Saunders Company: West Washington Square
Philadelphia, PA 19105

12 Dyott Street
London, WC1A 1DB

833 Oxford Street
Toronto, Ontario M8Z 5T9, Canada

Library of Congress Cataloging in Publication Data

Sagel, Stuart S

Special procedures in chest radiology.

(Saunders monographs in clinical radiology; v. 9)

Includes index.

1. Chest—Radiography. I. Title. [DNLM: 1. Thoracic radiography—Methods. WF975 S741]

RC941.S24 617'.54'07572 75-19855

ISBN 0-7216-7897-1

Special Procedures in Chest Radiology ISBN 0-7216-7897-1

Last digit is the print number: 9 8 7 6 5 4 3 2 1

DEDICATION

to

Beverlee
and to
Scott, Darryl and Brett

CONTRIBUTORS

JOHN H.M. AUSTIN, M.D.

Assistant Professor of Clinical Radiology
Columbia-Presbyterian Medical Center, New York, New York

JOHN V. FORREST, M.D.

Associate Professor of Radiology
Mallinckrodt Institute of Radiology
Washington University School of Medicine, St. Louis, Missouri

ROBERT C. McKNIGHT, M.D.

Assistant Professor of Radiology
Mallinckrodt Institute of Radiology
Washington University School of Medicine, St. Louis, Missouri

STUART S. SAGEL, M.D.

Associate Professor of Radiology
Mallinckrodt Institute of Radiology
Washington University School of Medicine, St. Louis, Missouri

ROGER H. SECKER-WALKER, M.B., M.R.C.P.

Associate Professor of Medicine and Physiology
St. Louis University School of Medicine, St. Louis, Missouri

GARY D. SHACKELFORD, M.D.

Assistant Professor of Radiology
Mallinckrodt Institute of Radiology
Washington University School of Medicine, St. Louis, Missouri

ALLAN L. SIMON, M.D.

Professor of Diagnostic Radiology
Yale-New Haven Medical Center, New Haven, Connecticut

EDITOR'S FOREWORD

"Specialized knowledge will do a man no harm if he has common sense, but if he lacks this, it can only make him more dangerous to his patients."

Oliver Wendell Holmes

Chest x-ray interpretation represents some 35 per cent of the practice of diagnostic radiology. How often these films lead to recommendations for further diagnostic procedures in the chest is not known. However, it is apparent that there is an increasing array of diagnostic modalities available to further pursue abnormalities detected on the plain radiograph. As experience is gained in applying a wide variety of techniques to the diagnosis of lung disease, there is a need for a widespread appreciation of the relative merits of alternative diagnostic approaches. The indications for using tomography, bronchography, needle biopsy, bronchial brushing, pulmonary angiography, or even oblique films and high kv techniques have been the subject of considerable controversy.

With newer diagnostic methods moving from the centers of radiologic research to the clinical practice of radiology, more widespread appreciation of these methods, their realistic application, and potential misuse becomes increasingly important. Some, such as bronchography, have been shown to have less efficacy than their current use would suggest. Others, needle biopsy for example, have demonstrated promise as diagnostic techniques which can obviate the need for more radical diagnostic intervention, e.g., thoracotomy. Thus, it is timely to compile the available evidence, clarify the methodology, and disseminate the state of the art.

Stuart Sagel received his radiology training at Yale University and the University of California in San Francisco. He has risen to eminence as a chest radiologist at the Mallinckrodt Institute of Radiology, where he is currently co-director of the chest division. There he has developed a leading program to further the application of newer technologies in the diagnosis of chest disease. For this ninth volume of the Saunders Monographs in Clinical Radiology, Dr. Sagel has brought together several distinguished radiologists and chest physicians. Many of this group owe their radiologic lineage to the teachings of Dr. Richard Greenspan of Yale University, who has been a leader in advocating appropriate applications of new technology in the diagnosis of chest disease. Indeed, Dr. Greenspan has been responsible for much of the thought and innovation that are leading these young radiologists to new horizons in chest diagnosis.

It is with considerable enthusiasm that I welcome this book to the Saunders Monographs in Clinical Radiology and recommend it to every practicing radiologist and physician concerned with the care of patients with chest disease.

E. JAMES POTCHEN, M.D.

PREFACE

Although plain films of the chest are the most common examination in radiology, the use of adjuvant radiologic procedures in chest diagnosis has received relatively little attention. Two superb texts[1,2] are available depicting the role of the chest radiograph in clinical diagnosis, but the exact function of the ancillary diagnostic methods is not examined in depth. This monograph describes the complementary and supplementary roles of these techniques to the plain chest radiograph, also comparing them to other non-radiologic diagnostic methods; which technique to use, when, and why is scrutinized.

The monograph is intended to be useful for the radiologist both in clinical practice and in training, and the pragmatic and feasible is stressed. Some procedures, such as bronchial arteriography or azygography, considered to be of questionable clinical value, are not discussed. Research material or technical factors beyond practical application have not been included. Guidelines for the application of these special procedures are provided, but it is obvious that available time, equipment, and personal experience will modify the evaluation of any particular chest abnormality. Needle aspiration biopsy requires an experienced cytologist for completion of the study. Similar limitations apply to other procedures described in this book, and the individual radiologist must decide which procedure best meets the patient's needs in a given circumstance. Also, the radiologic equipment utilized for many of the special procedures will be dictated by what is available. Most of the special roentgenographic and fluoroscopic chest examinations in our department are done in a single room, equipped with a fluoroscopic unit that has an over-the-table x-ray tube and an under-the-table cesium iodide image intensifier. The radiographic table has tilting capabilities, and the fluoroscopic image is displayed on a television monitor with image inverting capabilities. Tomography and angiography are easily performed in the same location, and this equipment permits great flexibility in patient positioning and facilitates a wide variety of film formats.

Undoubtedly, this book will be iconoclastic to many older radiologists. As the practice of medicine has undergone revolutionary changes in recent years, so has radiology. Newer diagnostic modalities have greatly reduced the need for some older radiologic techniques. Attention is directed toward the need to abandon unproductive special radiologic examinations and to establish criteria for use as definitively as possible. Tomography and bronchography are techniques greatly over-utilized in most institutions. Neither provides a conclusive tissue diagnosis upon which therapy can be based, and their use should be restricted to specific circumstances rather than for every undiagnosed pulmonary lesion. While needle aspiration biopsy or bronchial brushing require more expertise and are potentially hazardous, in many patients they can provide the final and often only significant information about a lung lesion.

1. Fraser, R. G. and Paré, J. A. P.: Diagnosis of Diseases of the Chest. Philadelphia, W. B. Saunders Company, 1970.
2. Felson, B.: Chest Roentgenology. Philadelphia, W. B. Saunders Company, 1973.

STUART S. SAGEL, M.D.

ACKNOWLEDGMENTS

The following is a list of friends and colleagues who graciously offered their advice and constructive criticism to the authors in the preparation of this monograph:

Kristin Bergfeld	William McAlister
R. Edward Coleman	Heber McMahon
Kent Ellis	Harry Morgan
Norman Hente	Charles E. Putman
Laura Klonis	S. David Rockoff
Michael Kyriakos	Robert Scheible

Special indebtedness is owed to my associate, Jack Forrest, who constantly counseled me and generously assumed added clinical burden while I was preparing the book. Gratitude is also extended to my secretary, Ann Brock, for her continuous help and patience in typing the manuscript and checking the reference listings.

My thanks and appreciation are given to Dr. E. James Potchen, Consulting Editor of the Saunders Monographs in Clinical Radiology, and to Mr. Jack Hanley, Medical Editor of the W. B. Saunders Company, for the opportunity to produce this monograph and for their support and encouragement throughout its preparation.

Finally, I would like to acknowledge the huge debt of gratitude most of the authors owe to Richard H. Greenspan, who has guided and stimulated us through training and friendship over many years.

STUART S. SAGEL, M.D.

CONTENTS

Chapter 1

TOMOGRAPHY

by John H. M. Austin, M.D., and Stuart S. Sagel, M.D.

Properly applied, tomography can be of great assistance in the diagnostic management of patients with chest diseases. When the findings on plain chest roentgenograms are in question, tomography is advantageous as a non-invasive procedure which can provide information of three major types:

1. Improved characterization of ill-defined or complex densities.
2. Improved demonstration of the site or sites of disease.
3. Occasional demonstration of disease unsuspected or minimally suspected on the basis of plain radiographs.

In selecting patients for tomography, the physician must be mindful of certain disadvantages of the procedure. Tomography does not provide tissue for cytologic, histologic, or bacteriologic examination. In most patients whose plain chest radiographs show an obvious pulmonary mass, diagnostic procedures which provide tissue (e.g., cytologic examination of sputum or needle aspiration biopsy) are preferable, simply because those procedures often yield a definitive diagnosis. Furthermore, although the average radiation dose to the skin is only about 50 mrads per tomographic exposure, the potentially harmful effects of any examination involving radiation may not be negligible. Finally, tomography is relatively costly for the patient and time consuming for the radiographer and radiologist. In appropriate patients, however, the benefits of the technique eclipse these limitations, because the anatomic and pathological information that tomography provides may be invaluable in clinical management. In this chapter, we review the nature of this information and the role of the radiologist in the technical performance of the tomographic examination.

IMPROVED DEMONSTRATION OF THE CHARACTER OF A LESION

Because tomography limits radiographic focus to tissues in a single plane, it may greatly assist in the demonstration of densities which on plain chest radiographs are complex or ill-defined. Certain common examples of the improved characterization provided by tomography are worthy of detailed attention: calcification in a nodule or mass, cavitation, hilar and airway mass lesions, dilated bronchi, and certain vascular abnormalities.

CALCIFICATION AND THE SOLITARY NODULE IN THE LUNG. If the radiologist questions the presence or absence of calcification in a pulmonary nodule, tomography usually can resolve the question. To detect calcification, a critical technical consideration is radiographic kilovoltage, because x-rays demonstrate calcification best at low kilovoltage levels in the diagnostic x-ray range.[9] Often, however, contemporary plain chest radiography employs relatively high levels of kilovoltage (120–150 kVp). Therefore, plain chest roentgenograms or fluoroscopic spot films exposed at low kilovoltage levels occasionally demonstrate calcification sufficiently well that tomography becomes unnecessary. As a rule, if calcification is not suggested on technically adequate, low kilovoltage roentgenograms, then it is unlikely that it will be demonstrated by tomography.

Calcification in granulomas is usually central (Fig. 1–1). If a well circumscribed, solitary, pulmonary nodule contains laminated or central calcification, then the appearance is diagnostic of granuloma.[6] If a well circumscribed nodule contains central calcification which is solid, stippled, or slightly inhomogeneous, then the lesion is

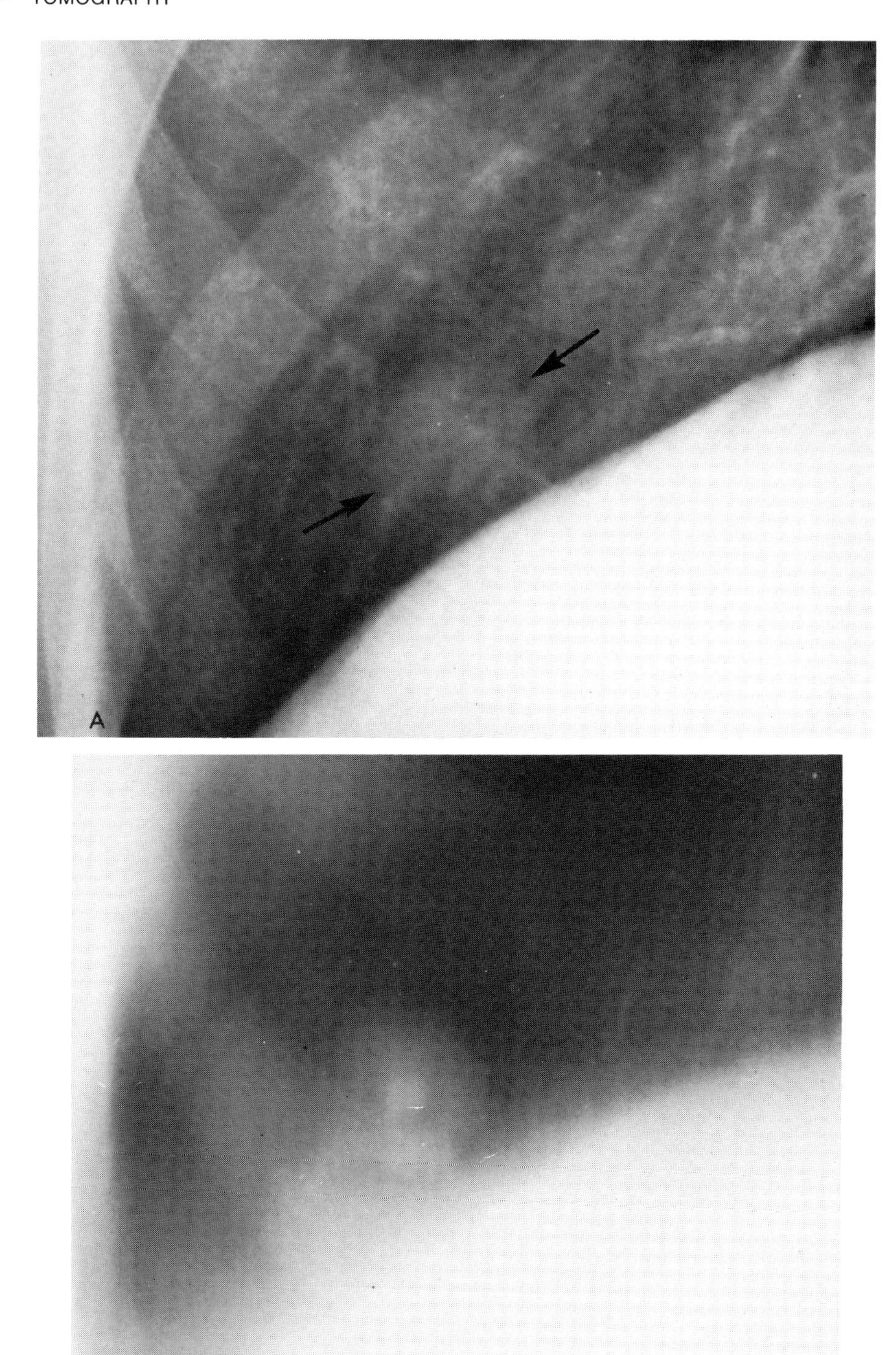

Figure 1–1. Tomographic characterization of a "coin" lesion. *A.* Detail of right lung base, posteroanterior roentgenograms, in a 58 year old man. A poorly defined nodule is present (arrows). *B.* Frontal tomogram demonstrates central calcification in a well circumscribed nodule. The lesion may confidently be interpreted as benign. (From Forrest, John V., and Sagel S.: Special procedures in pulmonary radiology. *In* Potchen, E. James, editor: Current Concepts in Radiology, vol. 2, St. Louis, 1975, The C. V. Mosby Co.)

benign and either a granuloma or hamartoma.[5, 15] If calcification is eccentric within a nodule, however, the diagnosis of benign disease must be questioned, because a carcinoma may rarely engulf or be adjacent to a calcified granuloma (Fig. 1–2). The occasional tomographic finding of inhomogeneity in density of a non-calcified, sol-

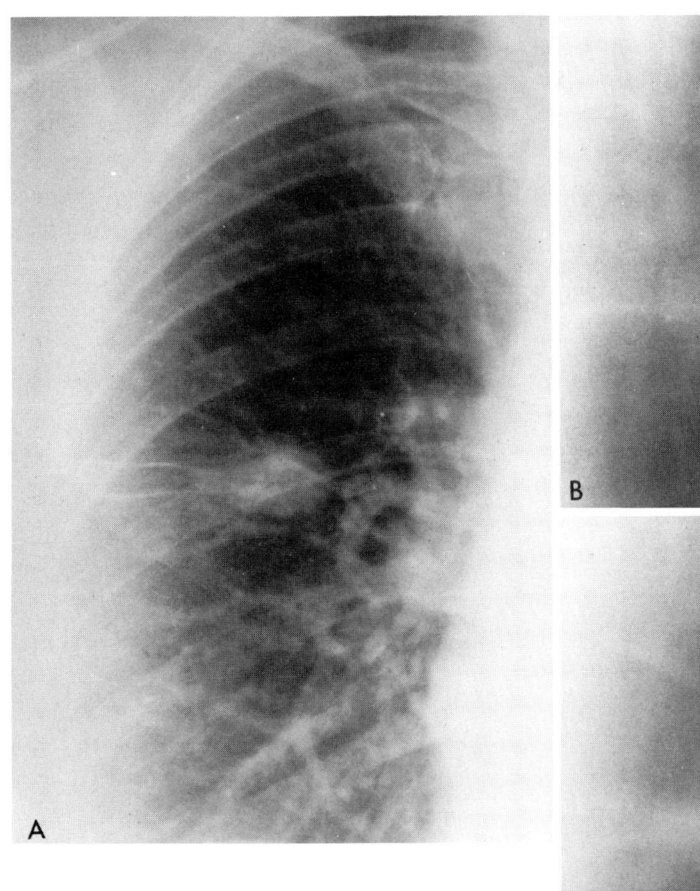

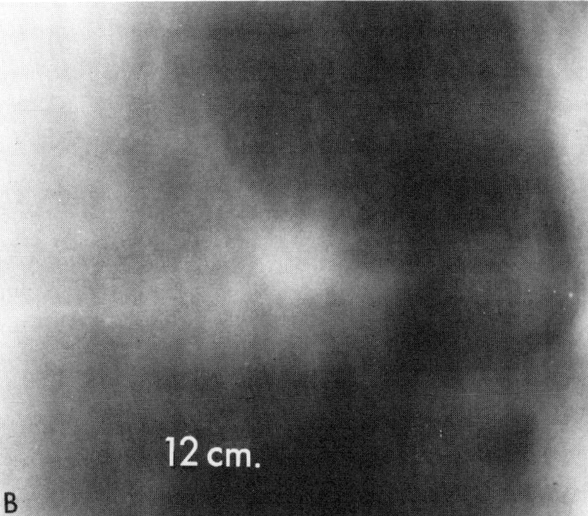

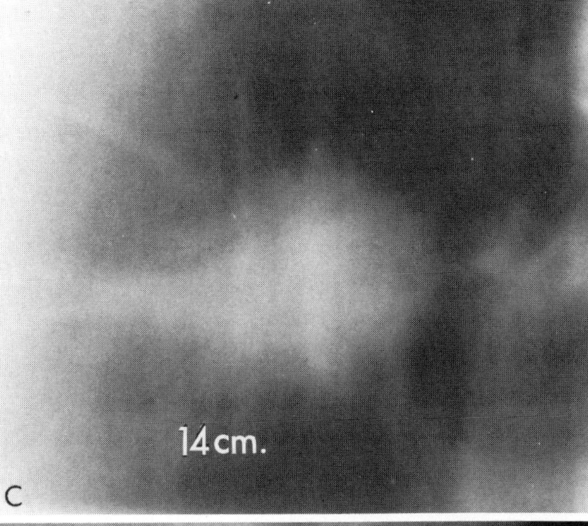

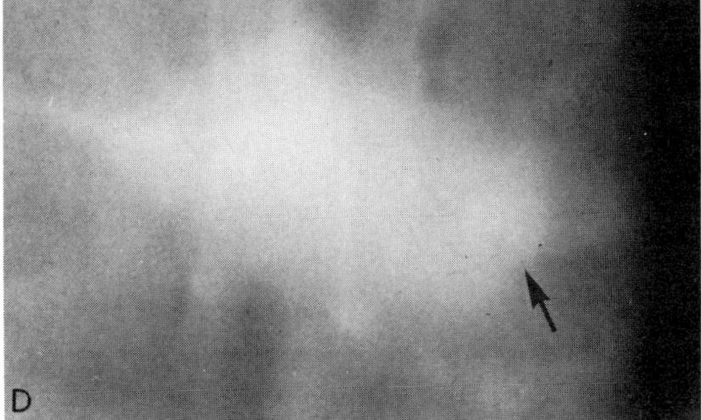

Figure 1–2. Tomographic characterization of a calcified mass. *A*. Detail of right mid lung field, posteroanterior roentgenogram, in a 68 year old woman. An irregular nodule, apparently containing calcification, is seen. *B* and *C*. Frontal tomograms show that the apparently central calcification and the mass density are seen best on different "cuts." *D*. Lateral tomogram demonstrates that the calcification (arrow) is within the periphery of the mass. Aspiration needle biopsy of the nodule disclosed adenocarcinoma cells.

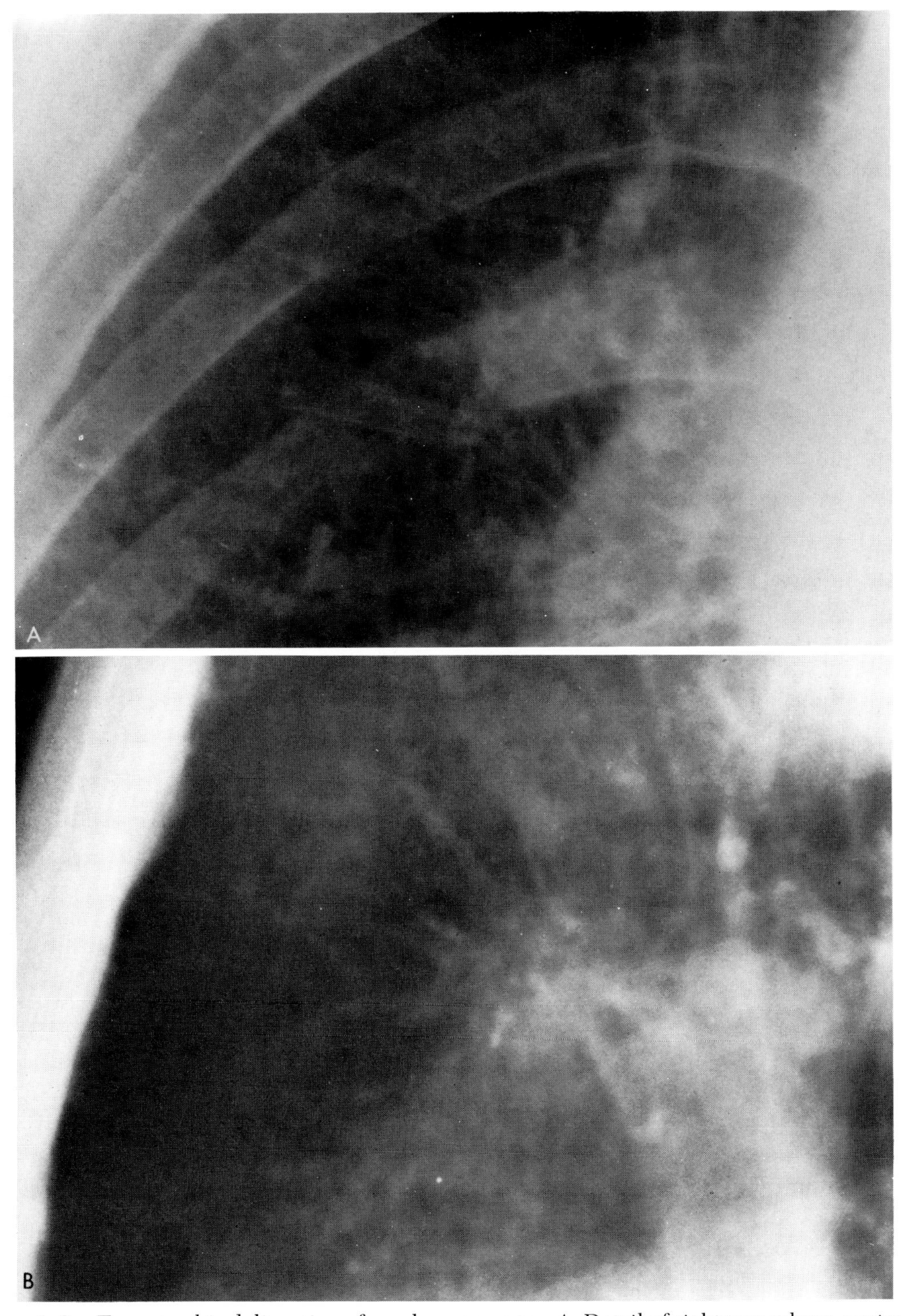

Figure 1–3. Tomographic delineation of a pulmonary mass. *A*. Detail of right upper lung, posteroanterior roentgenogram, in an asymptomatic 69 year old male smoker. An irregular mass is present medially. *B*. Detail of anterior upper chest, lateral roentgenogram (sternum to viewer's left). The mass questionably contains flecks of calcium.

Legend continued on the opposite page

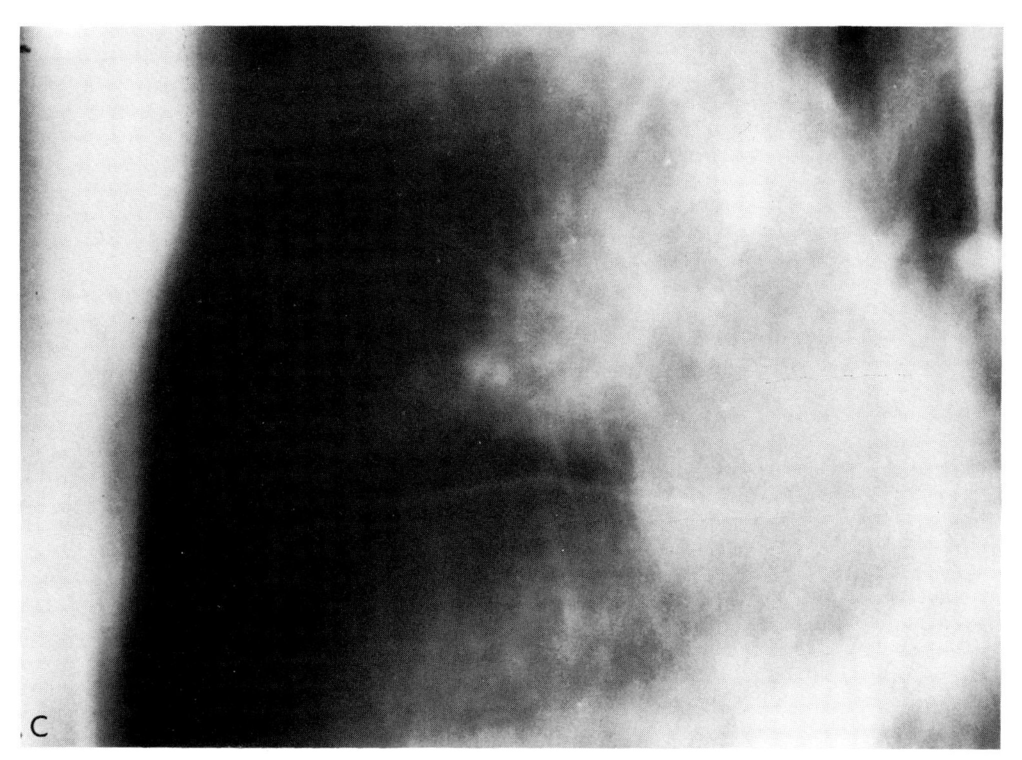

Figure 1–3 Continued. C. Lateral tomogram of the mass shows a spiculated border with central inhomogeneity. The lesion does not contain central calcifications, but several spicules seen end on mimic calcific densities. Pathologic diagnosis: squamous cell carcinoma.

itary, pulmonary nodule is useless in the differential diagnosis of malignant versus benign etiology.[14]

In the authors' experience, radiologists tend to err in diagnosing calcification in a lesion which later is proved to be a noncalcified carcinoma (Fig. 1–3). As a practical rule, if the radiologist is not absolutely certain of the tomographic diagnosis of calcification in a solitary pulmonary nodule, then the lesion should be considered noncalcified. If previous roentgenograms either do not show the identical lesion or are not available, and the patient is over the age of 30, then needle aspiration biopsy or surgical resection should be considered.[15]

Cavitary lung lesions. In the standard literature of several decades ago, radiologists encouraged the use of tomography whenever examination of plain chest roentgenograms raised the possibility of cavitation within a pulmonary lesion.[13] Currently, this use of tomography is only rarely of any clinical importance, although unquestionably tomography can demonstrate cavitation which is otherwise occult (Fig. 1–4). As no pathognomonic feature permits differentiation of neoplastic from inflammatory cavitation, definitive tissue or culture diagnosis is required even if cavitation happens to be demonstrated (Fig. 1–5). In pulmonary tuberculosis, the effectiveness of contemporary chemotherapy obviates the need to determine whether minimal cavitation is present. With the advent of modern diagnostic modalities that provide pulmonary tissue for appropriate analysis, such radiologic findings as cavitation in a mass, thickness of the wall of a cavity, or presence of fluid within a cavity should now be regarded as unreliable bases for diagnostic decisions.

On some rare occasions, however, demonstration of a cavity within an ill-defined pulmonary infiltrate may be of clinical value. As for example, in a patient with extensive pulmonary fibrosis caused by sarcoidosis, tomography may be necessary to demonstrate an intracavitary mycetoma. Even in such an instance, however, lordotic, oblique or lateral decubitus projections should initially be obtained, for these

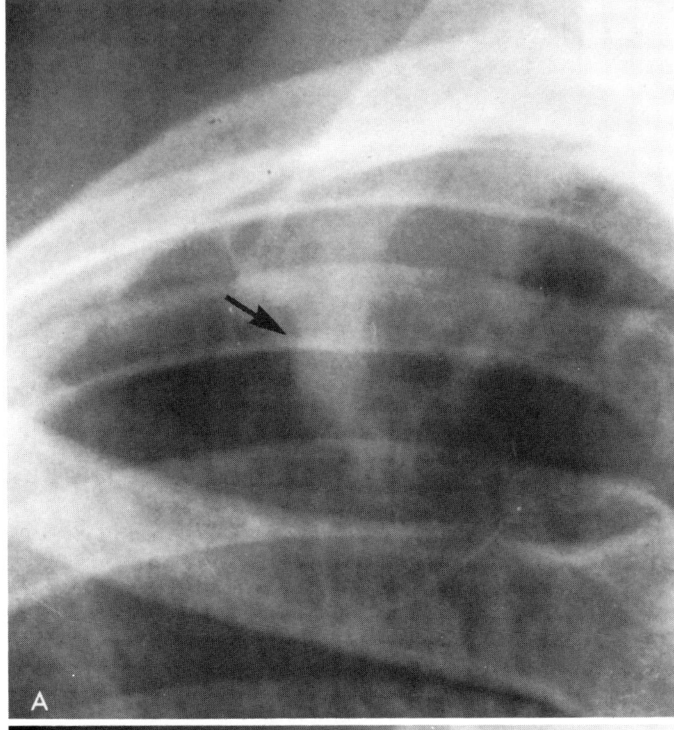

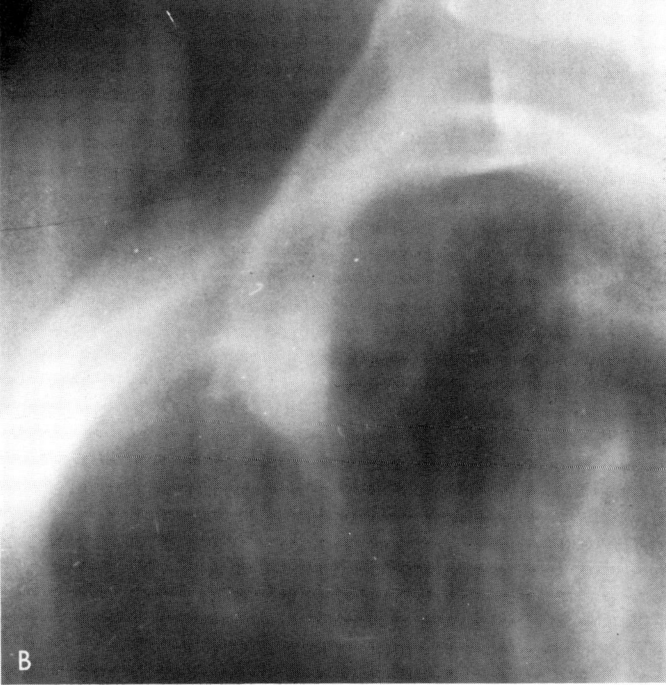

Figure 1–4. Tomographic documentation of cavitation. *A.* Detail of right lung apex, posteroanterior roentgenogram, in a 52 year old woman. A poorly defined density (arrow) is partially obscured by overlying ribs. *B.* Frontal tomogram reveals an irregular mass with cavitation. Tomography was of value in confirming the presence of the lesion and in providing information regarding location prior to subsequent needle aspiration biopsy, from which *M. tuberculosis* was isolated. The demonstration of cavitation had no effect on management of the patient.

views may demonstrate the cavity and fungus ball, obviating the need for tomography.

THE PROBLEM HILUM. Enlargement of a hilum may be caused by dilated pulmonary vessels, enlarged lymph nodes, or other mass lesions. Differentiation on plain films among these possibilities is a com-

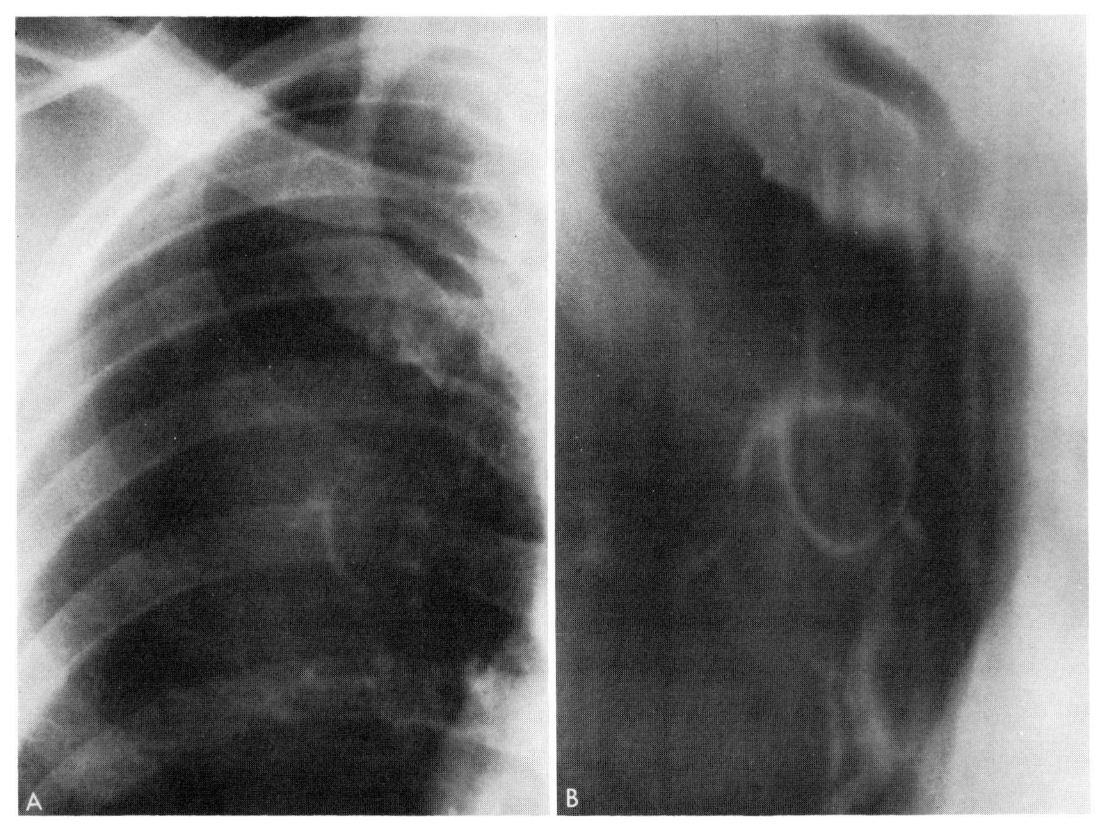

Figure 1–5. Tomographic demonstration of cavitation. *A.* Detail of right upper lung, posteroanterior roentgenogram, in a 63 year old man with back pain. Is there a cavitary lesion in the right upper lobe? *B.* Frontal tomogram shows a ring-shaped lesion with slightly irregular margins. Cytologic examination of sputum and biopsy of a lytic lesion in a lumbar vertebra disclosed squamous cell carcinoma.

mon and difficult problem, which tomography may resolve (Figs. 1–6, 1–7).

AIRWAY MASSES. For a patient with possible obstruction of a major bronchus, tomography may provide supplementary information or serve as an alternative to bronchoscopy (Fig. 1–8). The diagnosis of broncholithiasis must be considered whenever tomography demonstrates calcification in or adjacent to deformities of bronchial contour (Fig. 1–9).

BRONCHIAL DILATATION. Mucus may accumulate in dilated segmental and subsegmental airways, usually having a maximum diameter of about 1.0 to 1.5 cm. The diagnosis of bronchocele must be considered whenever a density is fusiform or cylindrical, tapers towards the hilum, and is located along the expected course of segmental or subsegmental bronchi (Fig. 1–10). If the patient is an asthmatic young adult, then the diagnosis of mucoid impaction in a dilated bronchus is virtually assured (Fig. 1–8). These appearances are sometimes evident on plain films, but are likely to be more distinct on tomograms.

ARTERIOVENOUS MALFORMATION. In the classic instance, an irregularly rounded density in the periphery of the lung with an obvious dilated artery entering the lesion and a dilated vein leaving it are pathognomonic. Often, however, the appearance as seen on plain chest roentgenograms is not diagnostic, and tomograms may be necessary to show the characteristic finding that the feeding artery does not taper between the hilum and the lesion (Fig. 1–11). The lesions may also be multiple, and tomography may reveal additional malformations which had not been suspected on the basis of the plain chest roentgenograms.[8]

VARIX. Venous varicosity in the lung may be suggested by tomography. In this entity, a pulmonary vein is aneurysmally

Text continued on page 11

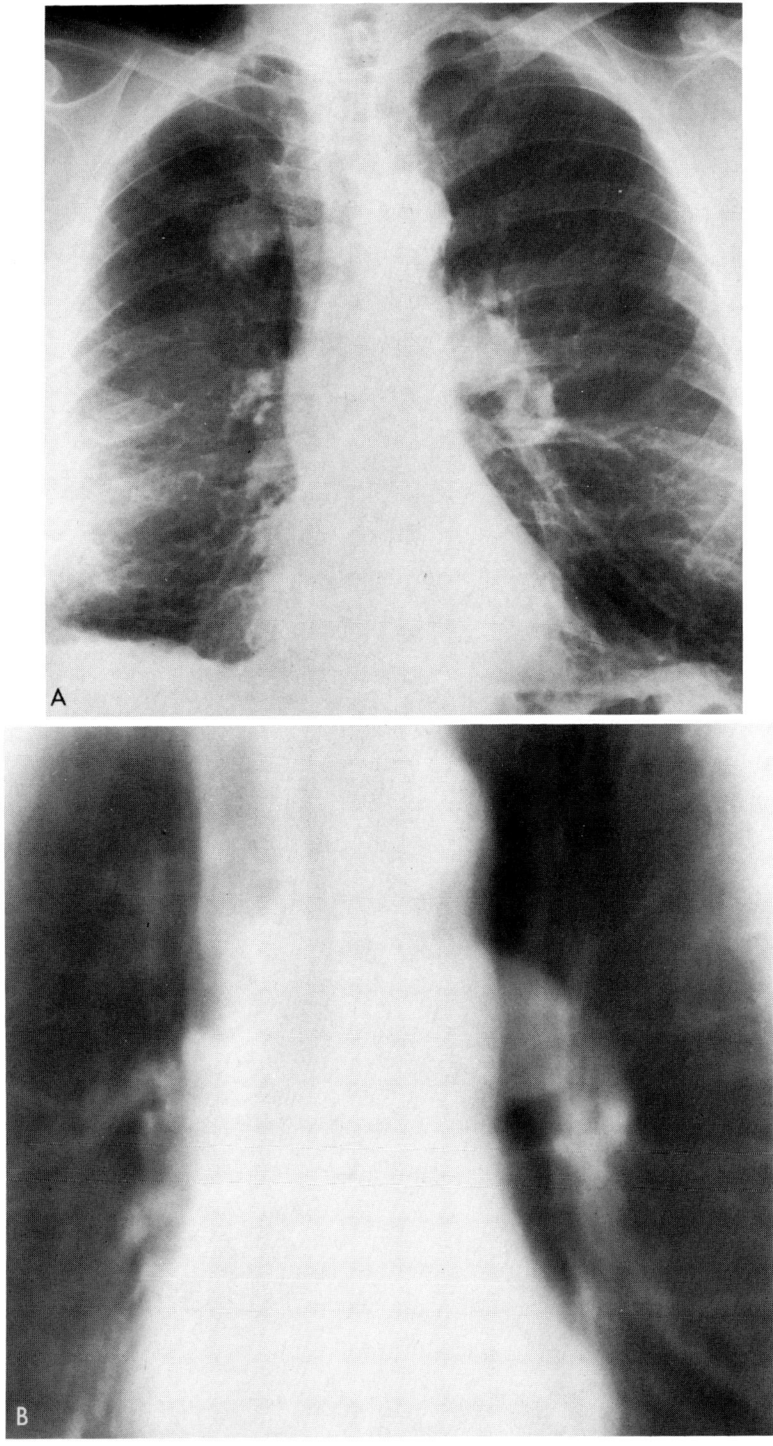

Figure 1–6. Tomographic evaluation of the "problem hilum." *A.* Posteroanterior chest roentgenogram of a 64 year old man with emphysema and a right upper lobe bronchogenic carcinoma shows a prominent left hilum. *B.* Frontal tomogram demonstrates characteristic configuration of an enlarged left pulmonary artery. (From Forrest, John V., and Sagel, Stuart S.: Special procedures in pulmonary radiology. *In* Potchen, E. James, editor: Current Concepts in Radiology, vol. 2, St. Louis, 1975, The C. V. Mosby Co.)

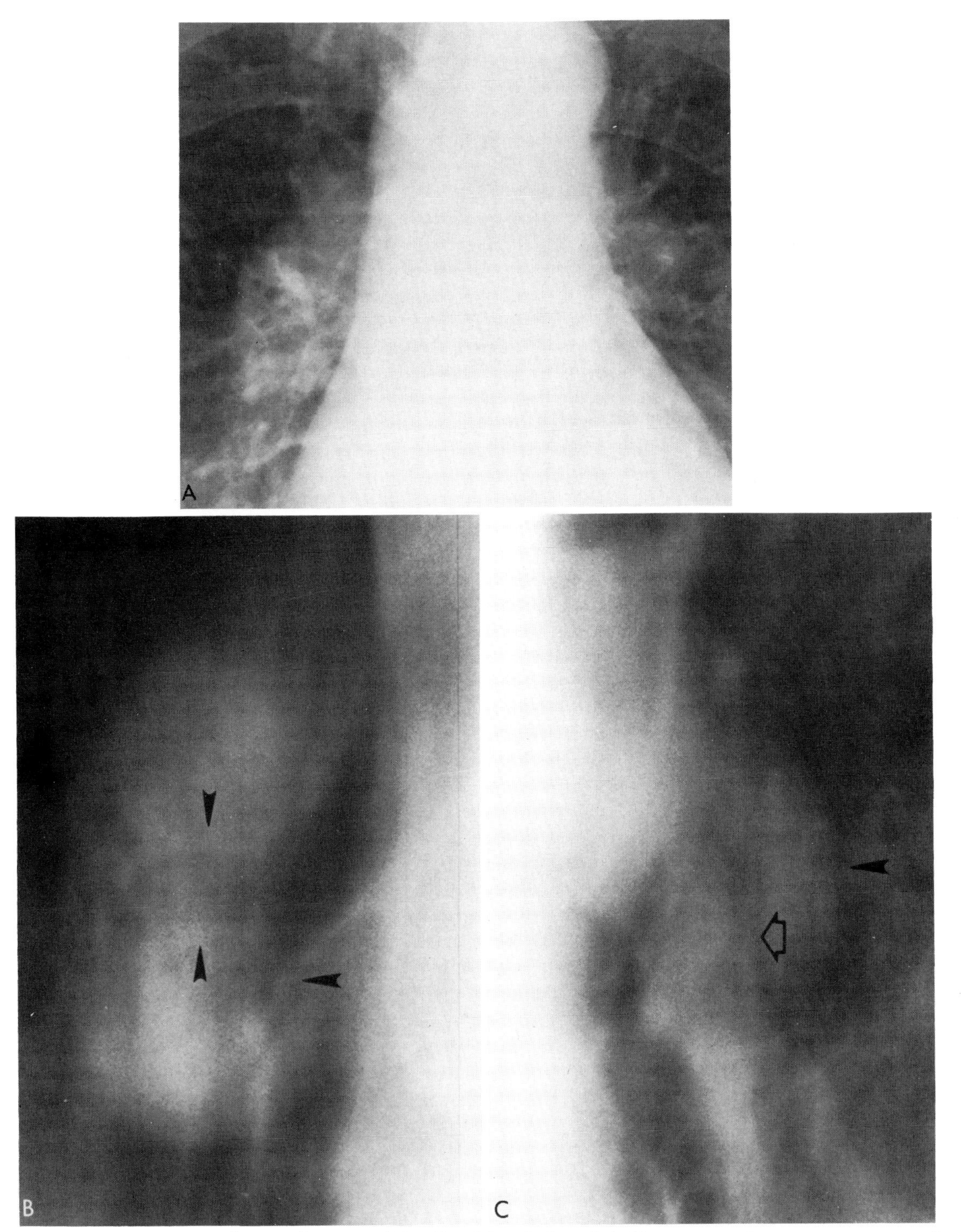

Figure 1–7. Tomographic evaluation of the "problem hilum." *A*. Posteroanterior roentgenogram of an asymptomatic 57 year old woman, interpreted as showing increased density at the inferior aspect of the right hilum and possible enlargement of the left hilum. *B*. Frontal tomogram of right hilum shows patent bronchi to the middle lobe (vertical arrows) and lower lobe (horizontal arrow). Rounded densities about the bronchi are consistent with enlarged lymph nodes. *C*. Frontal tomogram of left hilum reveals that the lateral aspect of the left descending pulmonary artery (open arrow) is distinct from a more lateral rounded mass (arrowhead). This rounded density was also interpreted as due to lymphadenopathy. These findings led to biopsy of a barely palpable, soft, supraclavicular lymph node, with pathologic findings consistent with sarcoidosis.

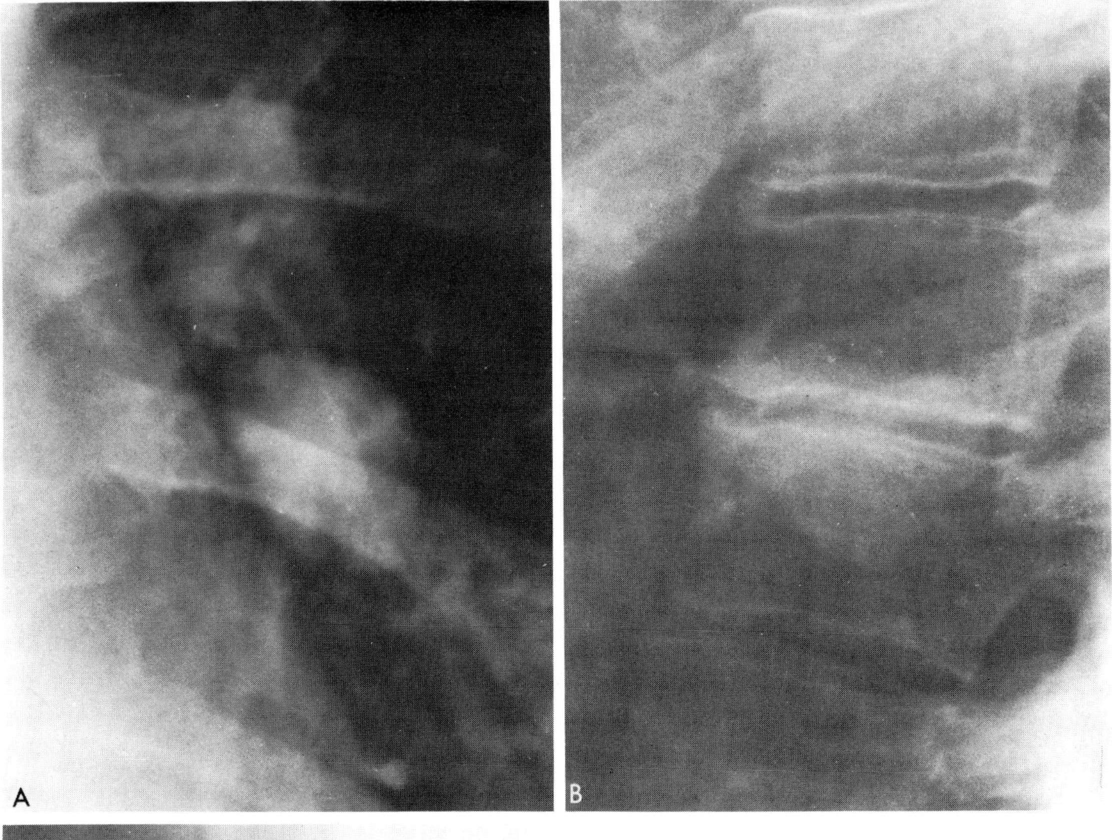

Figure 1–8. Tomographic characterization of airway mass. *A*. Detail of left mid lung, posteroanterior roentgenogram, in a 28 year old asthmatic woman. Lateral to the left heart border is an ovoid mass. *B*. Detail of mid posterior chest, lateral roentgenogram, demonstrates a lobulated mass overlying the spine. *C*. Lateral tomogram shows the mass to be heart-shaped, with the apex directed toward the hilum. Mucoid impaction in dilated superior and inferior subsegments (bronchocele) of the bronchus to the superior segment of the left lower lobe was the radiologic impression. The patient subsequently developed an abscess distal to the obstruction, and thoracotomy confirmed the radiologic diagnosis.

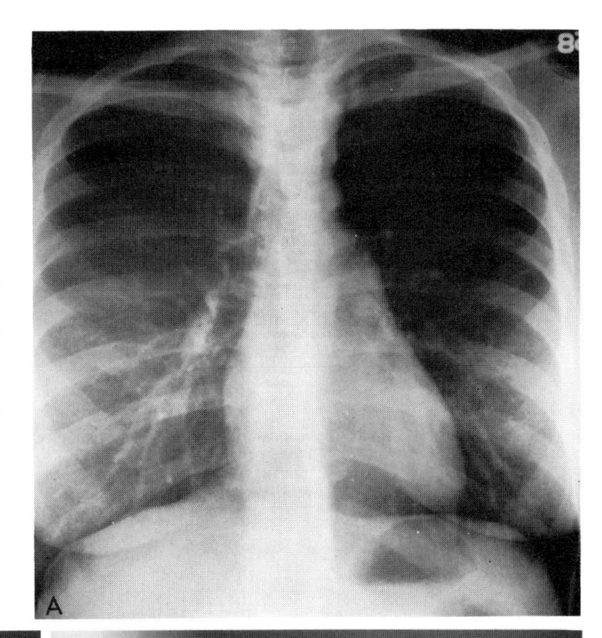

Figure 1–9. Tomographic localization and confirmation of broncholithiasis. *A*. Posteroanterior roentgenogram in a 14 year old girl with a history of coughing up "gravel" and one episode of hemoptysis. Calcifications overlie both hila. *B* and *C*. Frontal tomograms of the left hilar area demonstrate calcified lymph nodes in intimate association with the bifurcation of the left main stem bronchus, causing narrowing of the lingular and left lower lobe bronchi.

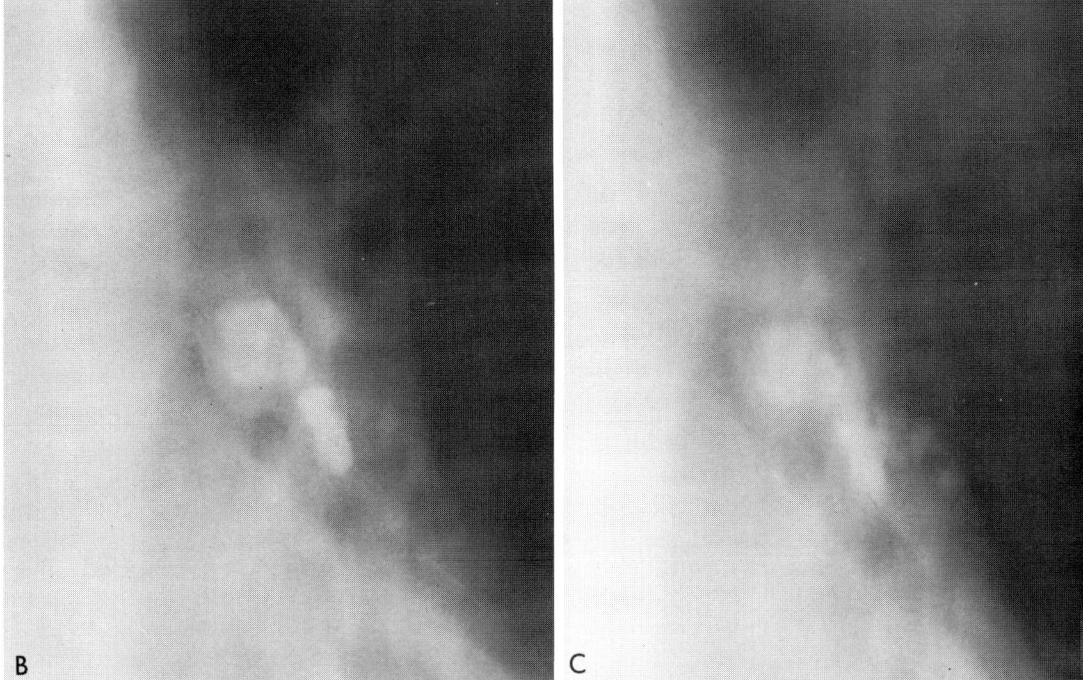

dilated, usually within 3 or 4 cm. of the entrance of the vein into the left atrium. Tomography demonstrates that the abnormal shadow is continuous with a pulmonary vein. Fluoroscopic documentation that the density is pulsatile and diminishes in size during a Valsalva maneuver makes the diagnosis of varix secure.[7] Also, tomography may be of value in distinguishing a prominent confluence of pulmonary veins from a pulmonary mass (Fig. 1–12).

ANOMALOUS PULMONARY VENOUS RETURN. Both the characteristic, inferiorly directed vein of the scimitar syndrome, and

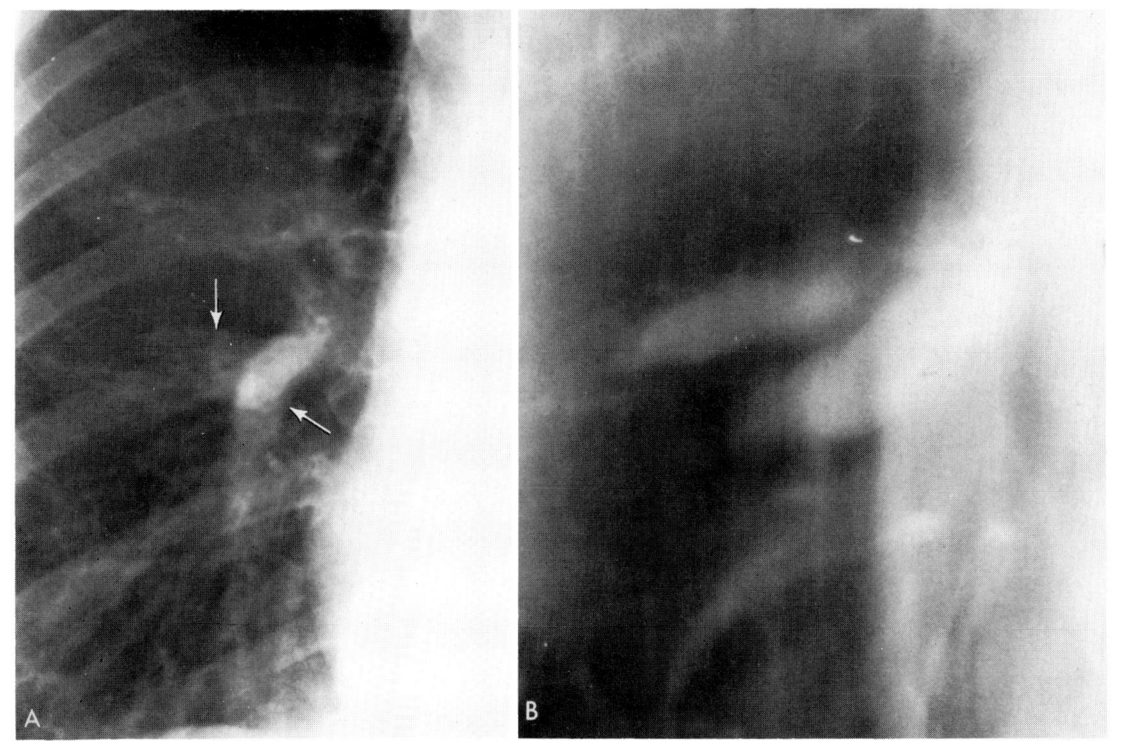

Figure 1–10. Tomographic demonstration of dilated bronchi. *A*. Detail of right mid lung, posteroanterior roentgenogram, in an asymptomatic 45 year old woman. An irregular density adjacent to the right hilum (arrows) is seen. *B*. Frontal tomogram reveals the characteristic branching tubular pattern of a bronchocele, in this patient due to congenital atresia.

other variants of anomalous pulmonary venous connections may on occasion be demonstrated to advantage by tomography[2] (Fig. 1–13).

IMPROVED DEMONSTRATION OF THE SITE OR SITES OF DISEASE

Pre-operative localization of a pulmonary lesion that is scheduled for resection or needle biopsy is occasionally an important indication for tomography. Before thoracotomy is performed, the thoracic surgeon must know in which lobe the lesion is situated in order to plan the suitable operative procedure (Fig. 1–14). Similarly, sometimes before needle biopsy is performed, the radiologist must know exactly where the lesion is situated in order to plan an appropriate approach. If plain chest radiographs or fluoroscopy do not show the lesion clearly in two projections at right angles to each other, then tomography may help the radiologist accurately locate the lesion (Fig. 1–4).

In some patients with doubtful localization of disease by plain roentgenograms, tomography may be utilized to establish which organ contains the lesion. For instance, a nodular density interpreted as probably located in the lung on plain roentgenograms may, on tomography, actually be shown to be situated in a rib (Fig. 1–15), on the skin, or in the pleura (Fig. 1–16). In a number of these cases, preliminary views of the ribs or inspection of the patient's skin will rule out any need for tomography.

OCCASIONAL DEMONSTRATION OF DISEASE NOT IDENTIFIED ON PLAIN CHEST ROENTGENOGRAMS

Tomography is a sufficiently powerful diagnostic tool that its use occasionally

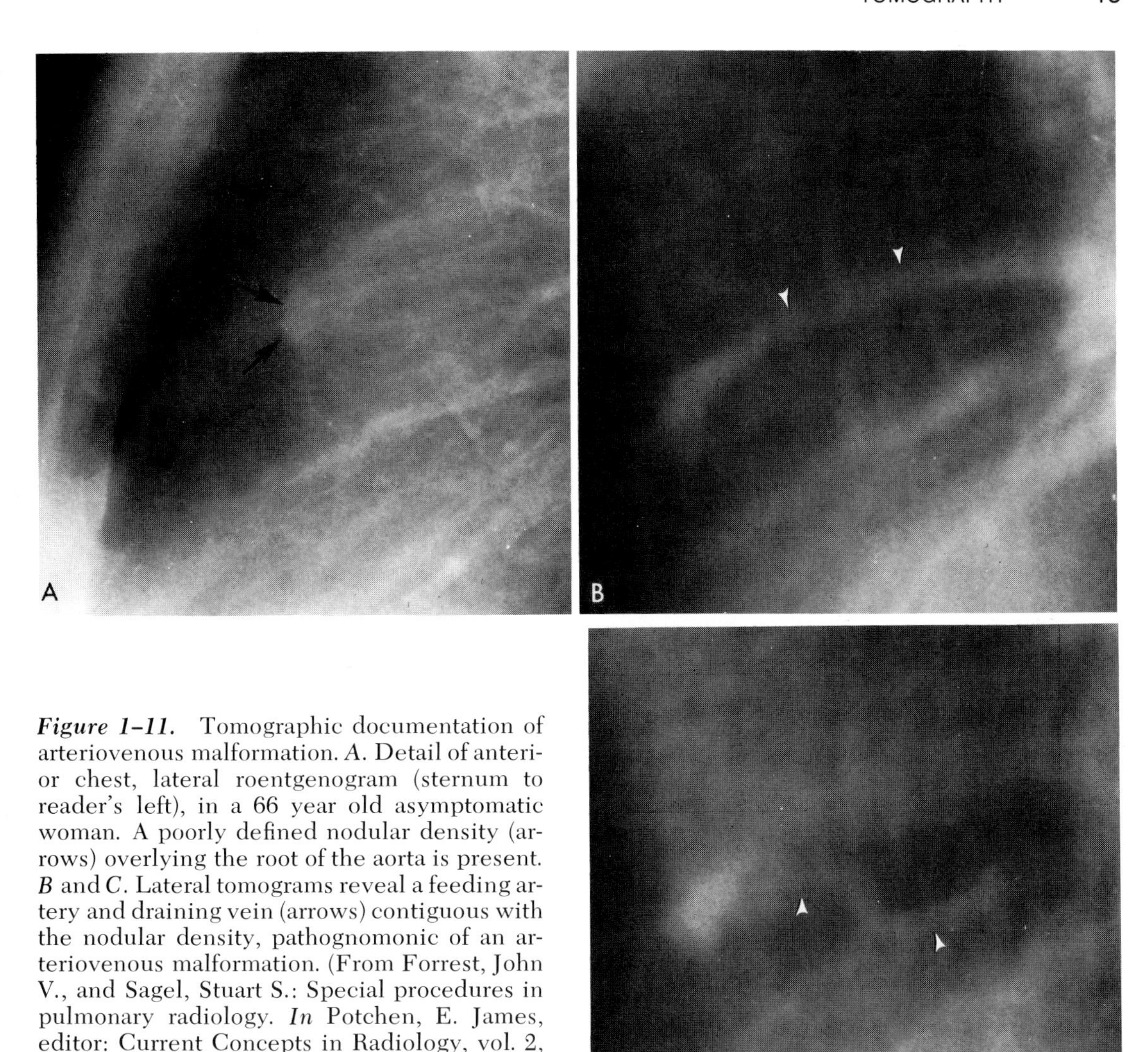

Figure 1–11. Tomographic documentation of arteriovenous malformation. *A*. Detail of anterior chest, lateral roentgenogram (sternum to reader's left), in a 66 year old asymptomatic woman. A poorly defined nodular density (arrows) overlying the root of the aorta is present. *B* and *C*. Lateral tomograms reveal a feeding artery and draining vein (arrows) contiguous with the nodular density, pathognomonic of an arteriovenous malformation. (From Forrest, John V., and Sagel, Stuart S.: Special procedures in pulmonary radiology. *In* Potchen, E. James, editor: Current Concepts in Radiology, vol. 2, St. Louis, 1975, The C. V. Mosby Co.)

yields findings which are not appreciated even upon retrospective analysis of plain chest roentgenograms. In the search for disease undetected by plain chest roentgenograms, the most prevalent use of tomography is to detect previously undiagnosed malignant disease in the lungs.

If a patient with an extrapulmonary primary cancer has no evidence of metastatic disease in the lungs on plain chest roentgenograms, should tomography of the chest be performed? Given good quality plain chest roentgenograms performed with high kilovoltage technique, the demonstration of unsuspected lesions by tomography is quite uncommon. Rarely, full chest tomograms at one centimeter intervals will disclose a nodule or nodules not seen on the routine plain chest radiographs (Fig. 1–17), especially if the patient is obese. Utilization of full chest tomography is generally restricted to those patients for whom radical surgery is proposed and for whom the detection of an occult pulmonary metastasis would markedly alter their care. To distinguish stable, healed granulomas

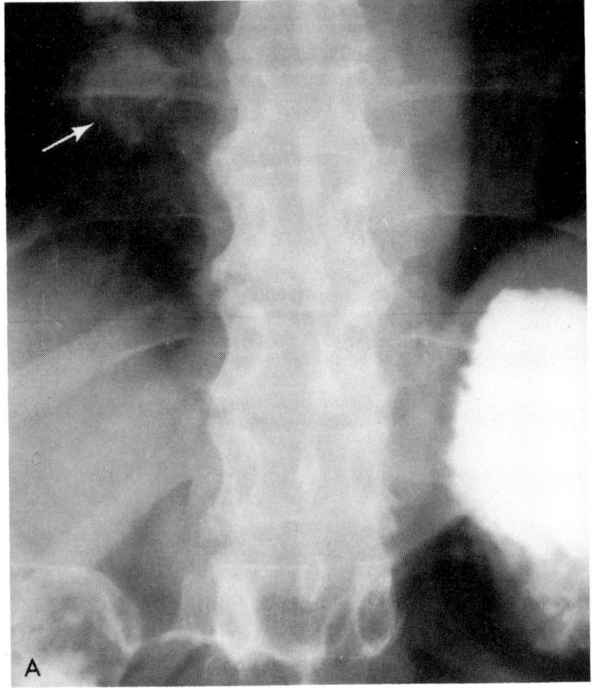

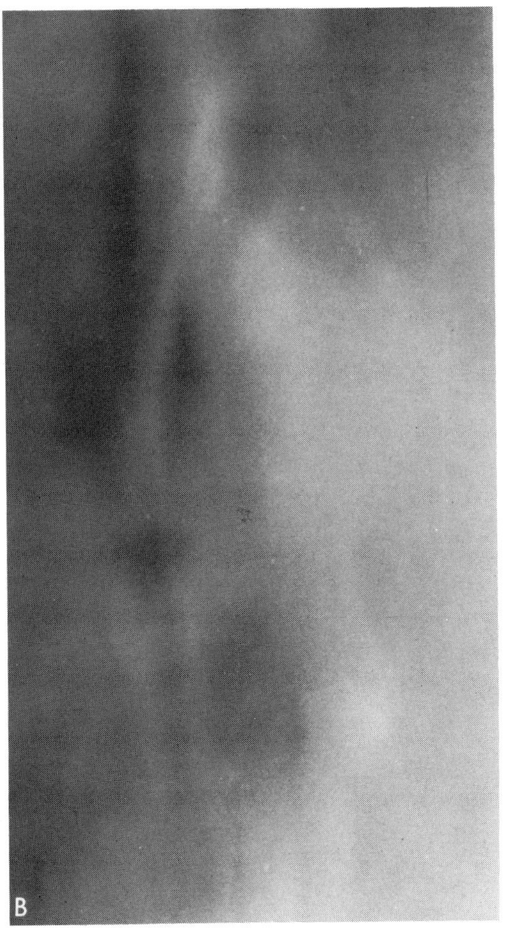

Figure 1–12. Tomographic documentation of the confluence of pulmonary veins. *A.* Detail of frontal roentgenogram obtained during an upper G.I. series in a 61 year old man. A poorly defined nodule at the right lung base (arrow) is seen. *B.* Frontal tomogram demonstrates multiple vessels entering the nodular density, the typical appearance of a prominent confluence of pulmonary veins. (From Forrest, John V., and Sagel, Stuart S.: Special procedures in pulmonary radiology. *In* Potchen, E. James, editor: Current Concepts in Radiology, vol. 2, St. Louis, 1975, The C. V. Mosby Co.)

from enlarging, small metastases, repeat laminagrams after a suitable interval (e.g., 4 to 6 weeks) are advisable (Fig. 1–18).

If a patient with one or more pulmonary metastases is a candidate for resection of the metastases, then tomography is useful to confirm the location of the lesions as well as their number.[4, 12]

TECHNIQUE

The diagnostic value of tomography depends upon skillful radiography.[1, 10] To obtain technically adequate radiographs, radiographer and radiologist must collaborate in the performance of the examination. The following important, practical considerations of technique are recommended.

Obtain adequate preliminary plain chest roentgenograms. The radiologist should accept a patient for chest tomography only after reviewing technically satisfactory, current roentgenograms of the patient. Oblique plain chest roentgenograms and/or fluoroscopy with spot films should be strongly considered. Often these studies provide sufficient localization and characterization of an abnormality that tomography becomes unnecessary. Common examples are fluoroscopic spot films at low kilovoltage demonstrating central calcification in a nodule, and oblique roentgenograms revealing that a "pulmonary" nodule is actually a fracture or bone island in a rib.

Talk with the patient before exposing tomograms. This simple courtesy has multiple benefits: the radiologist not only acquires a first-hand sense of the clinical situation, but also is able to stress to the patient the importance of holding still during the examination. Motion of the patient between exposures may inadvertently exclude portions of the lung from the examination, and is a common cause of technically unsatisfactory examinations. The radiologist also must continually be alert to the possibility that inspection of the patient's skin may reveal a cutaneous lesion as the cause of an apparent pulmonary density. Many patients express fears about the extent of radiation exposure from tomography, and the radiologist is well advised to reassure the patient that the total exposure is quantitatively rather small (e.g., 20 exposures at approximately 50 mrads per exposure add up to a total skin dose of 1 rad).

Consult with the radiographer. The radiologist can interpret only that information which the radiographer provides on the films. Before any tomograms are exposed, the radiologist and technologist should review the following:

1. The findings on plain chest roentgenograms, and the clinical question which tomography is expected to resolve.
2. Initial tomographic projection, e.g.,

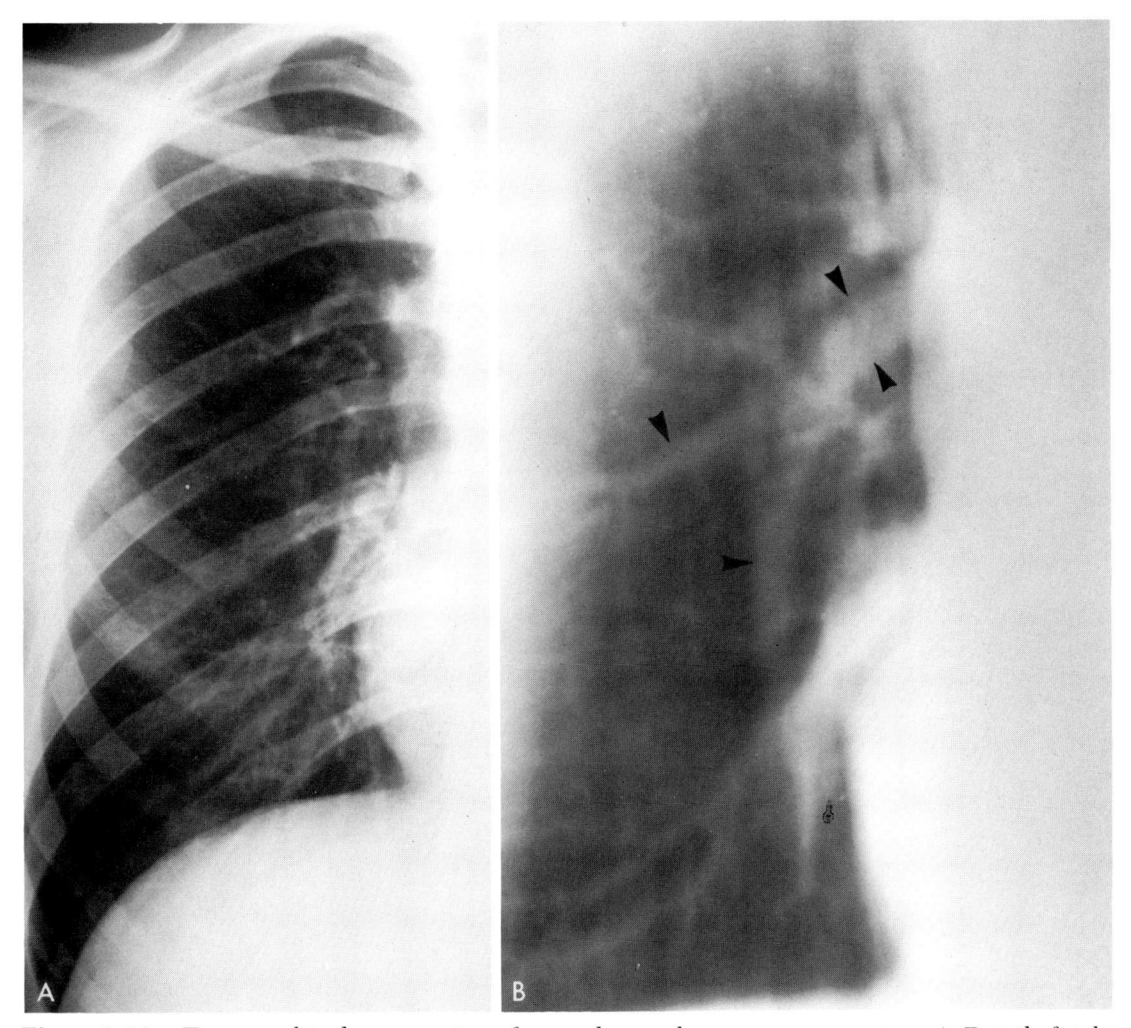

Figure 1–13. Tomographic demonstration of anomalous pulmonary venous return. *A.* Detail of right lung, posteroanterior roentgenogram, in an asymptomatic 18 year old man. An unusual, vertical, cylindrical density is seen lateral to the mediastinum. *B.* Frontal tomogram demonstrates that the tubular shadow (arrows) represents anomalous pulmonary venous drainage into the superior vena cava.

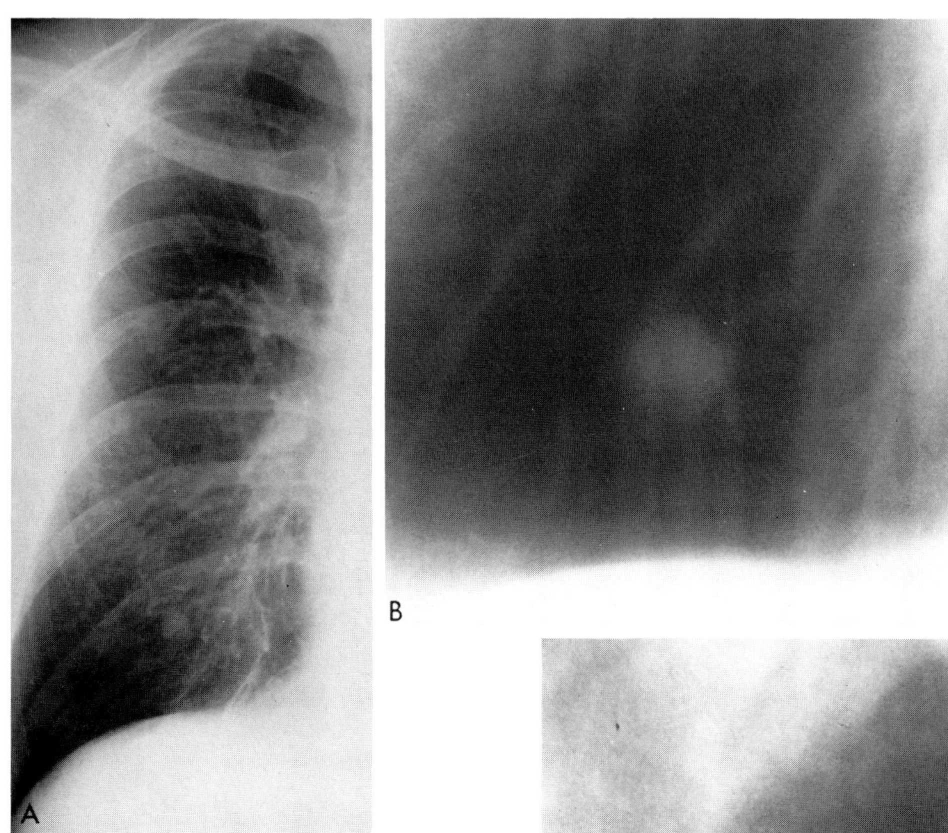

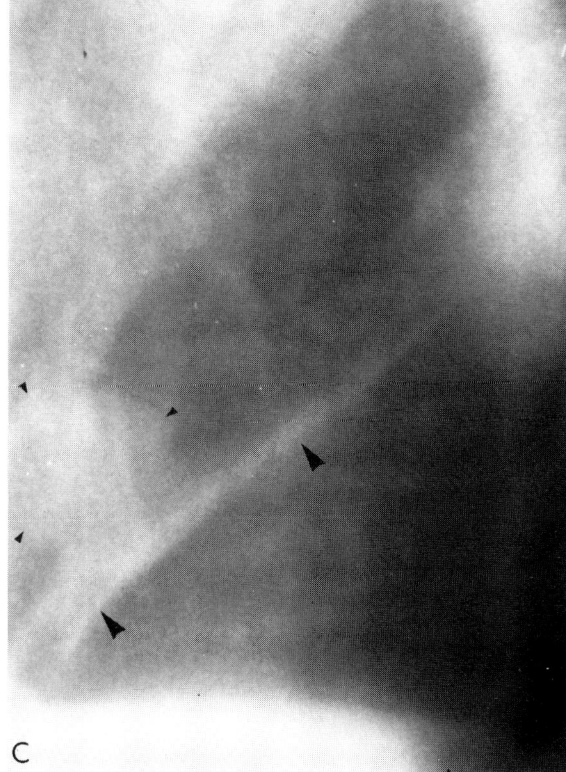

Figure 1–14. Tomographic localization of a pulmonary lesion. *A*. Detail of right lung, posteroanterior roentgenogram, in a 45 year old man. A small nodular density in the right lower lung field is demonstrated. A lateral plain chest roentgenogram was normal. *B*. Frontal tomogram demonstrates that the mass is non-calcified and situated in the mid chest, but does not reveal in which lobe the lesion is. *C*. Lateral tomogram discloses that the nodule (small arrowheads) is in the middle lobe, just anterior to the major fissure (large arrowheads), a finding which permitted ready localization of the lesion during surgery.

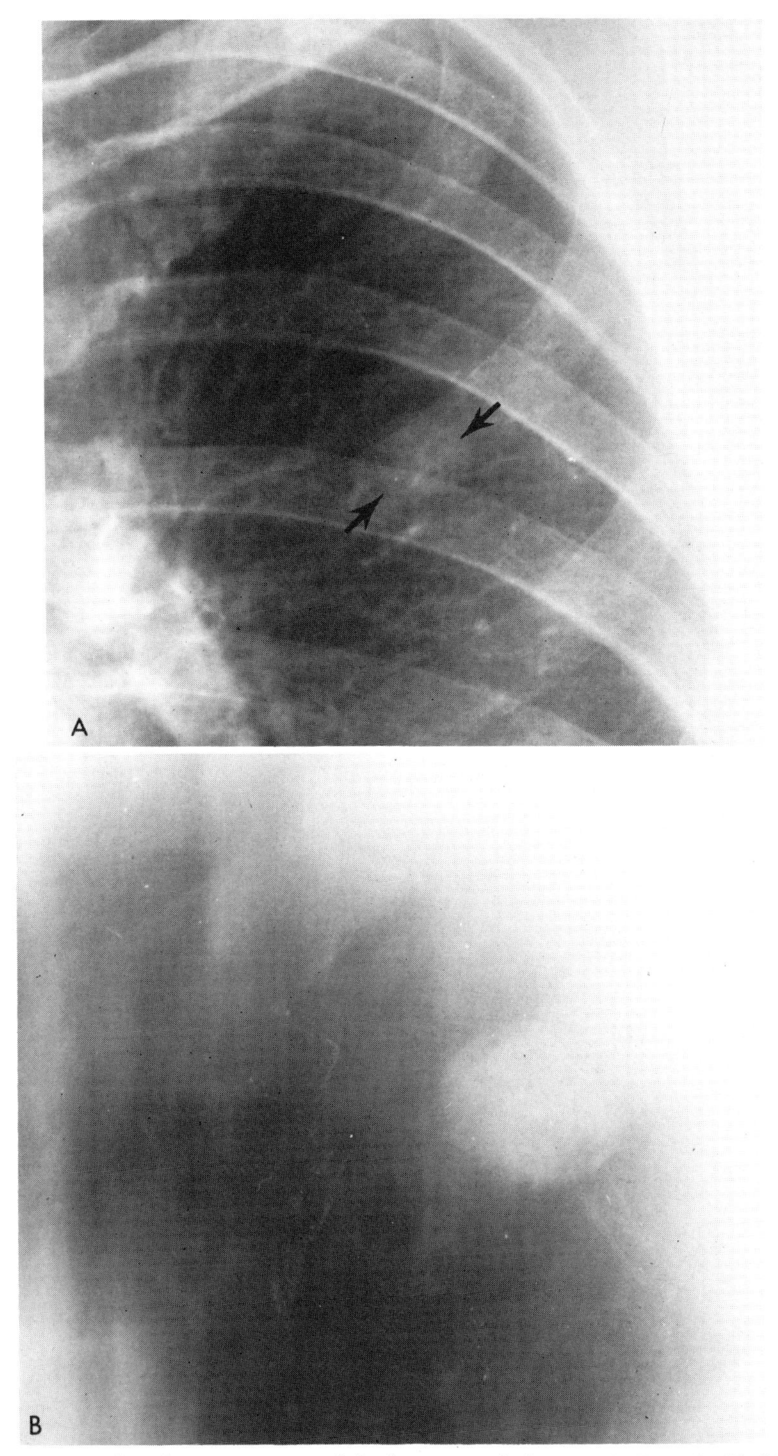

Figure 1–15. Tomographic demonstration of the location of a lesion. *A*. Detail of left mid lung field, posteroanterior roentgenogram, in a 41 year old man shows an ill-defined nodular density (arrows). *B*. Frontal tomogram discloses the far anterior location of this nodular density, contiguous with an anterior rib. The apparent soft tissue density is irregularly calcified, characteristic of a healing rib fracture.

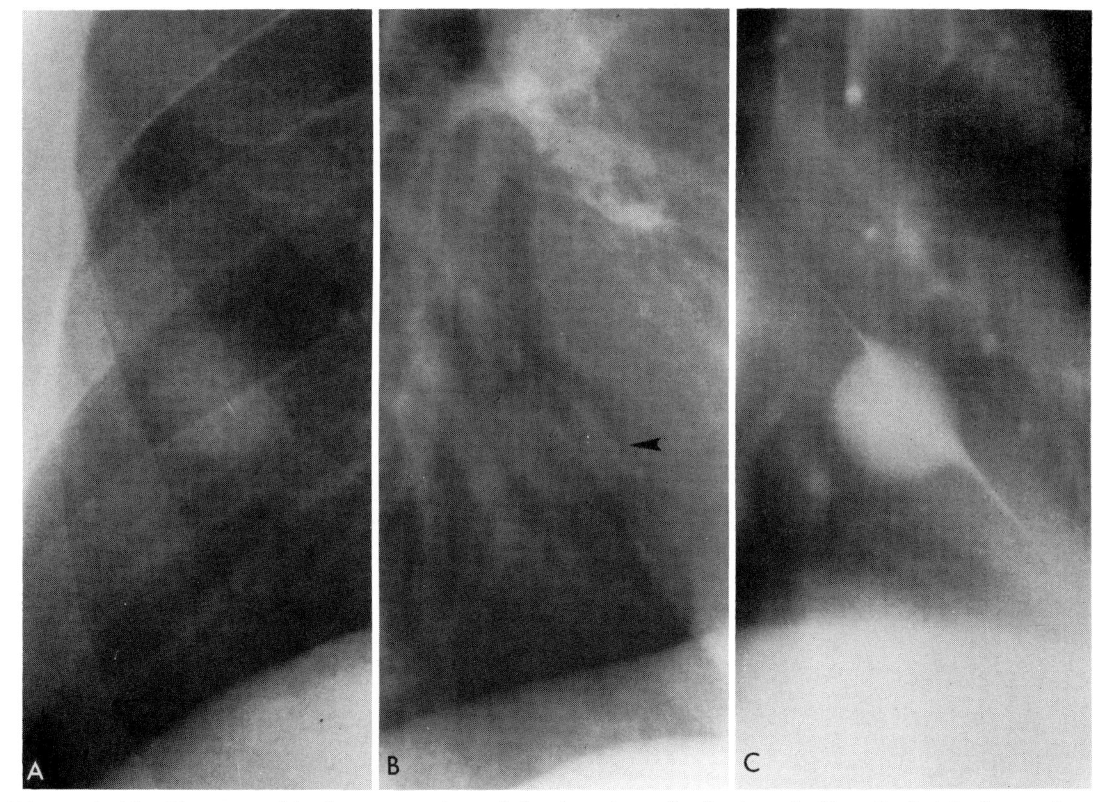

Figure 1–16. Tomographic demonstration of the location of a lesion. *A*. Detail of right lower lung zone, posteroanterior roentgenogram, in a 34 year old man. An ill-defined rounded density is seen. *B*. Detail of mid lower lung zone, lateral roentgenogram, shows that the ovoid density (arrow) overlies the posterior margin of the heart. Where is the abnormality? *C*. Lateral tomogram reveals that the lesion is situated within the major fissure. The patient had sustained a crush injury to the chest in an automobile accident ten weeks earlier, and a presumptive diagnosis of intrafissural hematoma was made. Subsequent roentgenograms showed the lesion was decreasing in size.

frontal or lateral. A useful guideline is to begin tomography in the same projection which best showed the lesion on plain chest films. For determining the relationship of a parenchymal lesion to the fissures, the lateral projection is usually preferred (Fig. 1–16). Rarely, oblique tomography may be helpful: the left posterior oblique projection is excellent for demonstrating the major bronchi on the left, and both oblique projections are recommended for showing the pulmonary veins entering the left atrium.[3] To detect masses in an airway, the best projection is perpendicular to the course of the airway in question. For example, the bronchus to the superior segment of each lower lobe courses posteriorly, so tomography with the x-ray beam at right angles to the bronchus, i.e., in the lateral projection, is usually ideal to demonstrate lesions of this specific bronchus (Fig. 1–8). Similarly, lateral tomography is usually preferable over frontal tomography for lesions of the middle lobe bronchus and the anterior segmental bronchi of the upper lobes. The patient is usually placed in the supine or the lateral decubitus position for tomography, as these positions are most easily maintained without moving.

3. Centering and coning of the x-ray beam. Careful centering and coning are critical. In tomography, as in general radiography, optimal detail of small lesions can be obtained only by appropriate coning to reduce photographic blur from scattered radiation. Furthermore, an excessive number of films covering the entire chest or uninvolved areas adds to the risks of x-ray exposure, and wastes the availability of the

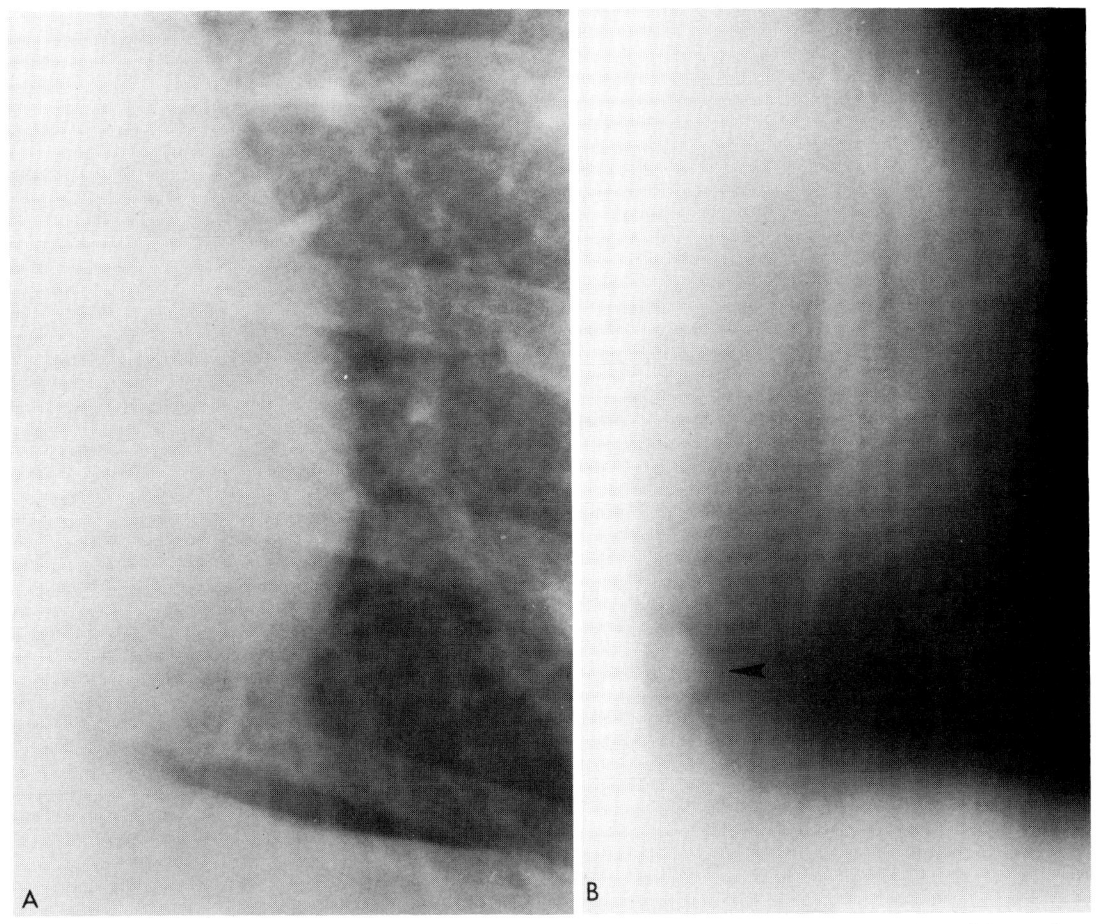

Figure 1–17. Tomographic demonstration of an unsuspected lesion. *A*. Detail of left mid lower lung field, posteroanterior projection, in a 12 year old boy with an osteosarcoma of the right tibia. No abnormal density is evident. *B*. Detail of a full chest frontal tomogram discloses a rounded density (arrow) inferior to the heart, compatible with metastatic osteosarcoma.

room and the time of the radiographer. Full chest laminagraphs taken routinely are unjustifiable.

4. Wedge filter on frontal views.[11] For optimal exposure of mediastinum and lungs on full chest tomograms, a filter that permits less radiation to penetrate the lungs than the spine and mediastinum is strongly advised.

Obtain a scout tomographic exposure, and review it for technical adequacy. Specify to the radiographer a level for the preliminary exposure, e.g., the midcoronal plane for frontal tomography of both lungs. After the scout film has been developed, review it with the technologist, analyzing exposure factors, centering, and coning. Appropriate alteration of the kilovoltage from that of the initial scout exposure is usually a necessity. Peak kilovoltage employed for frontal tomograms of the lungs is ordinarily 70 to 85 kVp; for lateral tomograms, 80 to 95 kVp. Linear motion with an arc of 30° to 40° is standard technique in chest tomography. The in-focus layer of a 30° arc is about 2 mm.[10] Linear motion is standard because arcuate motions produce rounded artifacts, simulating cavities. Also, exposure time for linear motion is relatively short (usually between 0.5 and 1.0 second). While hypocycloidal movement has its advocates,[16] this equipment is not

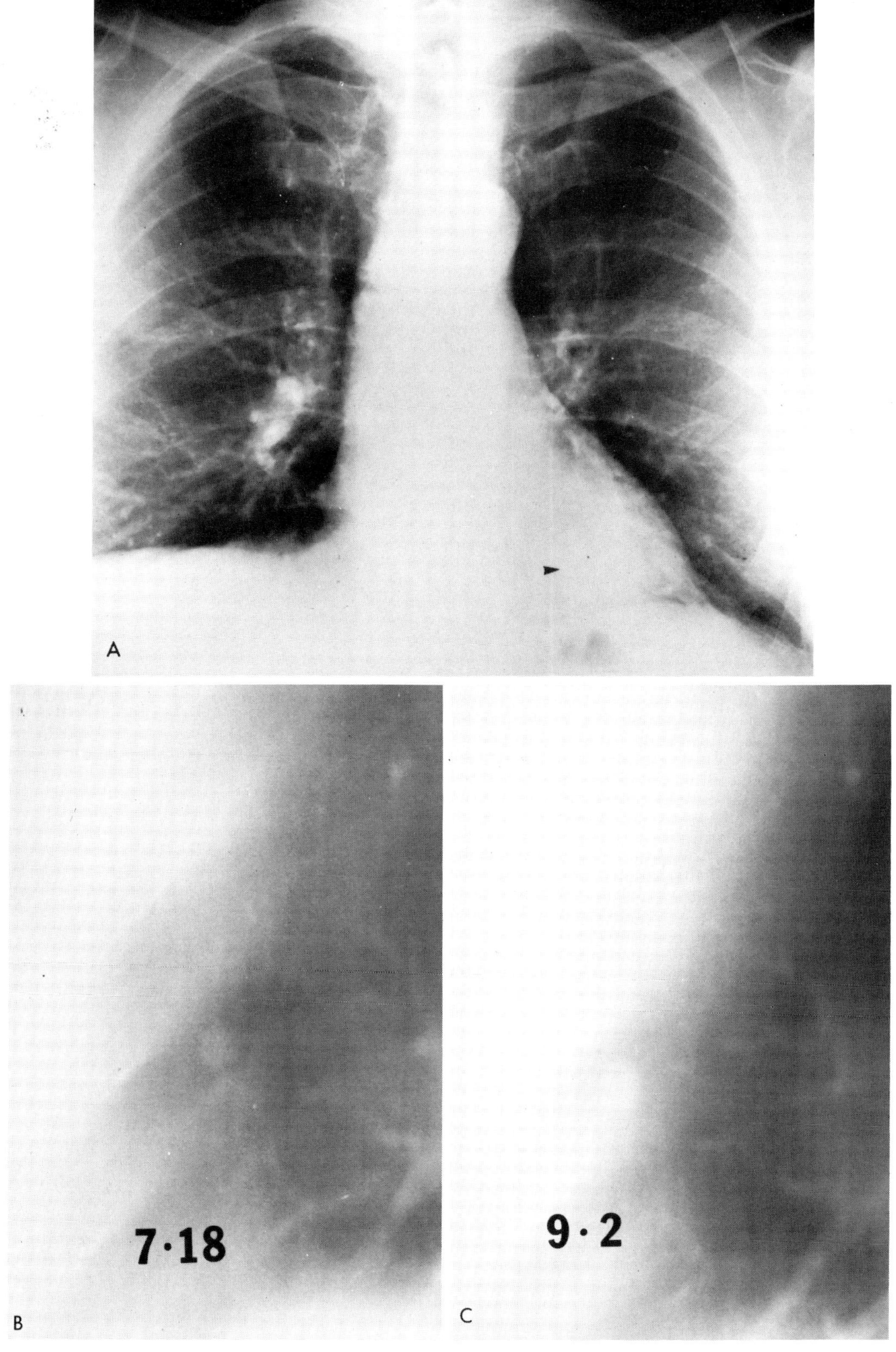

Figure 1–18. *See opposite page for legend.*

generally available, and the long tube cooling period necessary for chest tomography limits its practicality.

Order a series of exposures, carefully specifying the levels required. Usually, a series of tomographic exposures is obtained at levels 1 cm. apart. This interval is sufficient for general surveys of the chest, but further roentgenograms at closer intervals for details of specific structures may be helpful. For example, in a series of exposures 1 cm. apart, if a coin lesion 1.5 cm. in diameter is best seen on one exposure, then further exposures of the lesion at 0.5 cm. or even 0.3 cm. intervals will improve radiographic demonstration of the lesion. For characterization of solitary nodules, cone down views produce better definition than do exposures of the full lungs. If the exact location of calcification within a nodule as seen on one tomographic projection is in question, then it may be advisable to obtain tomograms in the perpendicular projection to resolve whether the calcification is central or eccentric (Fig. 1–2).

Discharge the patient only after reviewing all the roentgenograms obtained, arriving at a considered diagnostic impression, and concluding that further tomograms or other roentgenograms are unnecessary. More often than they would like to admit, the experience of the authors in reviewing roentgenograms after a patient has been discharged has been to find that specific, further tomographic exposures would have been useful. To avoid this situation, the radiologist should always carefully review the complete examination while the patient is still in the department. After this review, if the radiologist can think of no possible further views that might influence the final roentgenologic diagnosis, then the patient should be discharged from the department. Only by closely monitoring the performance of the tomographic examination can the radiologist provide optimal service to the patient.

BIBLIOGRAPHY

1. Cullinan, J. E.: Body section radiography. *In* Cullinan, J. E.: Illustrated Guide to X-Ray Technics. Philadelphia, J. B. Lippincott Company, 1972, pp. 144–166.
2. Dalith, F., and Neufeld, H.: Radiological diagnosis of anomalous pulmonary venous connection: a tomographic study. Radiology, *74*:1–18, 1960.
3. Favez, G., Willa, C., and Heinzer, F.: Posterior oblique tomography at an angle of 55° in chest roentgenology. Amer. J. Roentgen., *120*:907–915, 1974.
4. Feldman, P. S., and Kyriakos, M.: Pulmonary resection for metastatic sarcoma. J. Thorac. Cardiovasc. Surg., *64*:784–799, 1972.
5. Felson, B.: Thoracic calcifications. Dis. Chest, *56*:330–343, 1969.
6. Good, C. A.: The solitary pulmonary nodule: a problem of management. Radiol. Clin. North Amer., *1*:429–438, 1963.
7. Hipona, F., and Jamshidi, A.: Observations on the natural history of varicosity of pulmonary veins. Circulation, *35*:471–475, 1967.
8. Lodin, H.: Tomographic analysis of arteriovenous aneurysms in the lung. Acta Radiol., *38*:205–211, 1952.
9. Meredith, W. J., and Massey, J. B.: Fundamental Physics of Radiology. Baltimore, Williams & Wilkins Company, 1972, p. 80.
10. Ibid., pp. 351–363.
11. Moro, J.: New variable-thickness filter for chest laminagraphy. Radiology, *92*:646–647, 1969.
12. Morton, D. L., Joseph, W. L., Ketcham, A. S., Geelhoed, G. W., and Adkins, P. C.: Surgical resection and adjunctive immunotherapy for selected patients with multiple pulmonary metastases. Ann. Surg., *178*:360–366, 1973.
13. Rabin, C. B.: Radiology of the Chest. *In* Robbins, L. L., editor: Golden's Diagnostic Radiology. Baltimore, Williams & Wilkins Company, 1952, Volume I, p. 93.
14. Rigler, L. G.: The roentgen signs of carcinoma of the lung. Amer. J. Roentgen., *74*:415–428, 1955.
15. Trunk, G., Gracey, D. R., and Byrd, R. B.: The management and evaluation of the solitary pulmonary nodule. Chest, *66*:236–239, 1974.
16. Westra, D.: Tomography of the lungs and mediastinum. *In* Berrett, A., Brünner, S., and Valvassori, G. E., editors: Modern Thin-Section Tomography. Springfield, Illinois, Charles C Thomas, 1973, pp. 271–282.

Figure 1–18. Tomographic demonstration of an unsuspected lesion. *A.* Posteroanterior chest roentgenogram of a 65 year old man who had a malignant melanoma resected two years previously. A mass, 4 cm. in diameter, is seen in the left lower lobe behind the heart (arrow). No other lesion was noted and surgical resection of a solitary metastasis was contemplated. *B.* Detail of right mid lung, from a full chest frontal tomogram, discloses a 6 mm. non-calcified nodule. *C.* Frontal tomogram performed six weeks later demonstrates that the nodule has increased in size to 1 cm. in diameter, and thus represents another metastatic deposit rather than a granuloma. Surgery was cancelled and chemotherapy substituted.

Chapter 2

FLUOROSCOPICALLY ASSISTED LUNG BIOPSY TECHNIQUES

by Stuart S. Sagel, M.D., and John V. Forrest, M.D.

INTRODUCTION

The determination of the etiology of a pulmonary infiltrate or mass lesion seen in the lung on a chest roentgenogram is a common clinical problem. In many instances the pulmonary disease cannot be diagnosed by the usual clinical work-up—sputum examination and culture (including transtracheal aspiration), bronchoscopy, serologic studies, and other procedures. Establishment of the cause of the lesion(s) then depends upon examination of tissue from the radiographically demonstrated pulmonary density.

The ideal diagnostic test, with 100 per cent yield and no risk, unfortunately does not exist. Thoracotomy is unquestionably the most reliable method of diagnosis. However, it is also the most costly, painful, and dangerous. A fundamental logic in medicine dictates that the procedure least likely to injure should be used first before progressing to the more hazardous, discomforting, and expensive technique. Using this philosophy, two non-operative fluoroscopically assisted lung biopsy techniques—percutaneous aspiration needle biopsy and transcatheter bronchial brushing—have proved to be highly accurate diagnostic modalities that maintain low morbidity and relatively low financial cost.

Short of thoracotomy, bronchoscopy is the most accurate diagnostic method when an endobronchial lesion can be seen directly and a biopsy is taken. With lesions in the middle third or periphery of the lung, beyond visualization of the fiberoptic bronchoscope, the two fluoroscopically assisted lung biopsy techniques are most advantageous. The availability of image intensification fluoroscopy has made it possible to guide a needle or brush to pulmonary lesions situated in virtually any portion of the lung with a minimum of difficulty. Either aspiration needle biopsy or bronchial brushing is capable of providing tissue for cytologic or microbiologic studies, usually enabling definitive diagnosis of a pulmonary lesion and often obviating the need for thoracotomy.

INDICATIONS

It should be emphasized that the fluoroscopically assisted lung biopsy techniques are only relatively innocuous and inexpensive when compared to thoracotomy. They are not employed primarily when simpler diagnostic tests will suffice. Generally, when neoplasm is suspected, three negative sputum cytologic examinations are required before a biopsy procedure is undertaken. In the evaluation of pulmonary infection, sputum study (and, when practicable, transtracheal aspiration) should be tried and found to be inconclusive before a biopsy procedure is performed.

Aspiration needle biopsy or bronchial brushing is usually restricted to localized pulmonary lesions. With diffuse interstitial lung disease, a limited thoracotomy with open lung biopsy or forceps biopsy through a fiberoptic bronchoscope is customarily recommended. The rare exception is the patient who is an extremely poor surgical candidate. In such a circumstance, a radiologically assisted biopsy technique is sometimes utilized, despite its low success rate with diffuse non-circumscribed pulmonary disease, because of its low morbidity and virtual absence of mortality.

Any persistent localized pulmonary lesion undiagnosed by conventional methods is an indication for needle aspiration biopsy or bronchial brushing.

The types of patients likely to benefit include:

1. *Clinically inoperable, lung neoplasm suspected.* Patients with a pulmonary mass(es) who are unsuitable for thoracotomy, because of either metastatic disease or severe associated medical disorder, in whom a definitive tissue diagnosis is required before radiotherapy or chemotherapy can be instituted (Fig. 2–1).
2. *Pneumonic infiltration suspected.* These techniques are useful in obtaining microorganisms from a pneumonic infiltrate in any patient whose condition is deteriorating despite antibiotic therapy (Fig. 2–2). The implication of a specific causative agent is extremely important in the immunologically deficient patient—whether the deficiency is due to immunosuppressive drugs (collagen disease, post-transplantation), underlying disease (hypogammaglobulinemia), or both (leukemia)—because of the large variety of opportunistic infectious agents that might be responsible. These patients are frequently critically ill and require prompt and accurate pursuit of a specific etiologic agent. A few organisms that are potentially susceptible to chemotherapeutic agents account for the majority of opportunistic pulmonary infections.[16] In many immunosuppressed patients with pulmonary infiltrates, aspiration needle biopsy[1] or bronchial brushing[16] can provide diagnostic material for smear and culture without resorting to thoracotomy in these often poor-risk surgical candidates (Fig. 2–3).

   The differentiation of opportunistic infection from neoplastic pulmonary infiltration is often possible through the use of the fluoroscopically assisted biopsy techniques (Fig. 2–4). This is commonly important because many organisms responsible for opportunistic infection and metastatic neoplastic cells are difficult to recover from sputum samples or bronchoscopic washings.
3. *Indeterminate solitary pulmonary lesion.* The patient with a pulmonary mass discovered on a chest radiograph may have a bronchogenic carcinoma, granuloma, benign tumor, or solitary metastasis from another primary tumor. The usual diagnostic methods, including sputum cytology and bronchoscopy, for a solitary pulmonary lesion, especially when it is less than 2 cm. in diameter, may not reveal a diagnosis. Tomography often cannot exclude and never can confirm malignancy. Exploratory thoracotomy with excision of the mass is diagnostic and possibly curative, but may expose many patients to an unnecessary major operation if the definite diagnosis of a benign or malignant process can be made by other means. It should be remembered that the incidence of carcinoma in peripheral nodules detected as part of a routine roentgenographic study is less than 20 per cent.[8, 29]

   In the past, it has been the general concensus that neither aspiration needle biopsy nor bronchial brushing is indicated for the patient in good clinical condition with a solitary lung lesion. Thoracotomy is usually planned regardless of the results of the diagnostic procedure because of the generally reported 15 per cent false negative rate for lung carcinoma with the fluoroscopically assisted biopsy procedures. Recently, however, several institutions,[42, 55] including our own, with abundant experience with needle aspiration biopsy, have achieved accuracy rates greater than 95 per cent with bronchogenic carcinoma in the middle third or peripheral lung field. Aspiration needle biopsy is now advocated at our hospital in almost all solitary indeterminate pulmonary lesions. A positive pre-operative diagnosis of malignancy usually expedites and simplifies the surgical approach, besides often convincing both patient and referring physician that thoracotomy is necessary. Ascertaining the cell type of a malignancy prior to thoracotomy may be

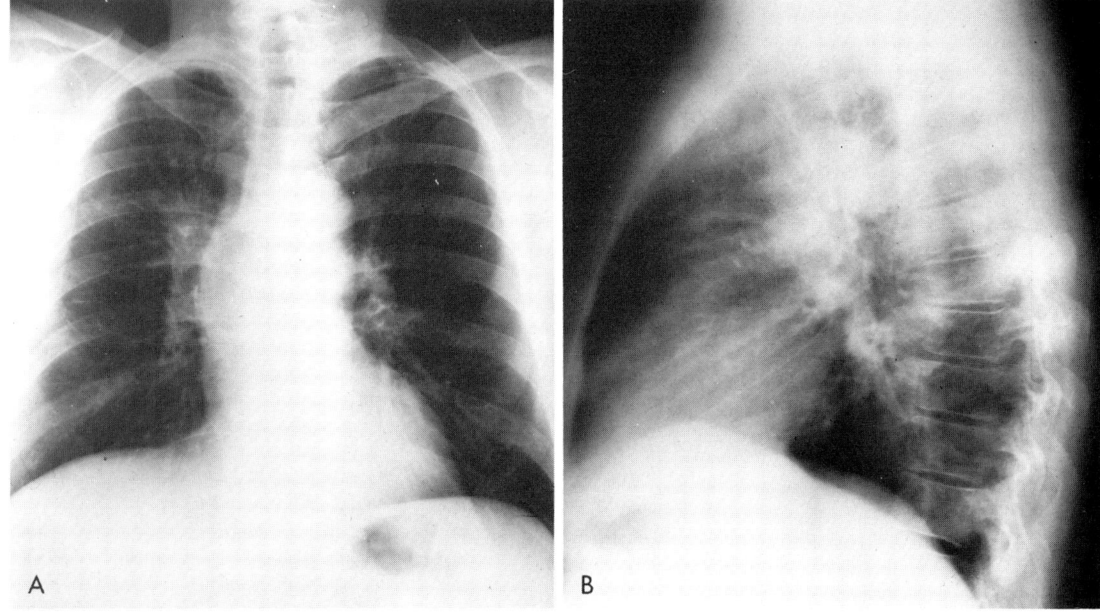

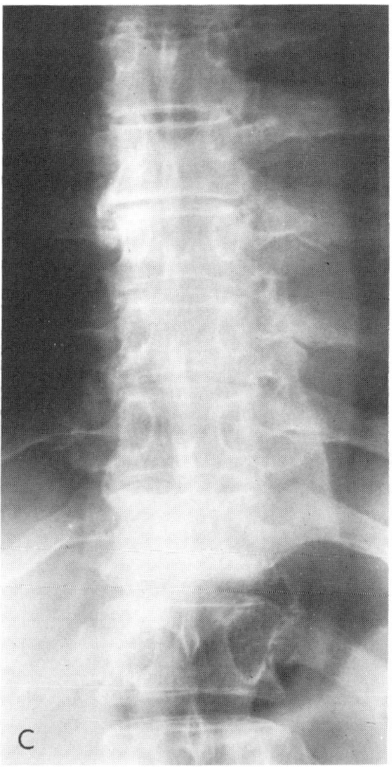

Figure 2–1. A 63 year old man with back pain. *A* and *B*. Posteroanterior and lateral chest radiographs demonstrate a mass lesion in the superior segment of the right lower lobe and right hilar lymph node enlargement. Sclerosis of the T-10 vertebral body is noted on the lateral projection. *C*. Frontal detail view of the lower thoracic spine shows a blastic lesion of the T-10 vertebral body associated with a left paraspinal mass.

Legend continued on the opposite page

worthwhile even when the lesion is almost certainly neoplastic, as resection in the presence of an oat cell carcinoma will almost certainly prove a useless adventure (Fig. 2–5). If a diagnosis of a granuloma or benign tumor is achieved by either cytologic or histologic study, then no further diagnostic procedures are necessary. If two aspiration needle biopsies have been negative in a patient with a solitary pulmonary nodule, the chance of malignancy is extremely low

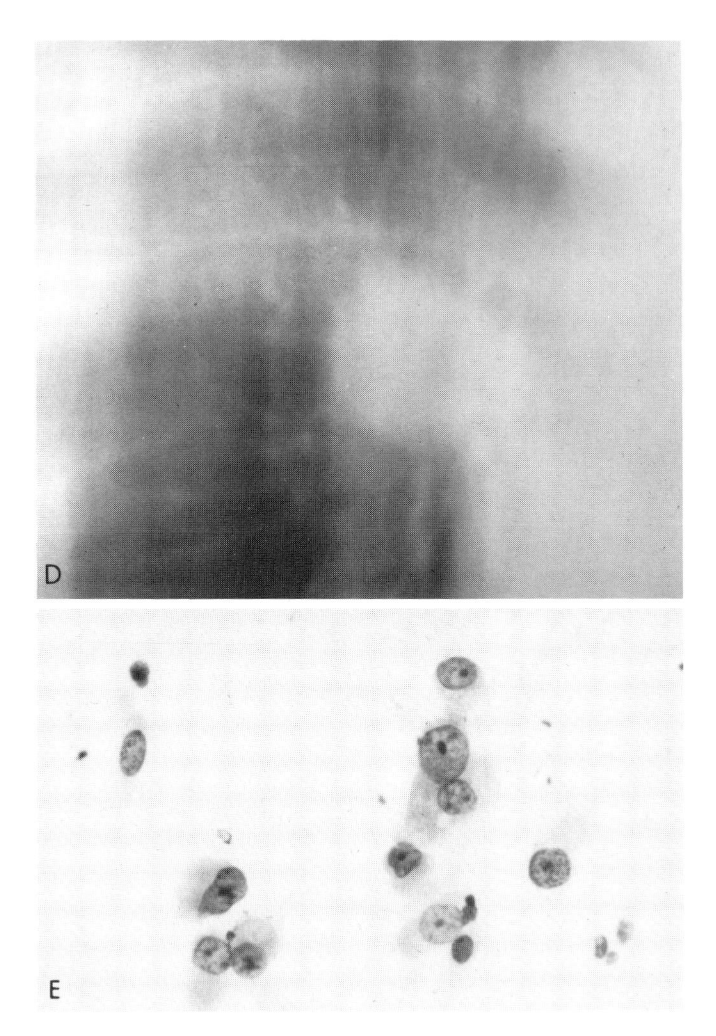

***Figure 2–1** Continued.* *D.* Frontal tomogram demonstrating mass in right lower lobe. Sputum examination and bronchoscopy were negative. *E.* Cytologic specimen of material obtained from aspiration needle biopsy of right lower lobe mass shows adenocarcinoma cells. (From Forrest, John V., and Sagel, Stuart S.: Special procedures in pulmonary radiology. *In* Potchen, E. James, editor: Current Concepts in Radiology, vol. 2, St. Louis, 1975, The C. V. Mosby Co.)

(<4%). Then only serial chest roentgenograms to observe for growth are recommended, assuming the patient is psychologically able to tolerate a period of watchful waiting (Fig. 2–6). This policy is especially advocated for older patients with solitary pulmonary lesions discovered incidentally on routine chest radiographs. No reliable data are available to suggest that this period of procrastination harms the patient whose lesion subsequently grows and proves to have a carcinoma, as early recognition appears to have little effect on ultimate post-surgical prognosis.[5] However, in hospitals where the radiologists' experience is limited, until expertise is acquired, it is certainly reasonable to initially employ this methodology of handling the solitary pulmonary nodule in the poor surgical risk patient.

In the patient with severe medical problems in whom thoracotomy may become justified if a definite diagnosis of lung carcinoma can be established, aspiration needle biopsy is routinely utilized. It is also performed in the patient with a suspected superior sulcus tumor,[47] to establish a definitive diagnosis before radiation therapy is administered, either prior to or instead of surgical resection (Fig. 2–7).

Generally, aspiration needle biopsy and bronchial brushing are considered complementary procedures, with each technique having its advantages and disadvantages.

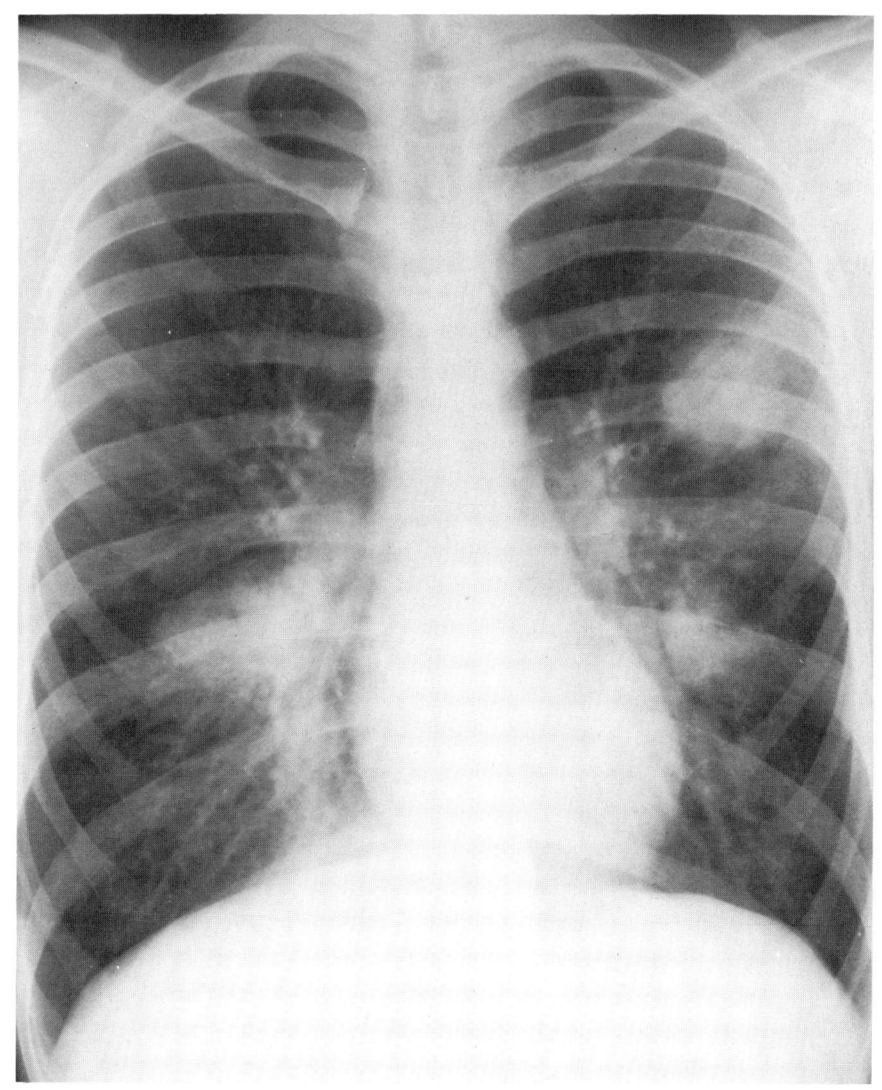

Figure 2–2. A 19 year old man, seriously ill with cough and high fever. Posteroanterior chest roentgenogram demonstrates bilateral pulmonic infiltrates, more extensive than on a radiograph obtained 5 days earlier despite interim treatment with tetracycline. Sputum examination was negative. Smears from percutaneous aspiration needle biopsy of the right lower lobe consolidation showed multiple cocci in clumps (subsequent cultures were positive for *Staphylococcus aureus*). Treatment with methicillin resulted in complete resolution of patient's symptoms and abnormal chest radiographic findings. (From Forrest, John V., and Sagel, Stuart S.: Special procedures in pulmonary radiology. *In* Potchen, E. James, editor: Current Concepts in Radiology, vol. 2, St. Louis, 1975, The C. V. Mosby Co.)

While the likelihood of significant complications occurring with bronchial brushing is virtually nil, it is often extremely time consuming (sometimes requiring up to 90 minutes). Aspiration needle biopsy is simpler to perform and rarely requires longer than 15 minutes of a busy radiologist's or sick patient's time. In addition, it has a much higher diagnostic yield than does brushing, and thus it usually is the initial procedure of choice.

Exceptions would be the patient with severe pulmonary emphysema or with an undiagnosed segmental pulmonary infiltrate in which an obstructing lesion beyond the reach of the bronchoscope is suspected. Also, bronchial brushing is the preferred procedure in any instance where broncho-

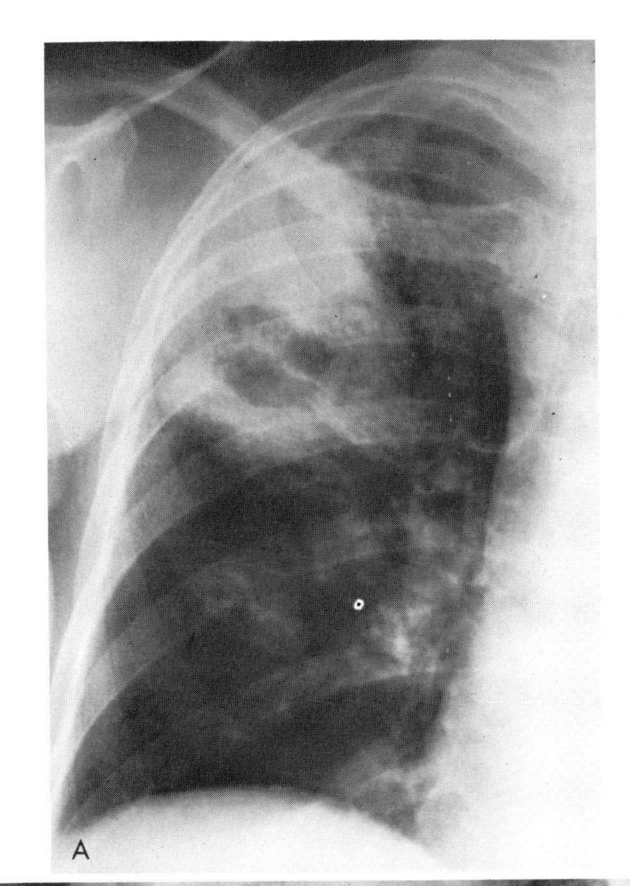

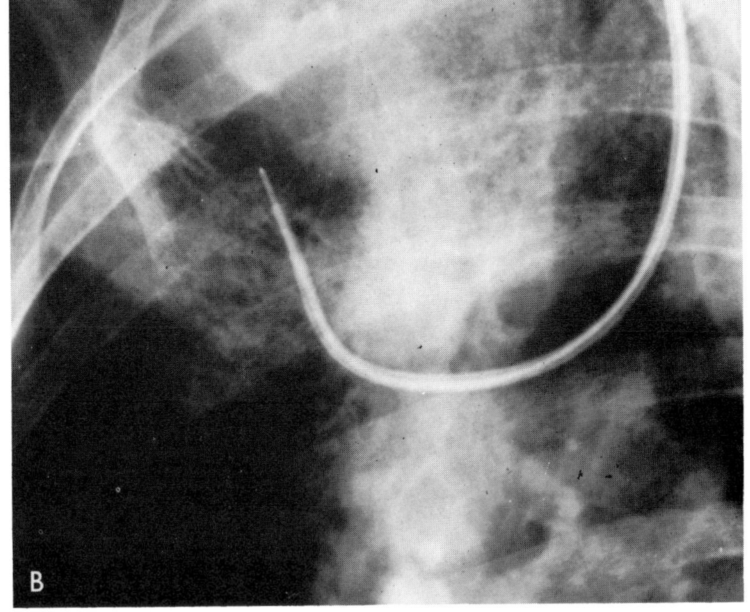

Figure 2–3. A 48 year old man with Hodgkin's disease, on treatment with chemotherapy, developed fever and a cough. *A.* Detail view from posteroanterior chest radiograph demonstrates a cavitary infiltrate within the right upper lobe. Sputum examination and transtracheal aspiration were negative. *B.* Fluoroscopic spot film demonstrating tip of brush within cavitary infiltrate. Culture of the brush scrapings yielded *Nocardia asteroides*.

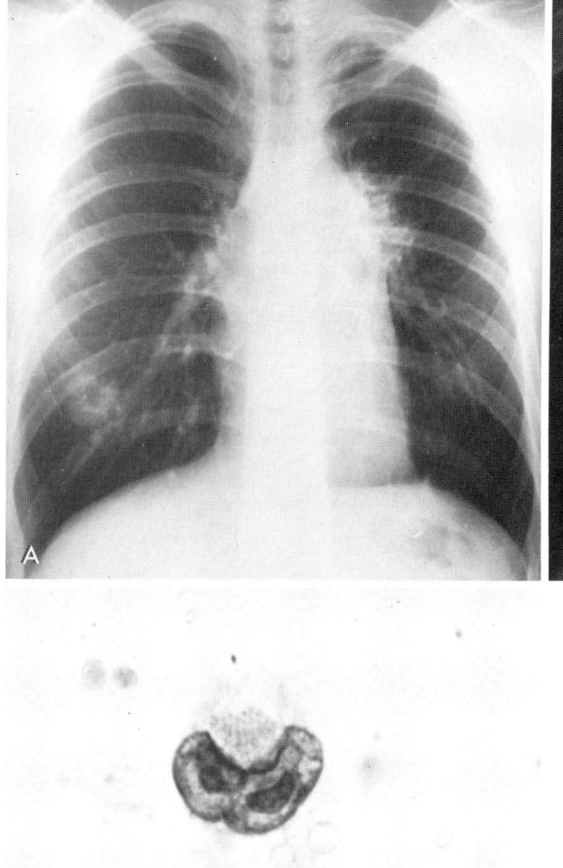

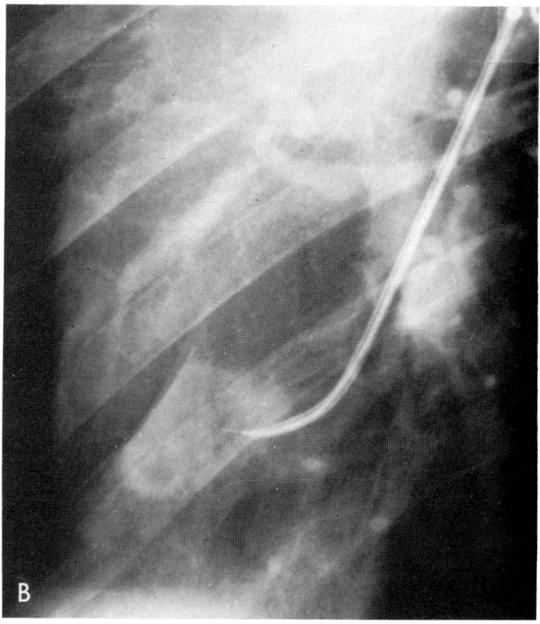

Figure 2–4. A 26 year old asymptomatic man treated with radiation therapy one year previously for mediastinal Hodgkin's disease. *A.* Posteroanterior chest roentgenogram demonstrates radiation fibrosis in the left upper lung field and a cavitary nodular infiltrate in the anterior basal segment of the right lower lobe. *B.* Oblique fluoroscopic spot film confirming tip of brush within the cavitary infiltrate. *C.* Cytologic preparation of brush scrapings showing neoplastic cell compatible with Hodgkin's disease. Culture of the brush specimen was negative. (From Forrest, John V., and Sagel, Stuart S.: Special procedures in pulmonary radiology. *In* Potchen, E. James, editor: Current Concepts in Radiology, vol. 2, St. Louis, 1975, The C. V. Mosby Co.)

graphic examination might yield important information in addition to obtaining samples from a suspicious pulmonary lesion (Fig. 2–8).

PERCUTANEOUS ASPIRATION NEEDLE BIOPSY

Percutaneous needle biopsy of the lung is not a new technique, having been described over a century ago before radiologic assistance was even available. The introduction of image intensification fluoroscopy, permitting the direction of needles to even very small pulmonary lesions with acceptable risk, along with the development of highly reliable cytologic techniques, has resulted in a revived interest in this diagnostic modality.[1,10,23,25,30,38,44]

Aspiration biopsy with a spinal type needle is a quick and simple method of diagnosis through which lesions situated in virtually any portion of the lung, or even in the mediastinum, may be aspirated. It is a relatively painless, safe, and easily learned procedure which can be accomplished in any hospital where image intensification fluoroscopy and good cytologic services are available. Lack of a cytopathologist is certainly no insurmountable problem, as tech-

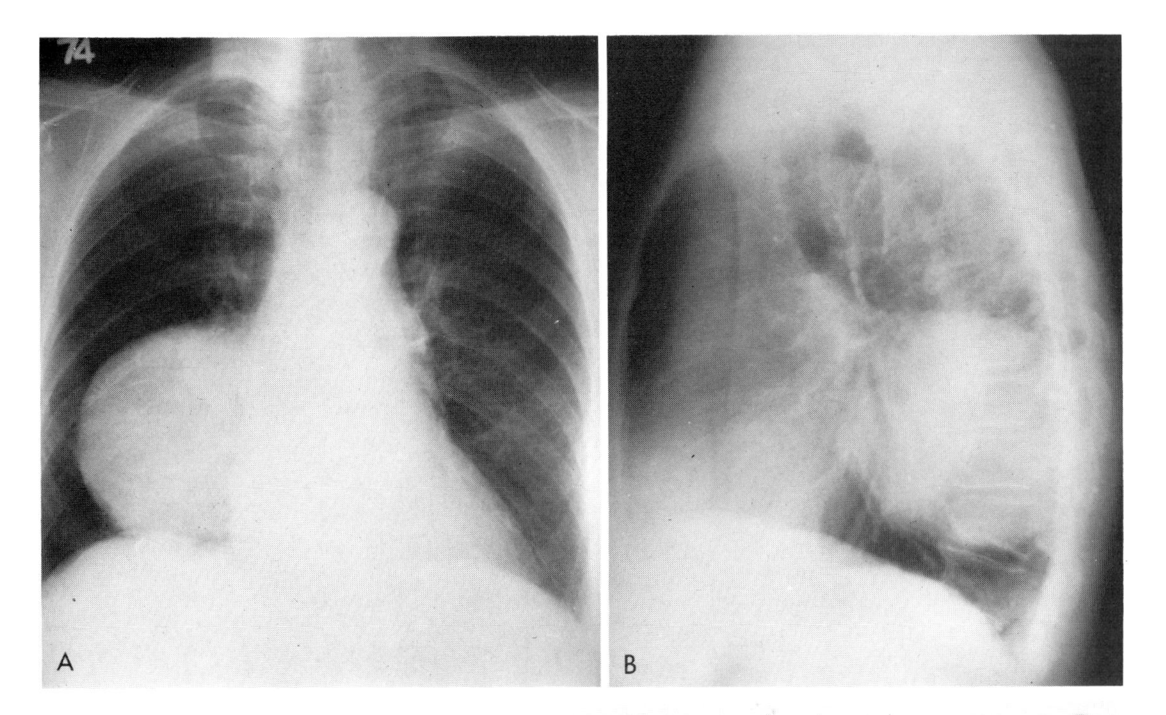

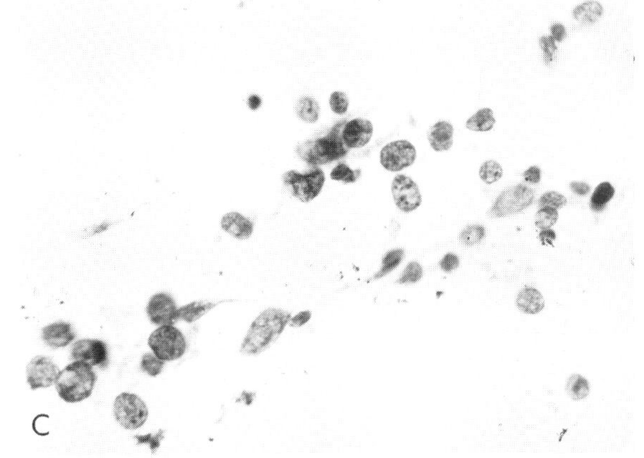

Figure 2–5. A 68 year old woman with weight loss. *A* and *B*. Posteroanterior and lateral chest radiographs demonstrate a large right lower lobe mass, which was not present three years previously. Sputum examination and bronchoscopy were negative. *C*. Cytologic preparation of needle aspirate, demonstrating oat cell carcinoma.

niques are available for preserving cells prior to transporting them to consultative laboratories.

Distinction between aspiration needle biopsy and cutting needle biopsy cannot be overemphasized. Aspiration needle biopsy is a relatively innocuous technique that generally deals with cellular material, rather than a core of tissue, and requires diagnosis by cytologic rather than histologic techniques. While cutting needle biopsy of the lung provides a tissue specimen for histologic rather than cytologic study, it is far more hazardous, having been associated with several deaths due to massive intrapulmonary hemorrhage at our institution as well as others.[28, 34] A cutting type needle[46] is almost never employed at our hospital for lung biopsy. The extremely rare exception is the case of a solid lung lesion (greater than 2 cm.) abutting upon or invading the chest wall,[51] in which the simple aspiration needle biopsy has been negative or non-diagnostic (Fig. 2–9). Percutaneous cutting needle biopsy should never be utilized in patients with diffuse pulmonary infiltrates. In this type of lesion the complication rate increases precipitously, and a limited thoracotomy with open lung biopsy or transbronchoscopic

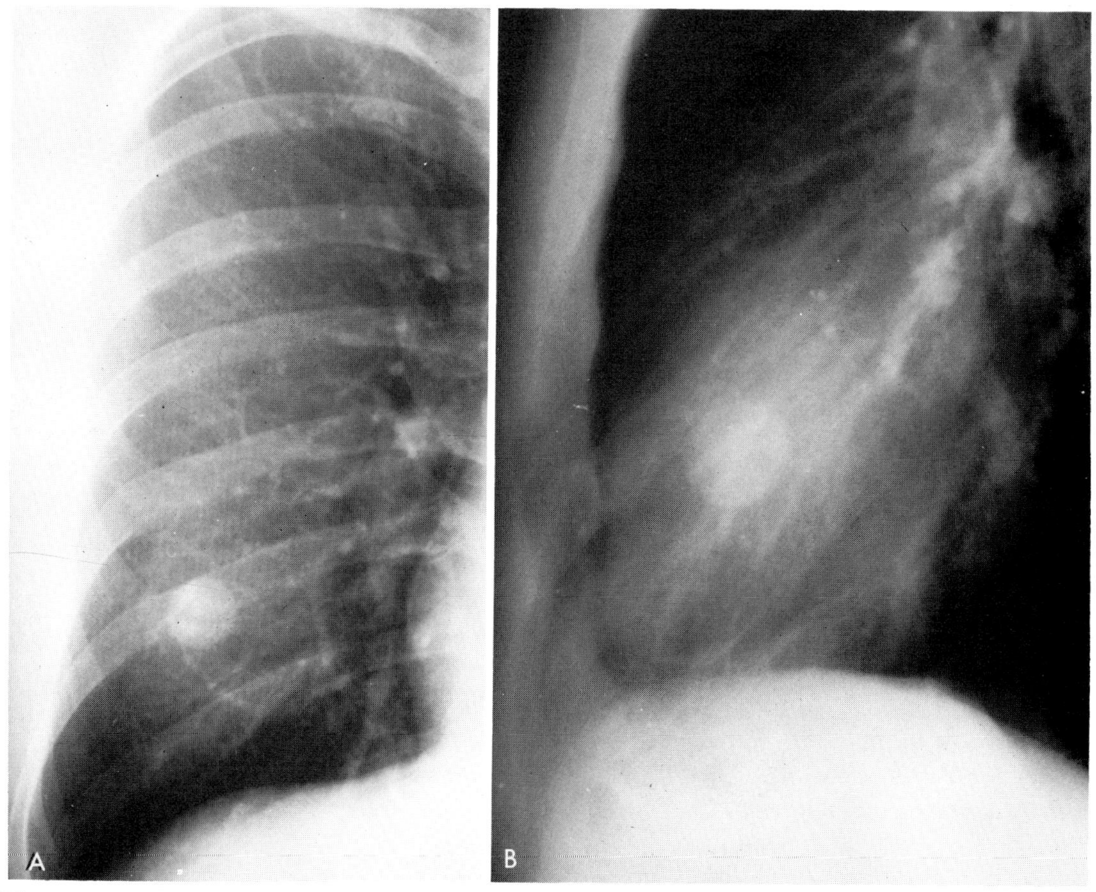

Figure 2–6. An asymptomatic 47 year old man. *A* and *B*. Detail views of posteroanterior and lateral chest radiographs demonstrate a well-circumscribed right middle lobe nodule. Aspiration needle biopsy performed on two separate occasions failed to yield malignant cells. The nodule is presumed to be a benign granuloma, and the patient is simply being followed with interval chest radiographs.

forceps biopsy are the preferred diagnostic procedures, as the complications are less frequent and a more satisfactory histologic specimen is obtained. A possible alternative method, with which no personal experience is available, is the trephine drill needle biopsy.[6]

Technique

No complex materials are needed for aspiration needle biopsy of the lung. An 18 gauge spinal type needle (Cook TB-18) whose inner cannula is sharp, making it possible to cut off some cellular material, is used.[45]

In order to assuage apprehension and reduce the minimal pain, 10 mg. of Valium or 75 mg. of Demerol is sometimes administered intramuscularly as a pre-medication, but this certainly may be omitted in the severely ill patient.

Prior to performing the actual biopsy, the patient is placed in a horizontal position on the fluoroscopic table with the affected area closest to the radiologist. The position of the patient is arranged so that the direction of thrust of the needle toward the lesion is parallel to the central X-ray beam (to avoid parallax error) and perpendicular to the radiologic table. The patient generally assumes a supine position for an anteriorly situated lesion and a prone position if the lesion is posterior. Rarely, oblique or lateral positioning is optimal for direction of the needle vertically along the X-ray beam. A posterior approach is always used for

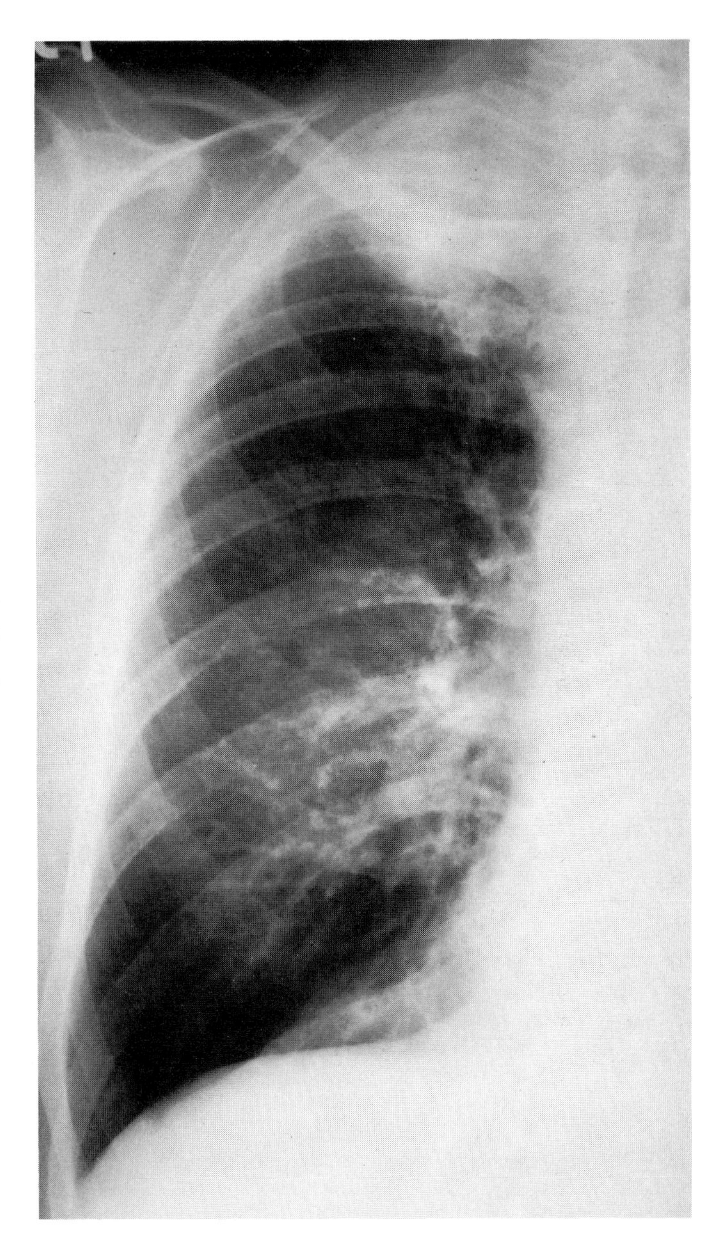

Figure 2–7. A 75 year old man with right shoulder pain of 7 months duration. Detail view from posteroanterior chest radiograph demonstrates a right apical lung mass. Cytologic preparation from a needle aspiration biopsy revealed squamous cell carcinoma.

apical lesions to avoid injury to subclavian vessels and the brachial plexus. Having the patient "hug" a large pillow which is placed under his thorax facilitates rotating the scapula out of the way. In the patient with multiple pulmonary lesions, the most peripheral accessible lesion is biopsied.

Occasionally, the bony skeleton may prove an obstacle to direct access to the lesion, making it necessary to use an oblique needle course. This occurs with small peripheral lesions located immediately adjacent to a rib or with mediastinal lesions.

To facilitate the use of long needles without breaking sterile technique by contacting the fluoroscopic equipment, an image intensification system with an over-the-table X-ray tube is preferred. Proper attention to X-ray protection with this type of apparatus is extremely important.

After optimal fluoroscopic positioning, the lesion is localized using the tip of a me-

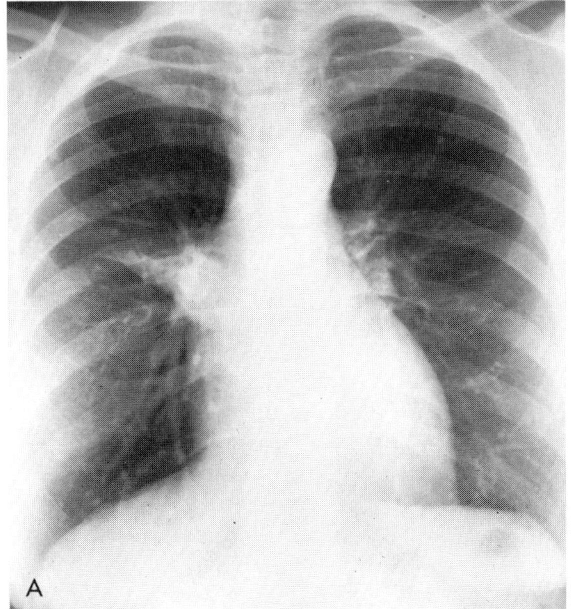

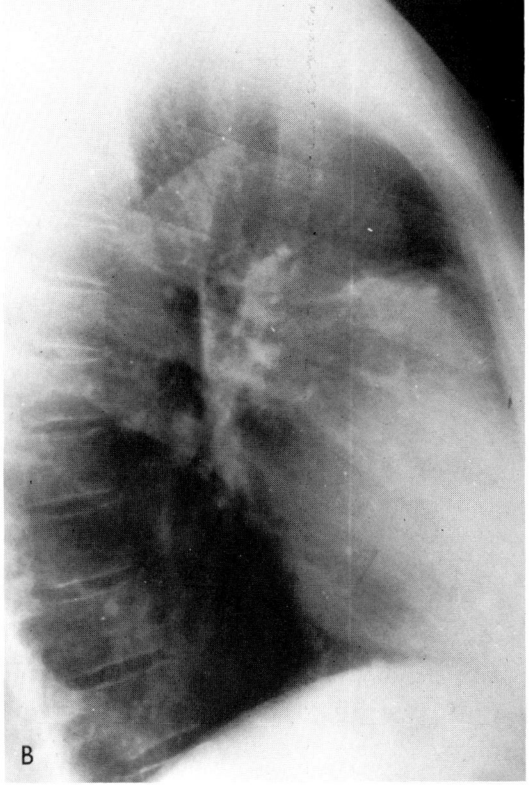

Figure 2–8. A 39 year old asymptomatic woman. *A* and *B*. Posteroanterior and lateral chest roentgenograms demonstrate an oblong mass density in the anterior segment of the right upper lobe and evidence of old healed granulomatous disease.

Legend continued on the opposite page

tallic pointer, and the skin over the lesion is marked, ideally in mid-expiration. Preferably, the site chosen should be such that the needle will pass over the superior aspect of the rib in its approach to the lesion, thus avoiding injury to intercostal vessels or nerves. The skin in the area is cleansed with disinfectant and draped with sterile towels, and then the skin and superficial soft tissues of the chest wall over the lesion are anesthetized. No attempt to infiltrate the pleura is made. A small incision is made in the skin and superficial subcutaneous tissue with a No. 11 scalpel blade to facilitate both advancing the needle through the chest wall, and aiding transmission of variations in lung consistency to the operator's fingers without interference from the skin.

The biopsy needle is now inserted into the skin and advanced over the rib. Proper position and direction of the needle is confirmed fluoroscopically while the needle is held by a long forceps with a jaw (Storz Instrument Co. N7175), thus avoiding irradiation to the hand. The biopsy needle with its contained stylet is then quickly thrust through the pleura while the patient is holding his breath, usually in mid-expiration. It is important that the parietal and visceral pleura be penetrated with one thrust, and that the sharp tip of the needle not linger in such a position that respiratory motion could result in a laceration of the visceral pleura. After penetration of the lung by the needle, if necessary, the patient may breathe shallowly when the needle is not being advanced. The needle tip is then guided to the periphery of the lesion by intermittent image intensification fluoroscopy (a television monitor is greatly preferable to mirror optics).

Determination of the depth of the lesion almost always can be accomplished using single plane fluoroscopy, which is much less cumbersome and certainly much more readily available than a biplane system. A fairly accurate estimate of the depth of the lesion can be calculated by study and measurement of the patient's posteroanterior

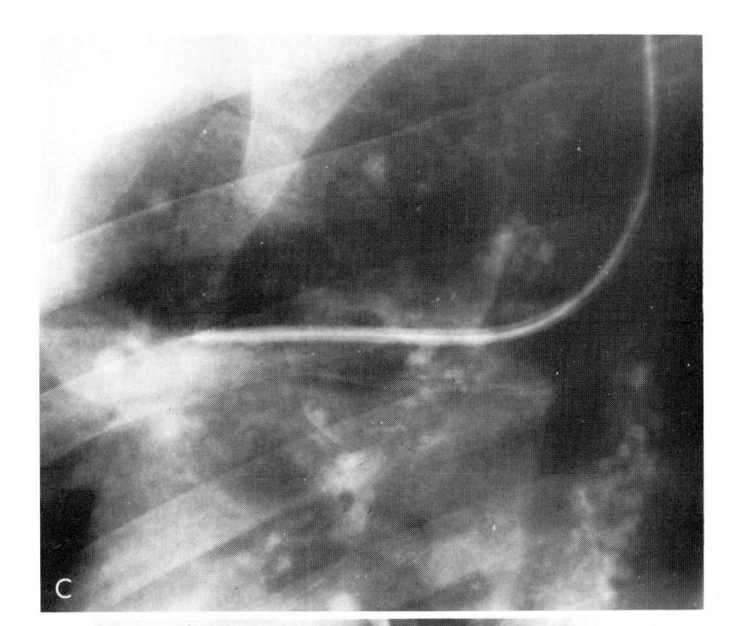

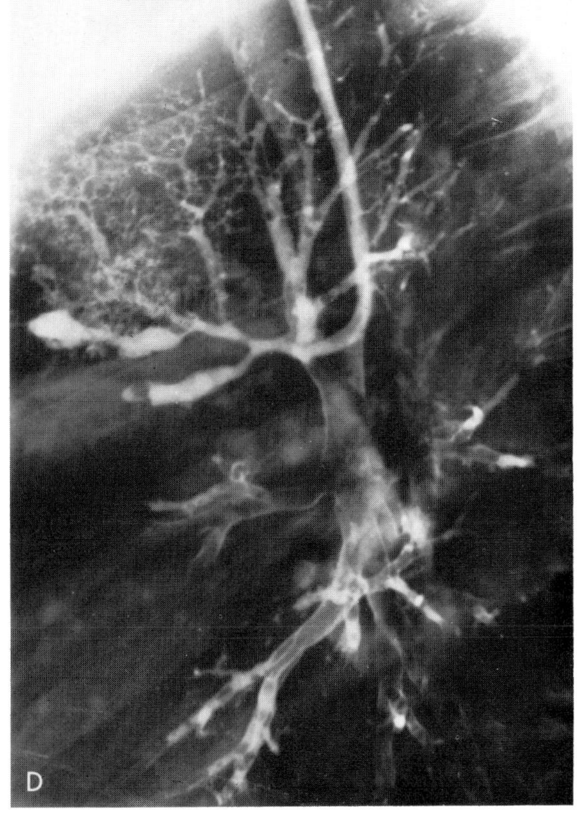

Figure 2–8 Continued. *C.* Fluoroscopic spot film confirming proper location of brush and catheter within the right upper lobe density. Culture and cytologic preparations of the brushings and washings were subsequently negative. *D.* Post-brush bronchogram demonstrates localized bronchiectasis in the anterior segment of the right upper lobe. The lesion was thought to be post-inflammatory in view of the negative brushings and bronchographic findings, and thoracotomy was averted. (From Forrest, John V., and Sagel, Stuart S.: Special procedures in pulmonary radiology. *In* Potchen, E. James, editor: Current Concepts in Radiology, vol. 2, St. Louis, 1975, The C. V. Mosby Co.)

and lateral chest radiographs. Occasionally, if it is necessary for better localization, oblique views or laminograms can be obtained; these are helpful in providing a more detailed assessment of the size and depth of the lesion (Figs. 2–1 and 2–10). Precise determination of the depth of the lesion prior to needle insertion is not necessary. Verification that the needle is in the periphery of the lesion is often achieved by

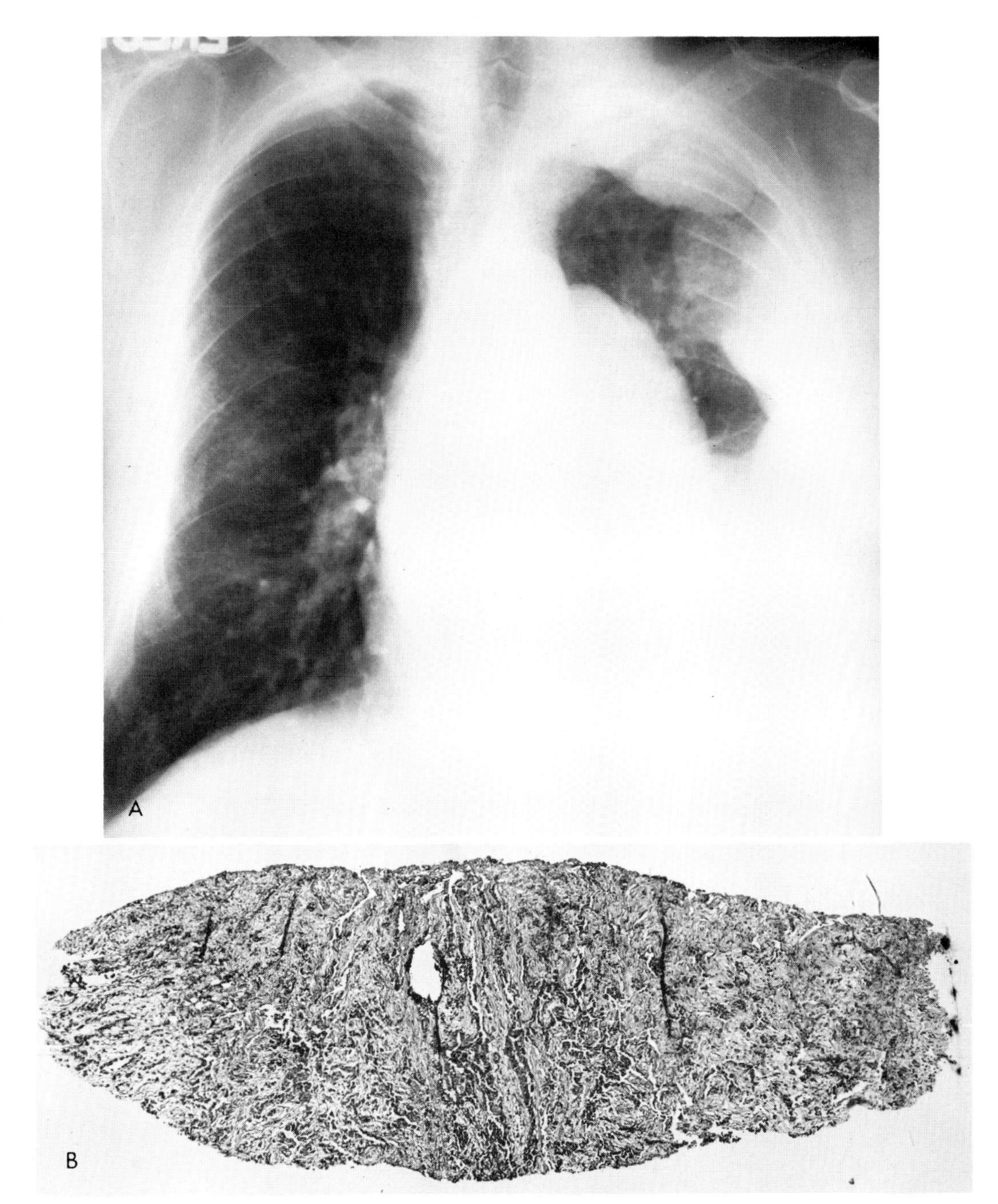

Figure 2–9. A 59 year old man with mild dyspnea and weight loss, and prior heavy asbestos exposure. *A*. Posteroanterior chest roentgenogram demonstrates multiple pleural-based masses throughout the left hemithorax. Cytologic preparation from a needle aspirate revealed unclassifiable malignant cells. *B*. Photomicrograph from histologic preparation (electron microscopy also performed) obtained by Vim cutting needle biopsy (original size 2 × 6 mm.) demonstrates malignant mesothelioma.

a feeling of increased resistance when the lesion is penetrated. This sensation usually occurs with solid neoplastic lesions. A short, quick jabbing motion is sometimes necessary to penetrate the mass, especially with small circumscribed lesions. If there is concern about the position of the needle tip relative to the lesion, fluoroscopy can

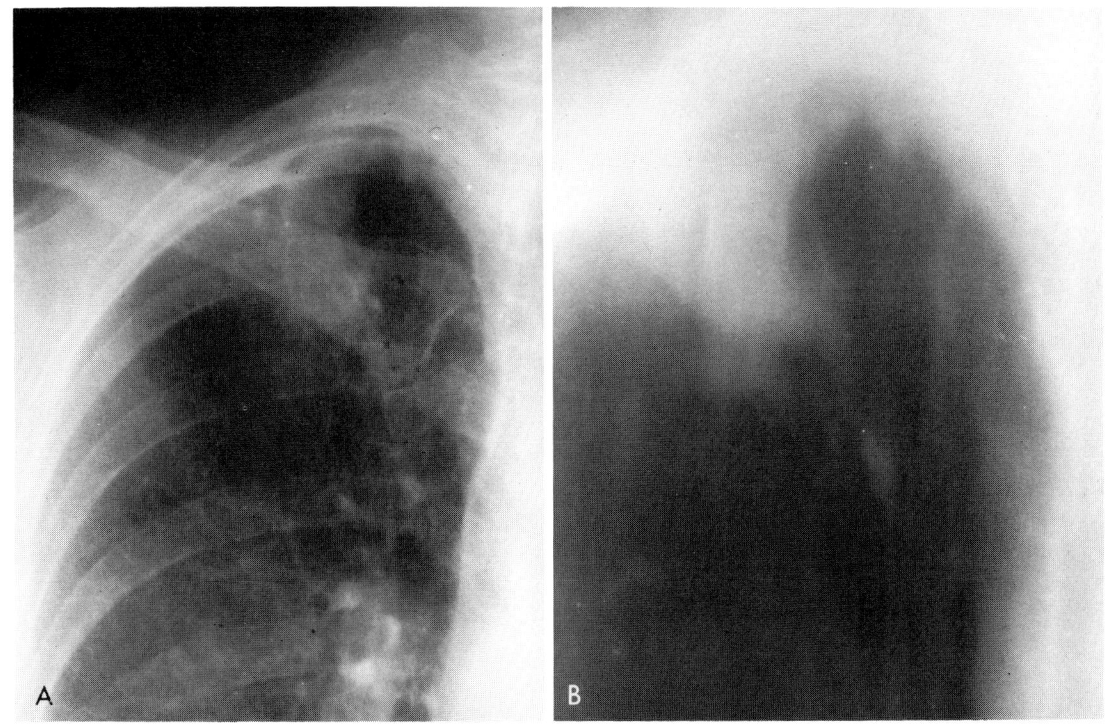

Figure 2–10. An asymptomatic 70 year old woman. *A*. Detail view of posteroanterior chest radiograph demonstrates an irregular right apical lung density. *B*. Frontal tomogram shows a mass-like apical infiltrate overlying the 3rd posterior interspace on the 8 cm. cut. The lesion could not be seen fluoroscopically. Therefore, a small metallic marker, to serve as a guide, was placed on the skin overlying the site of the density demonstrated tomographically. Marking the skin over apical lesions which are difficult or impossible to see fluoroscopically is valuable because respiratory motion has almost no affect on lesions in this location. Cytologic preparation of the needle aspirate from this location disclosed adenocarcinoma cells. (Comparison to Fig. 1–4 demonstrates the ability of needle aspiration biopsy to distinguish between similar roentgenographic densities.)

demonstrate whether movement of the tip of the needle and the lesion is synchronous during shallow respirations; if this is the case, penetration of the needle tip to the proper depth is confirmed. As a further check, if doubt still remains, the patient can be rotated slightly to an oblique position, and the tip of the needle with respect to the lesion can be checked fluoroscopically in this new projection.

If the mass to be biopsied is large, the specimen should be obtained from the periphery rather than the center of the lesion, since large neoplasms are often necrotic in the center. Cavitary lesions should be aspirated from both their inner and outer margins. If the lesion is neoplastic, the biopsy from the interior wall will often contain only necrotic material, while tissue obtained from the outer margin may establish the diagnosis. The converse is true when inflammatory cavities are biopsied.

On a few occasions, in patients with diffuse small nodular disease, we have done "blind" biopsies where a specific nodule could not be localized under the fluoroscope and have obtained positive results (Fig. 2–11). Similar success has been reported in cases of lymphangitic carcinoma.[26]

With the tip of the aspirating needle now placed optimally within the periphery of the lesion, fluoroscopy is discontinued and the patient is instructed to stop breathing. The stylet is removed, and a 20 cc. Luer-Lok syringe filled with 2 ml. of sterile balanced electrolyte solution (Polysal, Cutter Laboratories) is attached to the needle hub. (When the stylet is removed and before attaching the syringe, the radiologist should place his thumb over the hub of the needle

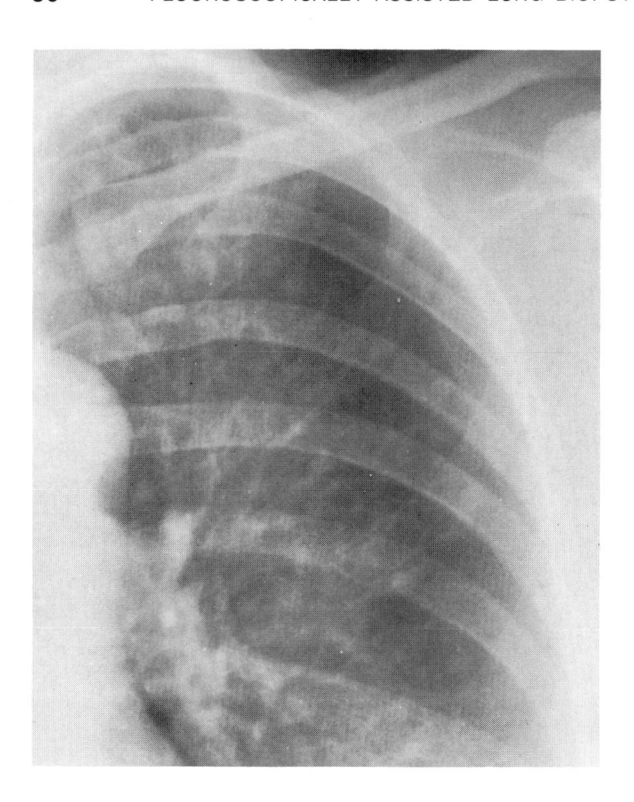

Figure 2–11. A 56 year old woman with cough and mild dyspnea. Detail view of left upper lobe from posteroanterior roentgenogram demonstrates small nodular densities throughout both lungs. Clinical evaluation was negative. Because of an inability to localize any specific nodule fluoroscopically, three "blind" aspirates were obtained from the left upper lobe. Cytologic preparation revealed adenocarcinoma cells.

to prevent the possibility of air embolism should the patient inadvertently breathe.) Constant suction is now applied to the syringe by withdrawing the plunger with the right hand. The barrel of the syringe is grasped with the left hand, and the syringe and needle are rotated clockwise and counterclockwise while being moved slightly forward within the lesion. With solid lesions this permits the sharp bevel of the needle to cut off very small fragments of tissue. With suction still applied, the needle is withdrawn from the thorax. The contents of the syringe and needle are then expressed into test tubes containing the balanced electrolyte solution. The syringe is then disconnected from the needle, and filled with about 3 ml. of sterile Polysal solution. The needle is then reconnected to the syringe and flushed through with the saline solution into test tubes. If a relatively large core of tissue is obtained, it is placed in formalin and sent for histologic study (Figs. 2–12 and 2–13). The biopsy procedure may be repeated two to three times until good specimens for all required studies are obtained. If a cystic structure is aspirated, this may be opacified with contrast media.[54]

The solutions in the test tubes are subsequently processed depending upon the clinical situation. Smears and cultures may be prepared for routine bacteriologic studies, mycobacterium, fungus, and so on (Fig. 2–14). If anaerobic infection is suspected, the aspirate is injected directly into a special "nitrogen-gassed" tube.

Material for cytologic study which was placed in the balanced electrolyte solution is immediately taken to the cytology laboratory, where smears and Millipore filters are prepared and then stained by the Papanicolaou technique. Any small tissue fragments are processed for histologic study after being placed in 5% agar to avoid loss during fixation and embedding. In addition to routine hematoxylin and eosin stains, a variety of special stains can be applied to the sectioned material when indicated (e.g., fungal, acid fast, mucin; Sudan III when a pleural based lipoma is suspected; melanin stains when metastatic melanoma is likely) (Figs. 2–13 and 2–15). Aspirates from suspected silicotic nodules may be studied via a polarizing microscope to search for the appropriate crystals.

Following completion of the needle aspi-

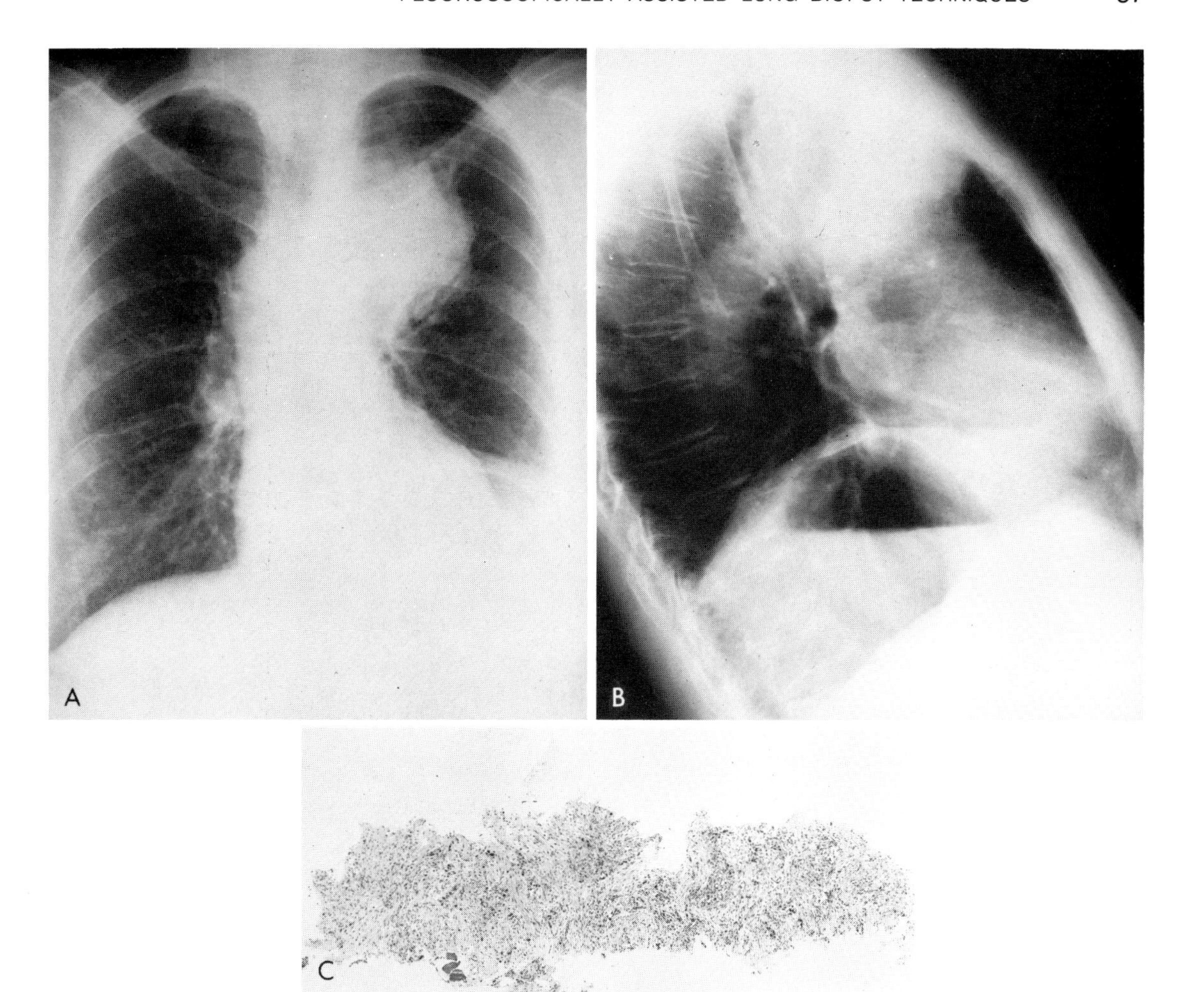

Figure 2–12. A 63 year old woman with hemoptysis and weight loss. *A* and *B*. Posteroanterior and lateral chest radiographs demonstrate a large left upper lobe mass extending into the mediastinum. Right paratracheal lymph node enlargement is present. The elevated left hemidiaphragm was confirmed by fluoroscopy as due to phrenic nerve paralysis. *C*. Histologic preparation of small tissue core (original size 0.8 × 3 mm.) obtained by percutaneous aspiration needle biopsy demonstrates poorly differentiated squamous cell carcinoma. (From Forrest, John V., and Sagel, Stuart S.: Special procedures in pulmonary radiology. *In* Potchen, E. James, editor: Current Concepts in Radiology, vol. 2, St. Louis, 1975, The C. V. Mosby Co.)

ration, the skin and subcutaneous tissues are gently massaged over the needle opening to prevent air from entering the pleural space, and a sterile bandage is then applied over the puncture site. An erect posteroanterior chest radiograph taken in expiration is obtained. (If the patient complains of dyspnea during the procedure, fluoroscopy is utilized to look for a pneumothorax.) Clinical observation of the patient for several subsequent hours is advised, along with the avoidance of intermittent positive pressure breathing (I.P.P.B.). If a small pneumothorax was detected on the postbiopsy film, a repeat chest radiograph is taken in 4 to 6 hours. Analgesia may be given for any associated pleuritic pain.

If results from the initial aspiration needle biopsy are negative, then the procedure is repeated (usually within 24 hours). Just as multiple sputum examinations improve the diagnostic yield, likewise multiple aspiration biopsies increase the chances for a correct diagnosis.

Complications

The possible complications of pulmonary aspiration needle biopsy are pneumothorax,

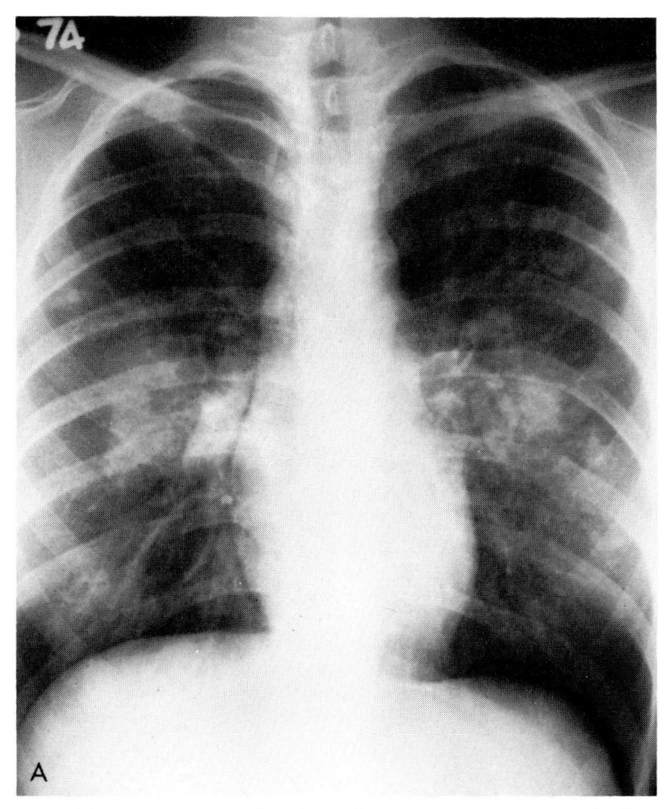

Figure 2–13. A 19 year old woman with pleuritic chest pain and low grade fever. *A.* Posteroanterior chest radiograph demonstrates patchy bilateral pulmonary infiltrates. Sputum examination and fungal serology were negative. The chest radiograph remained unchanged for two weeks.

Legend continued on the opposite page

pulmonary hemorrhage, empyema, and implantation of tumor cells in the needle tract.

In our series of 411 percutaneous aspiration needle biopsies, a pneumothorax has been by far the most common complication, developing in 78 cases (19%). As in other reported series,[10, 23, 44] in most instances the pneumothorax was small and resolved spontaneously. When the pneumothorax is large or dyspnea occurs, as happened in 32 (7.8%) of our patients, closed intercostal drainage was quickly instituted and maintained for about 24 hours. We have had no case in which a clinically significant pneumothorax developed when the immediate post-biopsy chest radiograph demonstrated no pneumothorax. The risk of a serious pneumothorax is much higher in patients with emphysema or stiff fibrotic lungs, and almost universal in patients requiring mechanical ventilation prior to biopsy. Utilization of a Teflon sheath to cover the aspirating needle and injection of blood after aspiration through the tract,[27] in our experience, has not greatly diminished the number of pneumothoraces nor decreased the number requiring treatment, and this technique is much more cumbersome to use.

Use of a simple catheter technique allows the radiologist to treat immediately any pneumothorax requiring therapy and thus prevent any complications that might arise from it. A No. 8 Teflon catheter (24 cm. in length) with multiple side holes near the tip is inserted via Seldinger technique into the second anterior intercostal space on the side of the needle biopsy.[39] The needle should be angled cephalad so that the catheter tip is subsequently placed near the lung apex. A three-way stop cock is attached to the hub of the catheter, to permit manual aspiration of air. The stop cock is then connected to a Heimlich valve,[3] which permits only unidirectional air flow (Fig. 2–16). The skin-catheter inter-

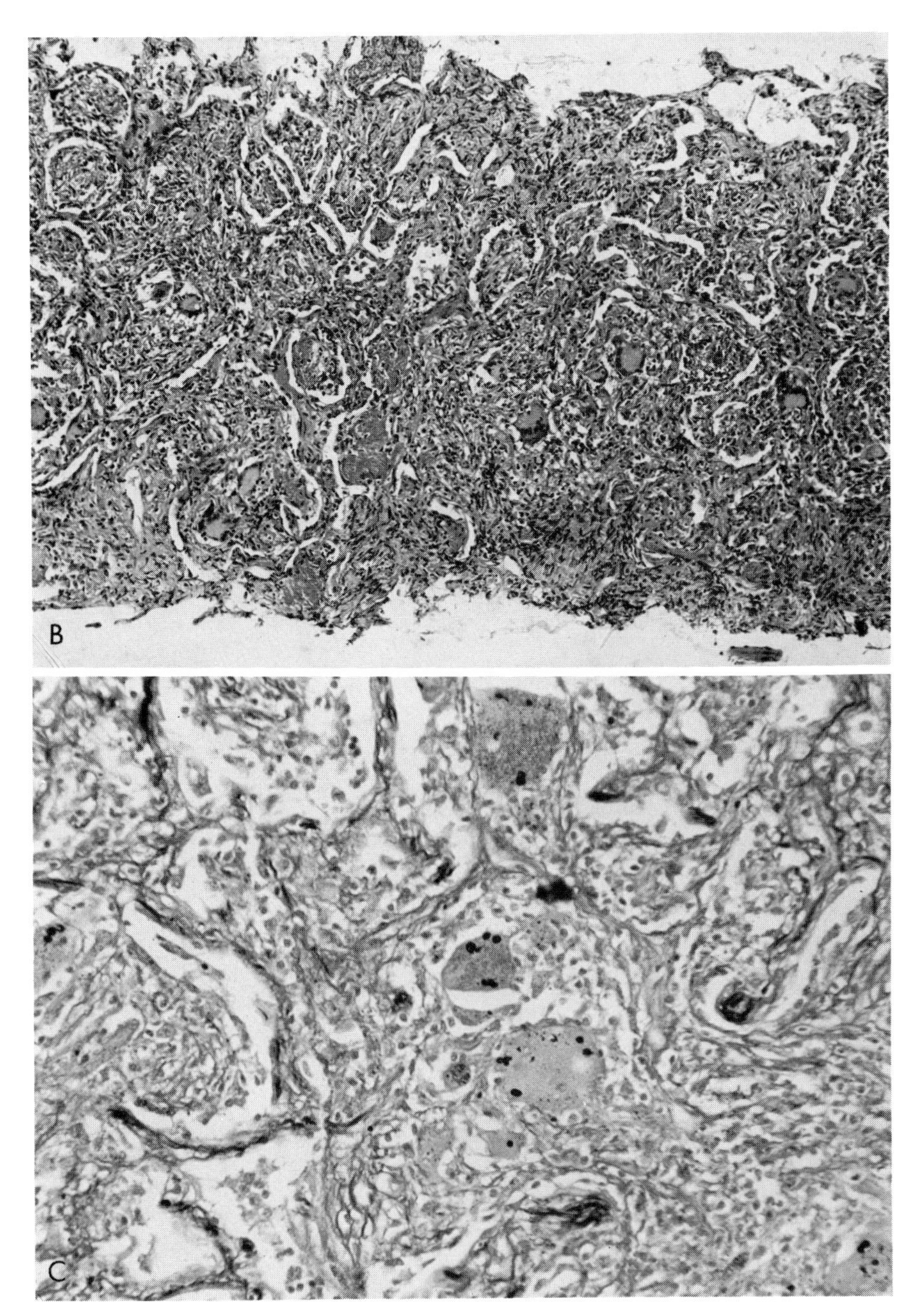

Figure 2–13 Continued. *B*. Hematoxylin and eosin stain of histologic preparation of a small core of tissue obtained from needle aspiration biopsy shows multiple granulomas. *C*. Gomori's methanamine silver stain discloses myriad *Histoplasma capsulatum* organisms.

face is sealed with Vaseline gauze, and the remaining connections with adhesive tape. Covering bandages are then applied. This apparatus suffices for most patients, allowing them complete ambulation (Fig. 2–17). If, after a period of 24 hours, the lung remains completely expanded, the catheter is withdrawn. Sometimes drainage is not rapid enough, and connection to an Emerson pump with suction or insertion of a larger chest tube by a surgeon is required. Certainly, the possible complication of a large pneumothorax is insufficient justification for preferring diagnostic thoracotomy

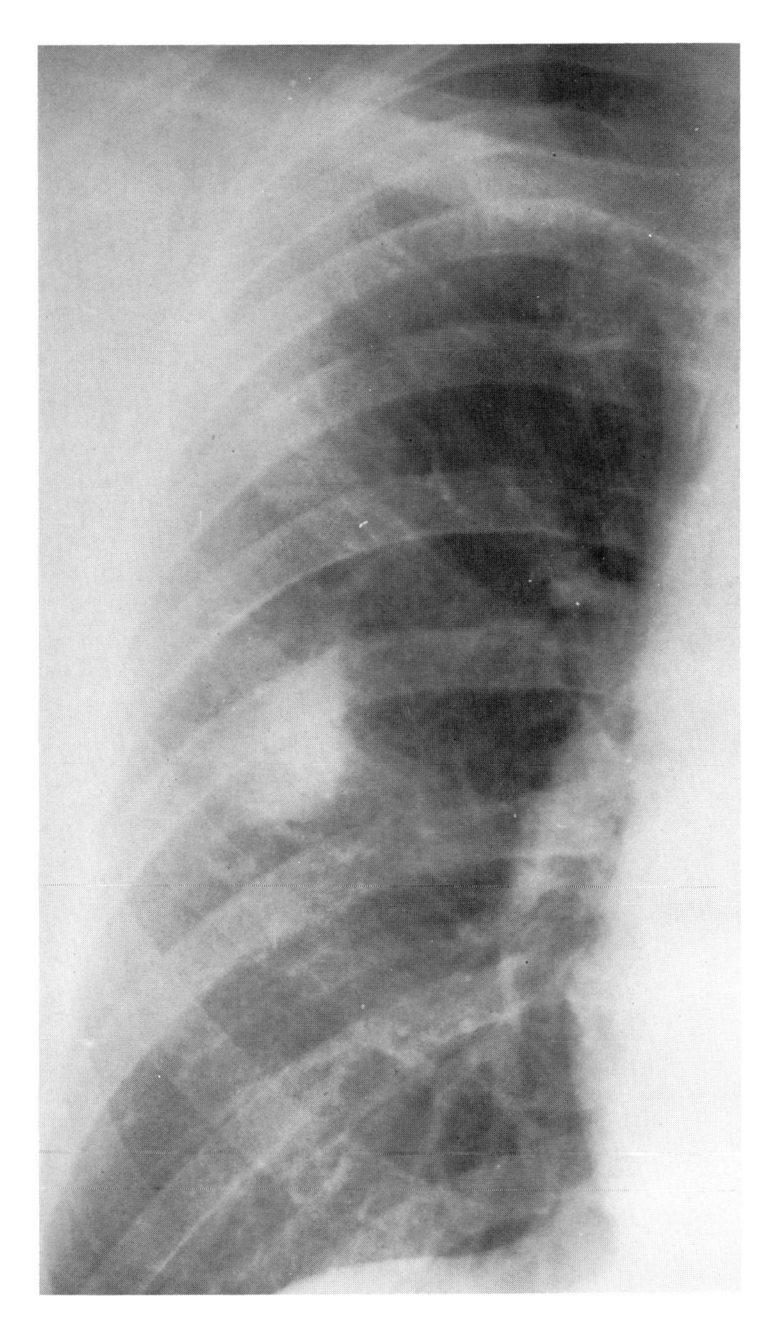

Figure 2–14. A 62 year old man with a "flu-like" illness. Detail view of posteroanterior roentgenogram demonstrates an irregular mass in the right mid lung field. The infiltrate persisted for three weeks, despite resolution of clinical symptoms. Sputum examination, fiberoptic bronchoscopic washings, and bronchial brushings were negative. Culture of material obtained from needle aspiration disclosed *Cryptococcus neoformans.*

over needle biopsy, since the insertion of a chest tube into the pleural space is no more difficult after needle biopsy than when it is inserted into 100 per cent of patients after surgery.

Hemoptysis is unusual, occurring in about 5 per cent of patients immediately following the aspiration biopsy. It is invariably mild and transitory, and none of our patients have ever required treatment. Two patients with clinically and radiographically severe pulmonary hypertension coughed up about 75 cc. of blood, but this stopped spontaneously within several minutes (Fig. 2–18). Bleeding into the lung parenchyma about a lesion occurs in about 10 per cent of patients, with about half experiencing the invariable mild hemoptysis. Four cases of small asymptomatic pleural effusions, presumably due to blood within

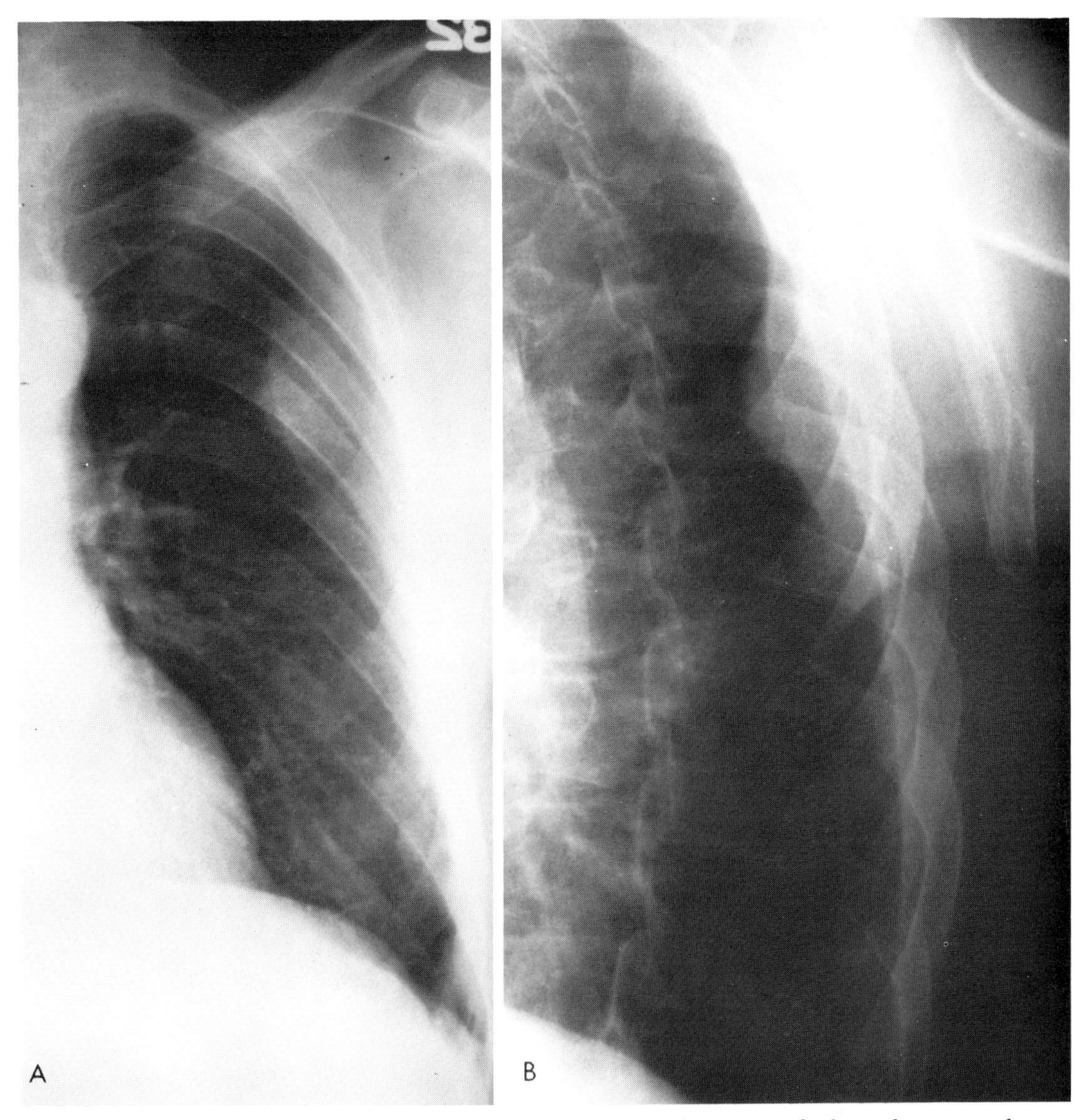

Figure 2–15. An asymptomatic 62 year old man, four years after removal of a malignant melanoma from his left leg. *A* and *B*. Detail views from posteroanterior and oblique radiographs demonstrate pleural-based masses in the left lateral hemithorax.

Illustration and legend continued on the following page

the pleural space, have occurred following the procedure.

The risk of spread of infection to the pleural space is small and more theoretical than actual.[22, 25] The incidence of empyema appears to be no greater than in comparable cases managed without needle biopsy.[30]

Implantation of tumor cells into the needle tract resulting in intrapulmonary, pleural, or subcutaneous dissemination occurs,[2, 25, 50] but is extremely rare.[4, 11] This complication usually is seen only in advanced malignant neoplasm, when the risk is of little clinical importance compared to the establishment of a diagnosis. In a series of 5,000 cases of aspiration needle biopsy, two instances of implantation metastasis (one to the pleura and one to the chest wall) are reported.[33] The overall survival rate of patients with lung cancer who had a prior aspiration needle biopsy was identical to a similar group who just had surgery.[42] It must be remembered that cutaneous or

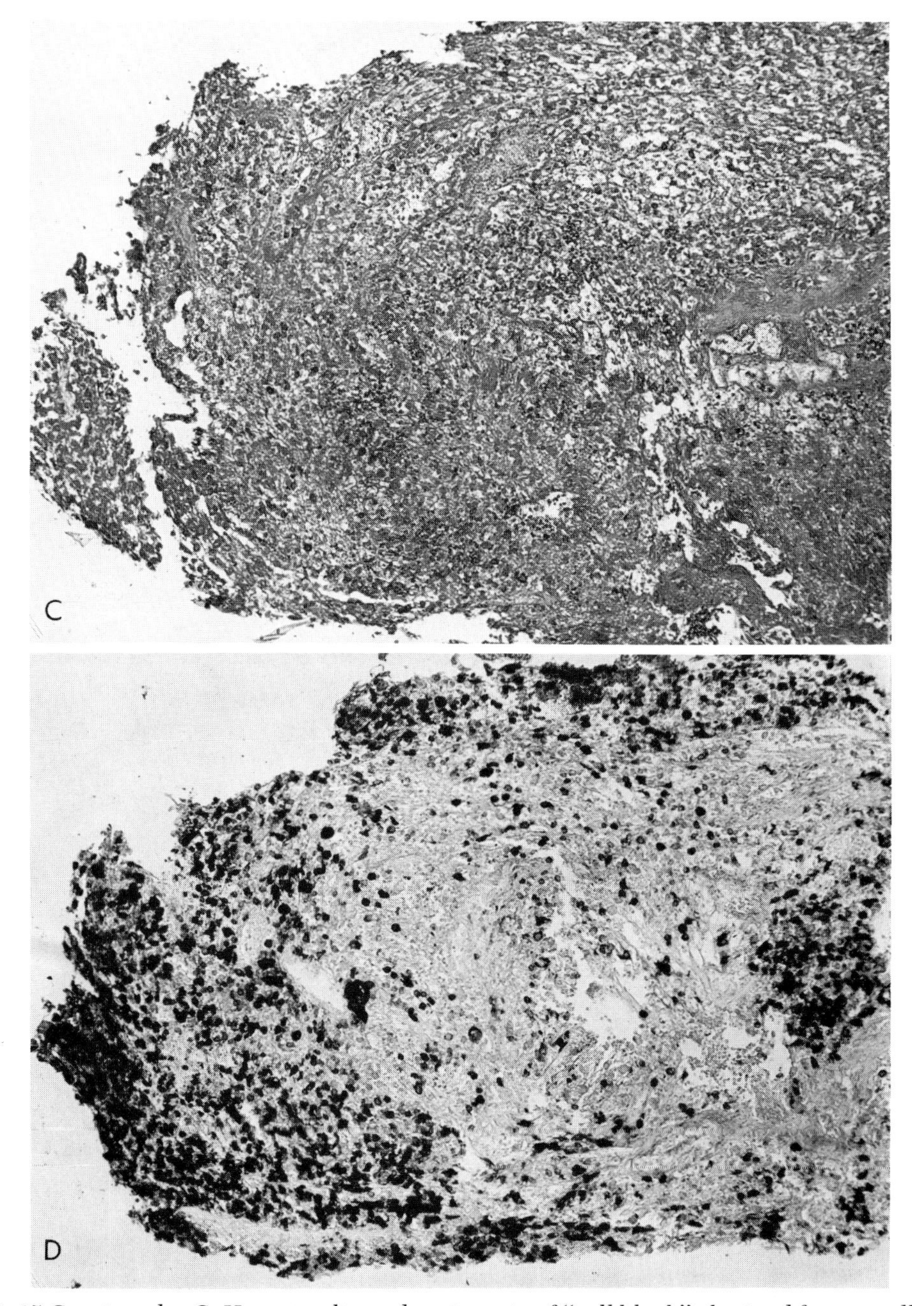

Figure 2–15 Continued. *C*. Hematoxylin and eosin stain of "cell block" obtained from needle aspiration biopsy demonstrates necrotic malignant cells. *D*. Application of Fontana-Masson stain reveals melanin within the malignant cells.

pleural implants are also a potential complication of thoracotomy performed for the diagnosis or treatment of bronchogenic carcinoma.[43] No case of this complication of aspiration needle biopsy has been encountered by these authors, and generally this risk is considered negligible.

In our experience, as with other large series,[24, 33] the mortality rate with aspiration needle biopsy has been zero. Fatal compli-

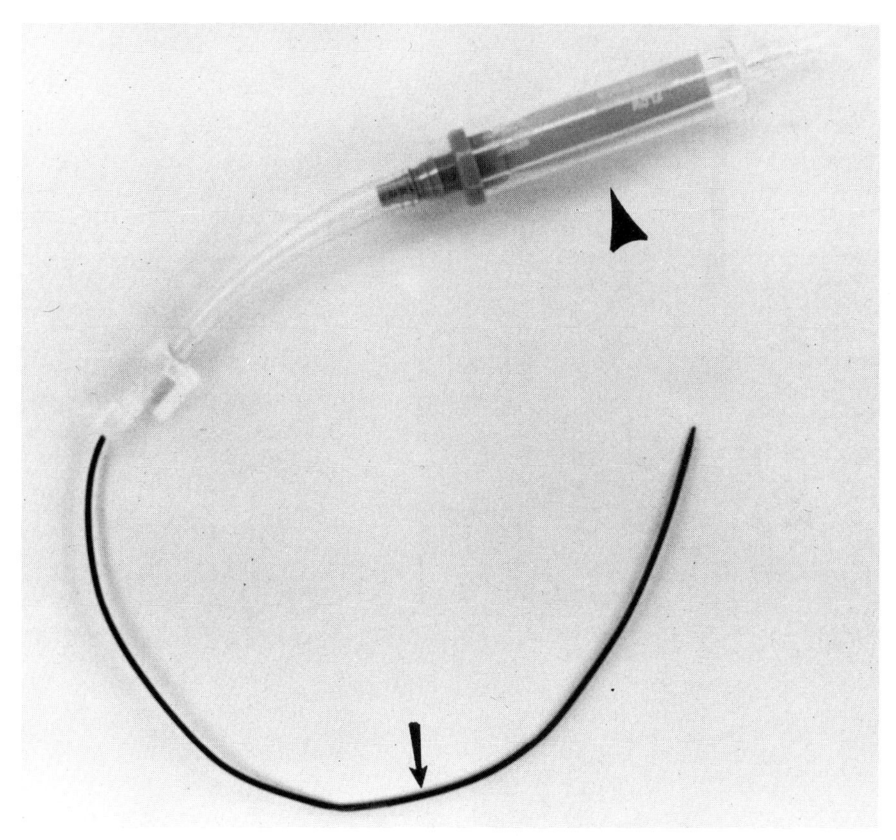

Figure 2–16. Catheter assemblage for simple treatment of pneumothorax. A number 8 F Teflon catheter (arrow) with multiple side holes near the tip is attached to a 3-way plastic stop cock (which facilitates manual aspiration). The stop cock is connected by a short segment of polyethylene tubing to the Heimlich one-way drainage valve (arrowhead).

cations are extremely rare, with cases due to air embolism[48] and tension pneumothorax[25] reported. If proper precautions are taken, neither of these complications should occur.

Contraindications

In reality, a potential candidate is anyone who can lie supine or prone without moving for about 10 minutes. If the patient has an uncontrollable cough, or if an echinococcal etiology of a pulmonary lesion is suspected, then needle aspiration is contraindicated. The presence of a systemic bleeding diathesis, clinically suspected pulmonary hypertension, severe emphysema, pneumonectomy on the contralateral side, or suspected vascular etiology of a pulmonary lesion are only relative contraindications to aspiration needle biopsy, which can be performed following platelet transfusion and when apparatus to treat a pneumothorax immediately are readily available (Fig. 2–19). Fear of puncturing vascular structures with an aspirating needle is generally unfounded (Fig. 2–20). Aspirating needles have been inadvertently placed in the thoracic aorta, right atrium, superior vena cava, and pulmonary artery and veins, all without ill effects.[24] All that is necessary is that the needle be withdrawn and appropriately redirected. The injection of contrast media through the aspirating needle has even been advocated if blood is aspirated from the needle to confirm an intrapulmonary vascular anomaly.[54]

Results

An overall accuracy with aspiration needle biopsy of about 80% is accepted in

Text continued on page 47

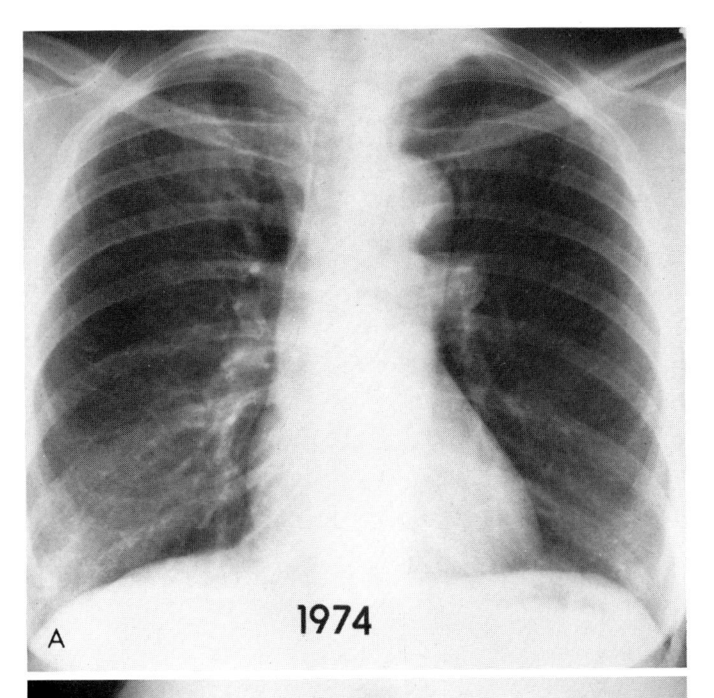

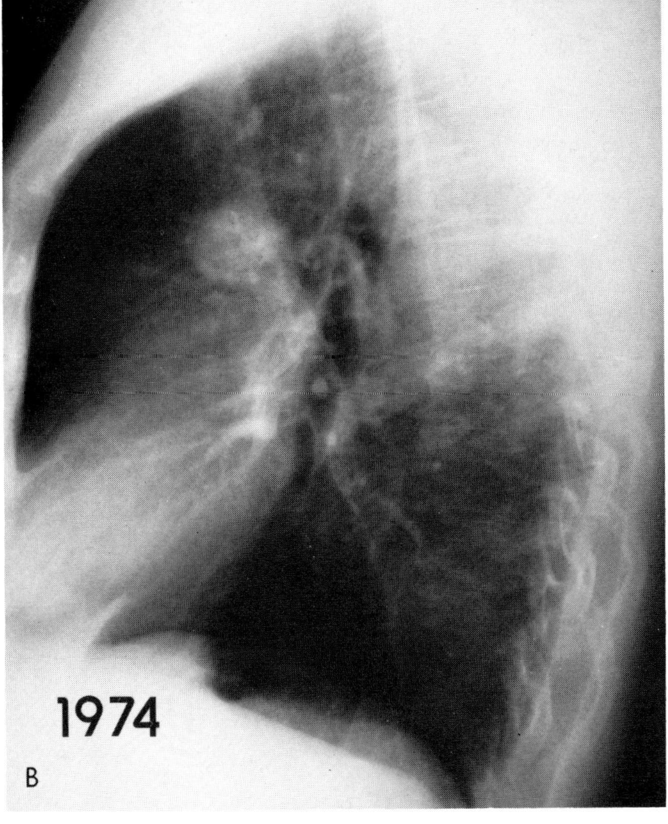

Figure 2–17. An asymptomatic 57 year old woman. *A* and *B*. Posteroanterior and lateral chest radiographs demonstrate an irregular 3 cm. mass in the anterior segment of the left upper lobe just anterior to the hilum. Cytologic preparation of needle aspirate disclosed oat cell carcinoma.

Legend continued on the opposite page

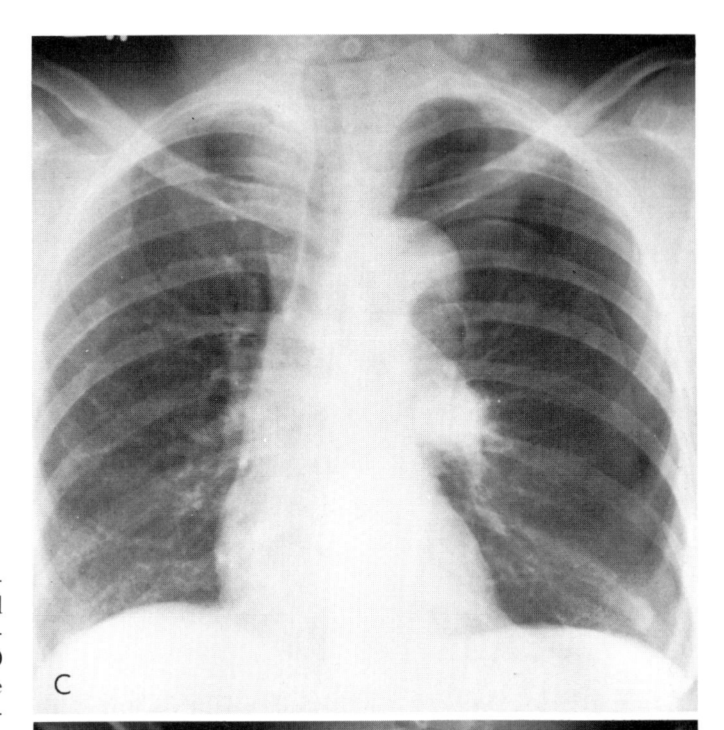

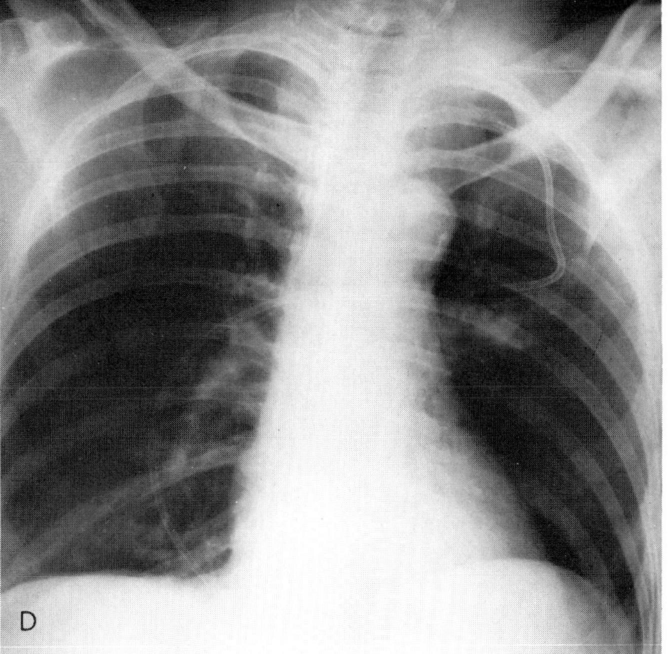

Figure 2–17 *Continued.* *C.* Posteroanterior chest radiograph obtained following the needle aspiration biopsy discloses an approximately 50 per cent left pneumothorax. The patient was mildly dyspneic. *D.* Anteroposterior chest radiograph obtained after insertion of Teflon catheters into the left pleural space demonstrates complete re-expansion of left lung.

Illustration and legend continued on the following page

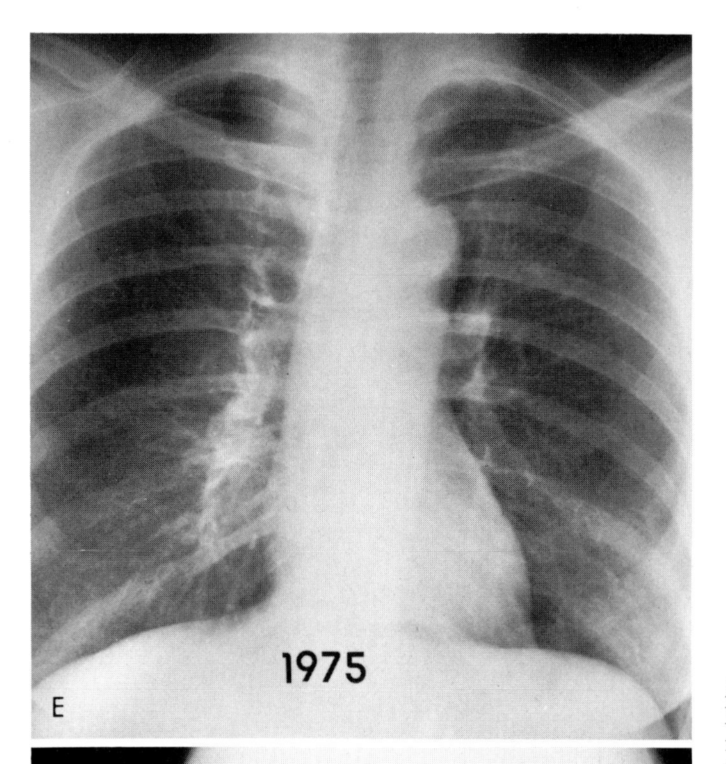

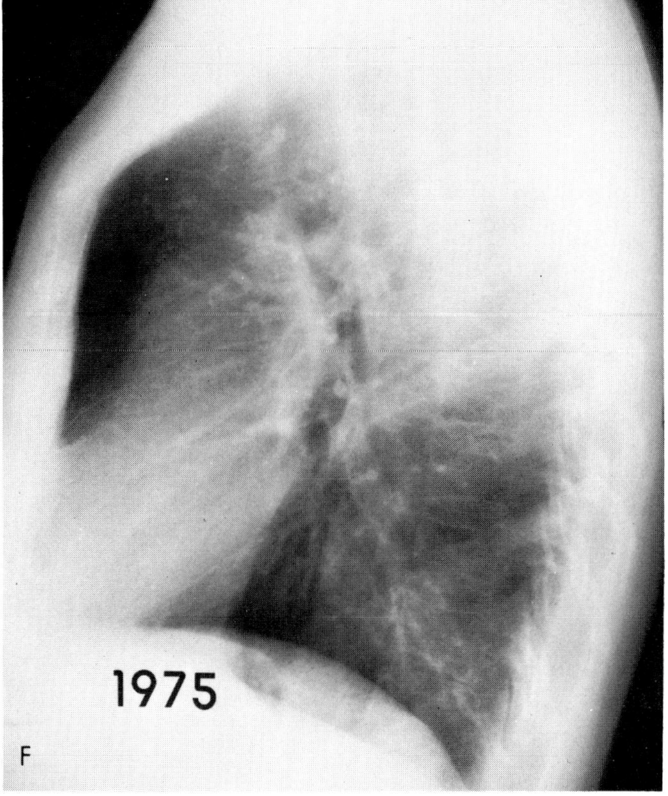

Figure 2–17 Continued. *E* and *F*. Posteroanterior and lateral chest radiographs ten months after radiation therapy to the left upper hemithorax demonstrates complete disappearance of the carcinoma.

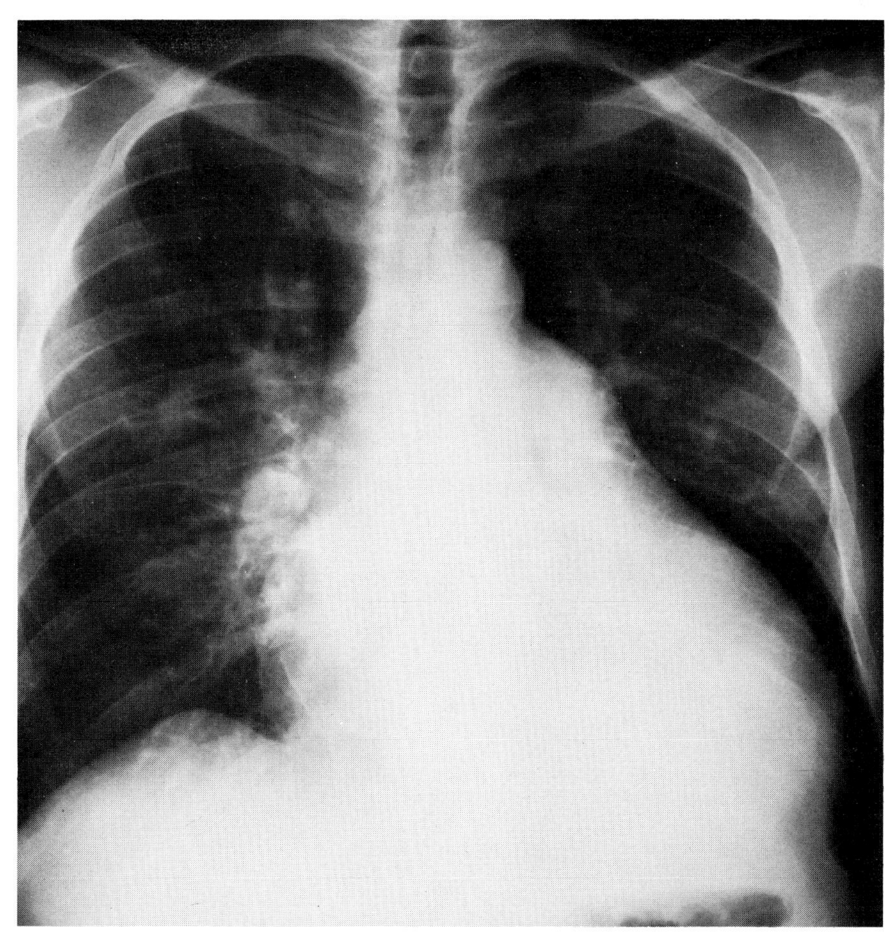

Figure 2–18. A 49 year old man referred for surgical correction of severe rheumatic heart disease. Posteroanterior chest radiograph demonstrates a nodular density in each lung, besides cardiomegaly and evidence of pulmonary arterial hypertension. Aspiration needle biopsy of the left mid lung field nodule was performed. The patient coughed up approximately 100 cc. of bright red blood in about a 3 minute period immediately after the procedure. The hemoptysis stopped spontaneously. Cytologic preparation of the aspirate disclosed adenocarcinoma cells, and surgery was cancelled.

the literature;[1, 25, 38, 44] these data correlate closely with our early experience in approximately 200 cases.[37] However, with increasing expertise, our success rate is greater than 95% during the past year (Table 2–1). Two negative aspiration biopsies, in our experience, are sufficient to exclude cancer with greater than 98% accuracy. These figures correspond to other recent reports of approximately 95% accuracy in neoplastic lesions.[42, 55] Thus, while the basic technique of aspiration needle biopsy is simple, it is obvious that (as in golf or tennis) increased practice leads to increased perfection. One false positive cytologic diagnosis has occurred in our series (Fig. 2–21). This is a somewhat lower rate than previously described[24, 42] and this problem is undoubtedly related to the expertise of the cytopathologist.

BRONCHIAL BRUSHING

Many techniques for bronchial brushing have been described[14, 49, 52, 53] and all are relatively simple and readily learned. Transcatheter bronchial brushing is an application of arteriographic techniques to the tracheobronchial tree, in which (under local anesthesia) the catheter is selectively

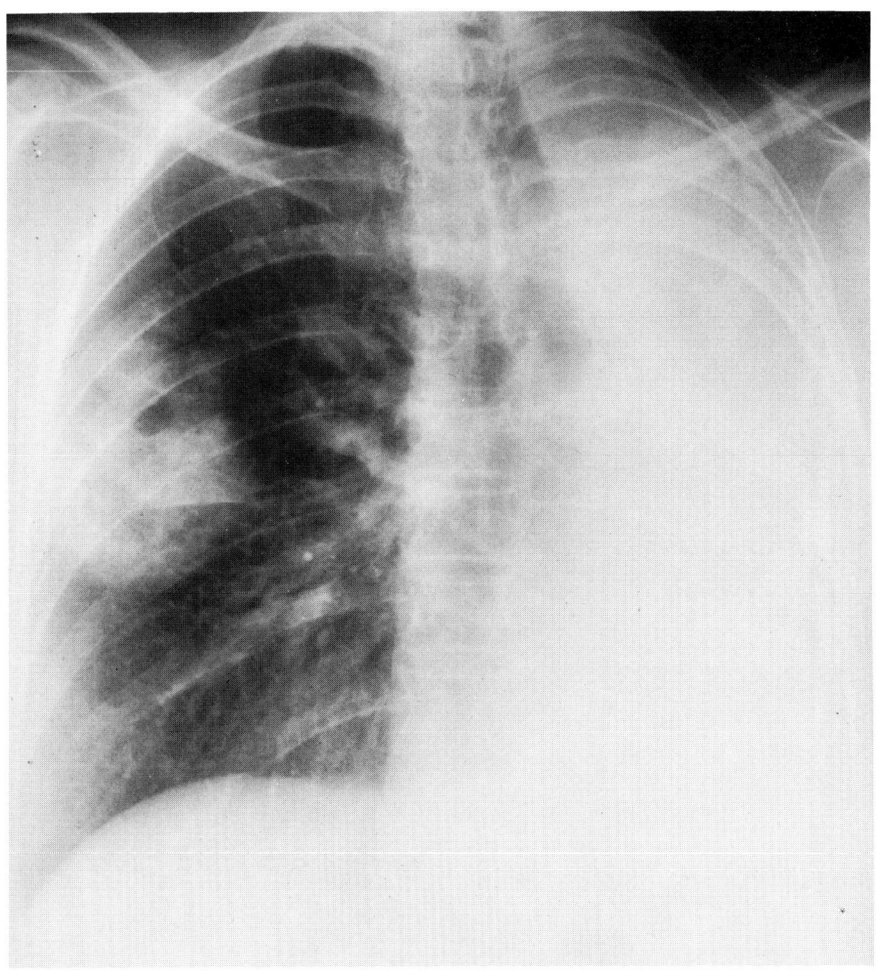

Figure 2–19. A 58 year old woman, two years after left pneumonectomy for alveolar cell carcinoma. Posteroanterior chest roentgenogram demonstrates a fluffy cavitary infiltrate in the right mid lung field. Sputum examination, bronchoscopy, and bronchial brushing were negative. Cytologic preparation of needle aspirate showed alveolar cell carcinoma. (From Forrest, John V., and Sagel, Stuart S.: Special procedures in pulmonary radiology. *In* Potchen, E. James, editor: Current Concepts in Radiology, vol. 2, St. Louis, 1975, The C. V. Mosby Co.)

positioned in the bronchial tree with the aid of image intensification fluoroscopy. The importance of fluoroscopy in brushing mid and peripheral lung lesions cannot be overemphasized. Brushings obtained through the fiberoptic bronchoscope are extremely accurate in central or mid-zone lesions when the brush can be applied directly to a visualized bronchial mass.[52] As with previous reports,[41, 52] we have found that fiberoptic bronchoscopic brushings of peripheral lesions beyond the reach of the scope produce results as accurate as the transcatheter technique of brushing only if the bronchoscopy is also done under fluoroscopic control to assure that the proper peripheral area was brushed. Fluoroscopy aids immeasurably in documenting the relationship of the instrument tip to a lesion beyond the segmental bronchus, ensuring that the proper peripheral area is brushed (Fig. 2–22). In our hospital, bronchial brushing of mid and peripheral lung lesions is almost always done by the radiologist as a separate procedure from bronchoscopy. This avoids tying up expensive fluoroscopic equipment for long periods of time, and alleviates invariable conflicts in busy clinicians' time and fluoroscopic room availability.

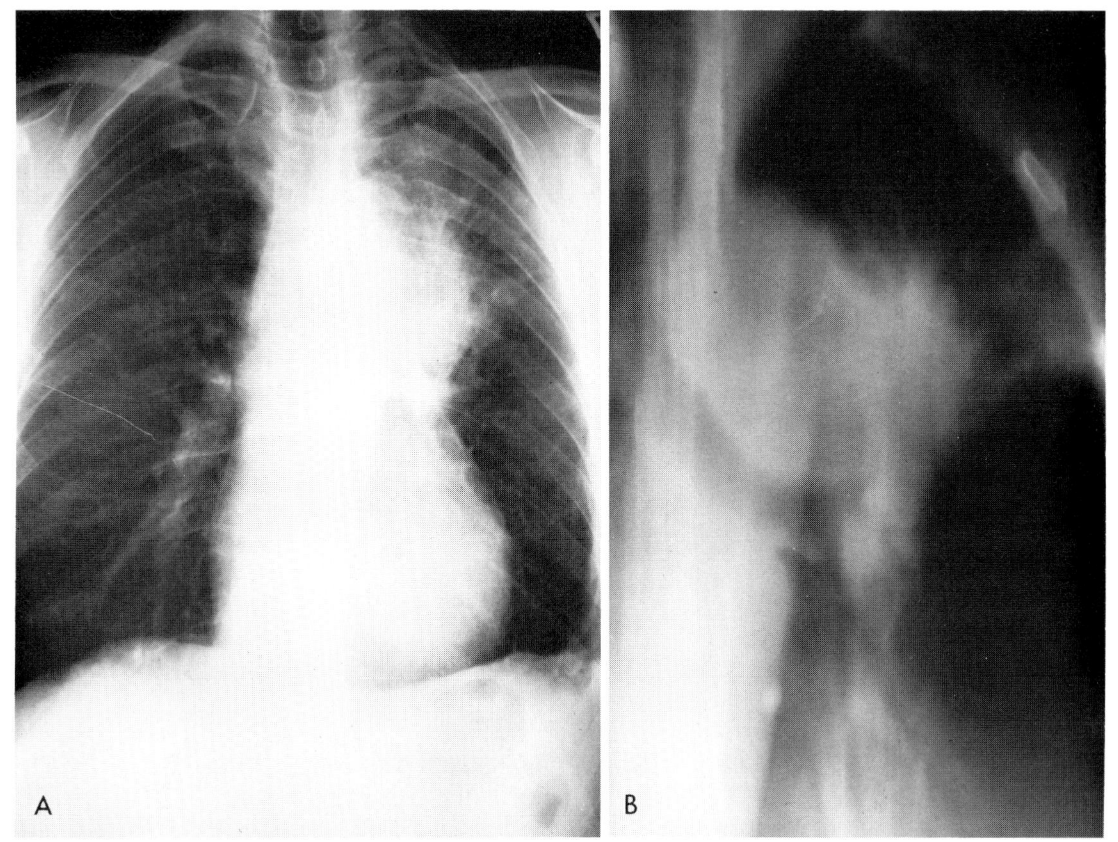

Figure 2–20. A 59 year old man with hoarseness (due to left vocal cord paralysis). *A*. Posteroanterior chest radiograph demonstrates an infiltrating lesion about the left hilum. *B*. Frontal tomogram demonstrates a mass filling the aorto-pulmonary window, with "cut-off" of the bronchus to the apical posterior and anterior segments. Sputum examination, fiberoptic bronchoscopy × 2, and bronchial brushing were negative. Needle aspiration biopsy, with the tip of the needle placed just lateral and inferior to the aortic knob calcification, disclosed epidermoid carcinoma cells.

TABLE 2–1. Aspiration Needle Biopsy, 1974 Results

	Total	PATHOLOGIC DIAGNOSIS					
				MALIGNANT NEOPLASM			
		Definitive Diagnosis	*Positive Micro-biology*	*Positive*	*False Negative*	*False Positive*	*Negative, being followed*
Patients	132	112	16	96*	4†	1	11

*Two biopsies required in 7 patients.

†2 patients with bronchogenic carcinoma, neither of whom had a second study.

1 patient with a fibroxanthosarcoma (in which a positive cytologic diagnosis is probably impossible).

1 patient with multiple small pulmonary nodules (subsequently proved by thoracotomy to be metastatic carcinoma).

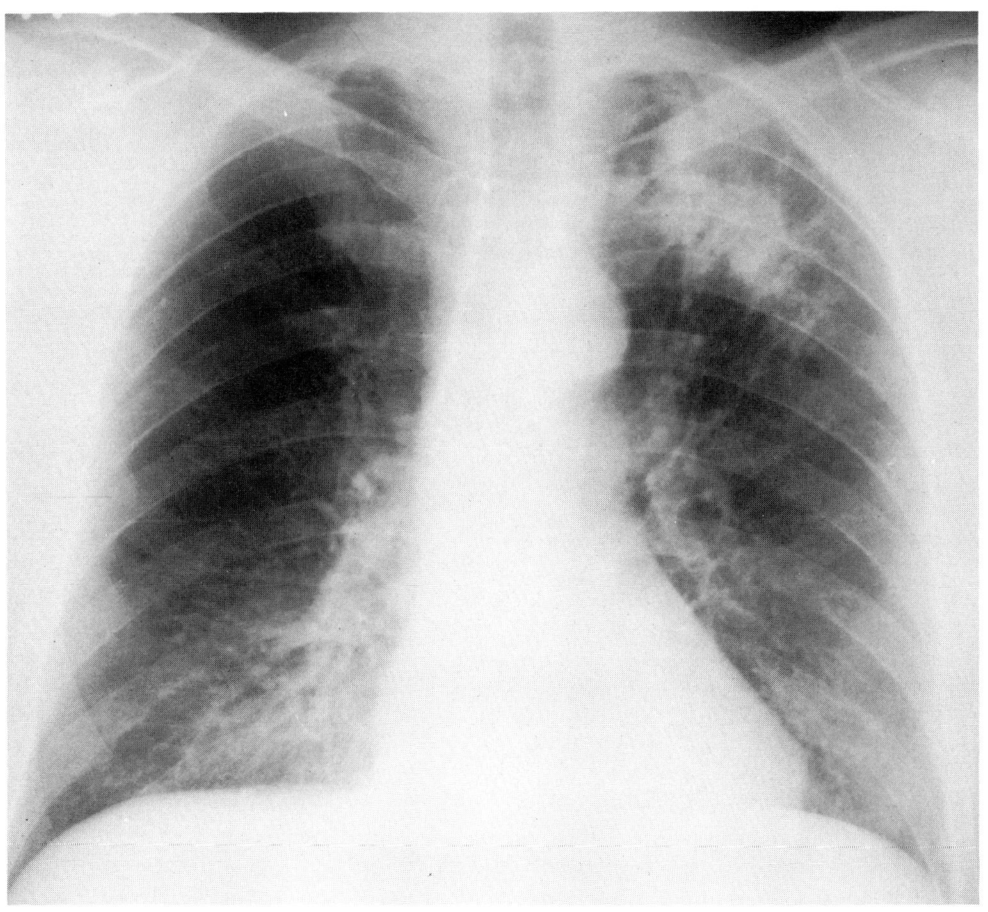

Figure 2–21. A 63 year old man with cough and weight loss. Posteroanterior chest radiograph demonstrates an irregular left upper lobe infiltrate. Sputum examination and bronchoscopic washings were negative. Cytologic preparation from needle aspirate was interpreted as demonstrating squamous cell carcinoma. No microorganisms were seen on special stains. Examination of specimen from left upper lobectomy disclosed only active tuberculosis, without any neoplasm. (Subsequent culture of the needle aspirate grew out *Mycobacterium tuberculosis.*)

Technique

We generally employ catheter technique for brushing mid and peripheral lung lesions. Occasionally, in lesions in which bronchial obstruction is considered as a possible cause of peripheral density, fiberoptic bronchoscopy and brushing are done as a combined procedure under local anesthesia in the radiology department. The catheter technique utilized in our department is to introduce pre-shaped arterial catheters (USCI–4608) through the cricothyroid membrane using the Seldinger technique.[7] This approach is easy, and permits optimal control of the catheter and guide wire for positioning. By diminishing the distance, as opposed to oral or nasal introduction, torque control problems are greatly reduced and local anesthesia is more easily managed. This approach also better facilitates the diagnosis of pulmonary infection, as the catheter is not contaminated with upper respiratory tract organisms which might result in confusion with pulmonary pathogens. Specific curves are put in the distal tip of the catheter for selective placement in the desired bronchial segment (Fig. 2–23).

Fasting before the examination reduces the possibility of aspiration of gastric contents during the procedure, but this is not a problem with a generally healthy cooperative patient. Patients are usually premedi-

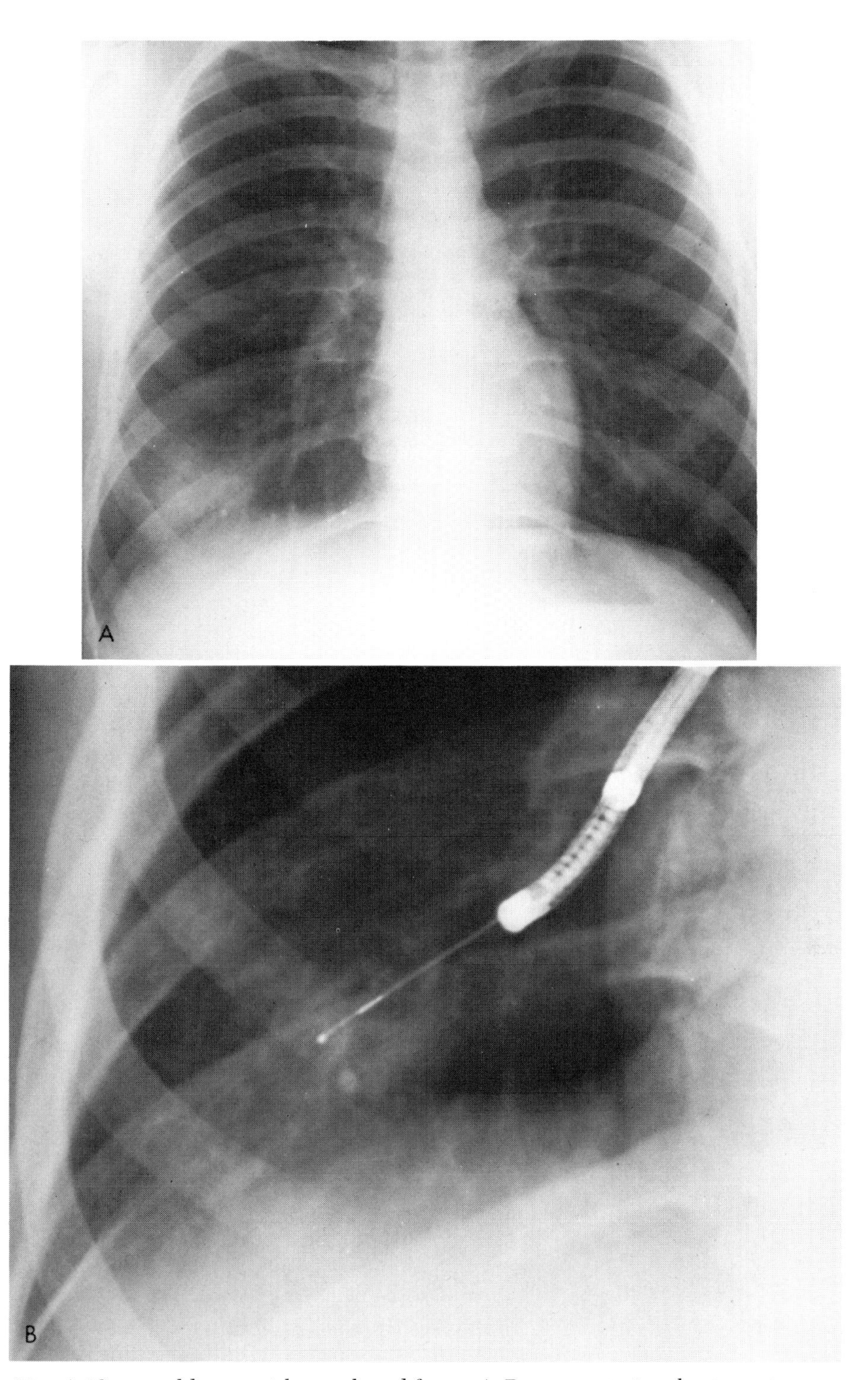

Figure 2–22. A 19 year old man with cough and fever. *A.* Posteroanterior chest roentgenogram demonstrates consolidation within the anterior basal segment of the right lower lobe. *B.* Fluoroscopic spot film obtained following insertion of brush through fiberoptic bronchoscope, confirming tip of brush within the lesion. Subsequent culture of brush scrapings revealed anaerobic streptococci. (From Forrest, John V., and Sagel, Stuart S.: Special procedures in pulmonary radiology. *In* Potchen, E. James, editor: Current Concepts in Radiology, vol. 2, St. Louis, 1975, The C. V. Mosby Co.)

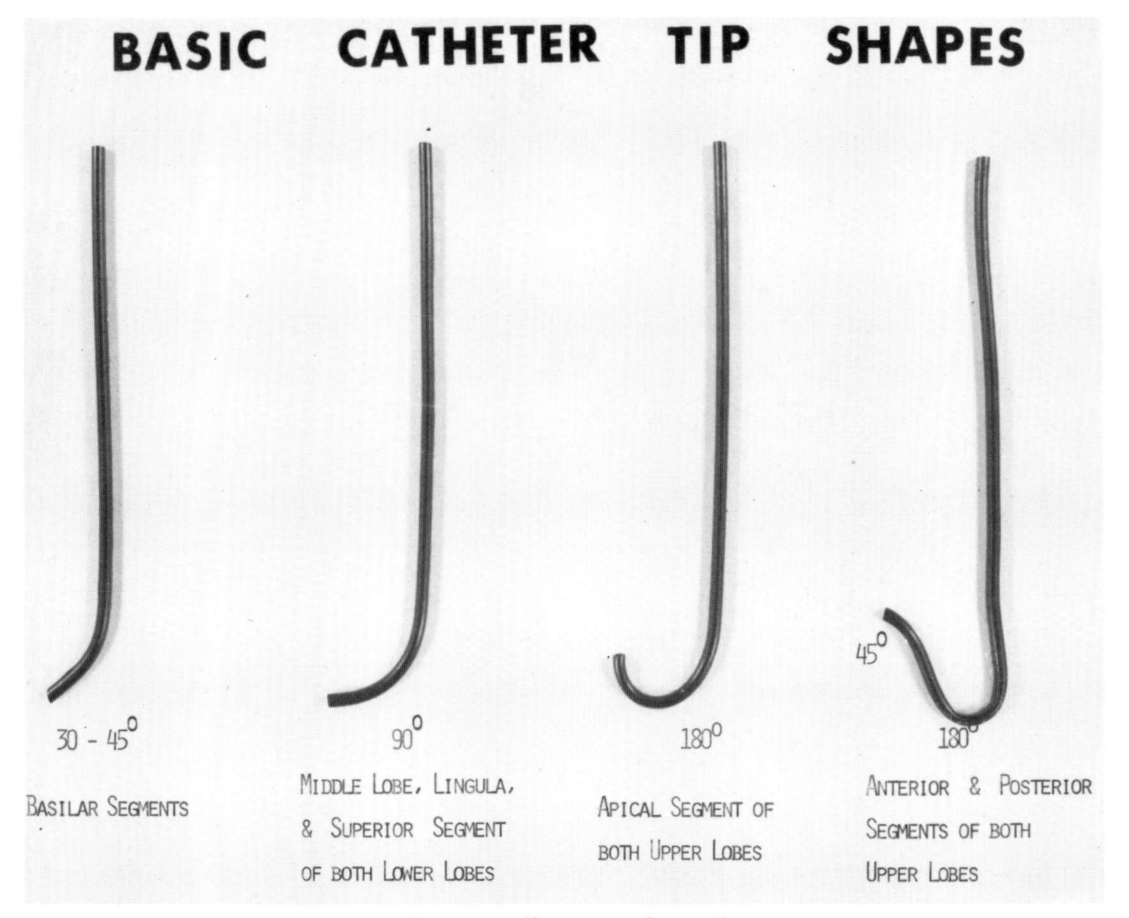

Figure 2–23. Shape of tip of the catheter usually required for selective catheterization of the orifices of the segmental bronchi.

cated with 0.4 mg. of atropine subcutaneously to decrease secretions, 30 to 60 mg. of codeine to dull the cough reflex, and 5 to 10 mg. of Valium as a sedative. The patient is placed supine on the fluoroscopic table, with a small pillow beneath the shoulders to hyperextend the neck, and the anterior neck is cleansed and draped. A syringe containing 1 per cent Lidocaine with a 25 gauge needle is used to raise a small skin wheal over the cricothyroid membrane and then to infiltrate the subcutaneous tissues. The membrane is then punctured and 2 cc. of anesthetic is injected into the larynx and upper trachea. The needle is removed, and a 2 mm. puncture in the skin over the membrane is made with a No. 11 scalpel blade. A curved 16 gauge needle (Cook BN-16) is then inserted through the cricothyroid membrane with the tip pointing distally. An additional 3 cc. of local anesthesia is injected, followed by inspiration. A guide wire (Cook TSF-35-65) is next inserted through the needle, and the needle is then withdrawn. The pre-shaped catheter is then placed over the guide wire and inserted into the lower trachea.

After an additional 3 cc. of local anesthetic is injected, the tip of the catheter is advanced under television image intensification fluoroscopic control into the segmental or subsegmental bronchus in which the lesion is situated. Peripheral bronchi can be probed with the flexible end of the guide wire or a controllable brush (USCI-2701) as the catheter is manipulated, until the bronchus leading to the lesion is entered. A catheter tip deflector (Cook TDH-100) may be used when the lesion is not readily reachable. The catheter is generally

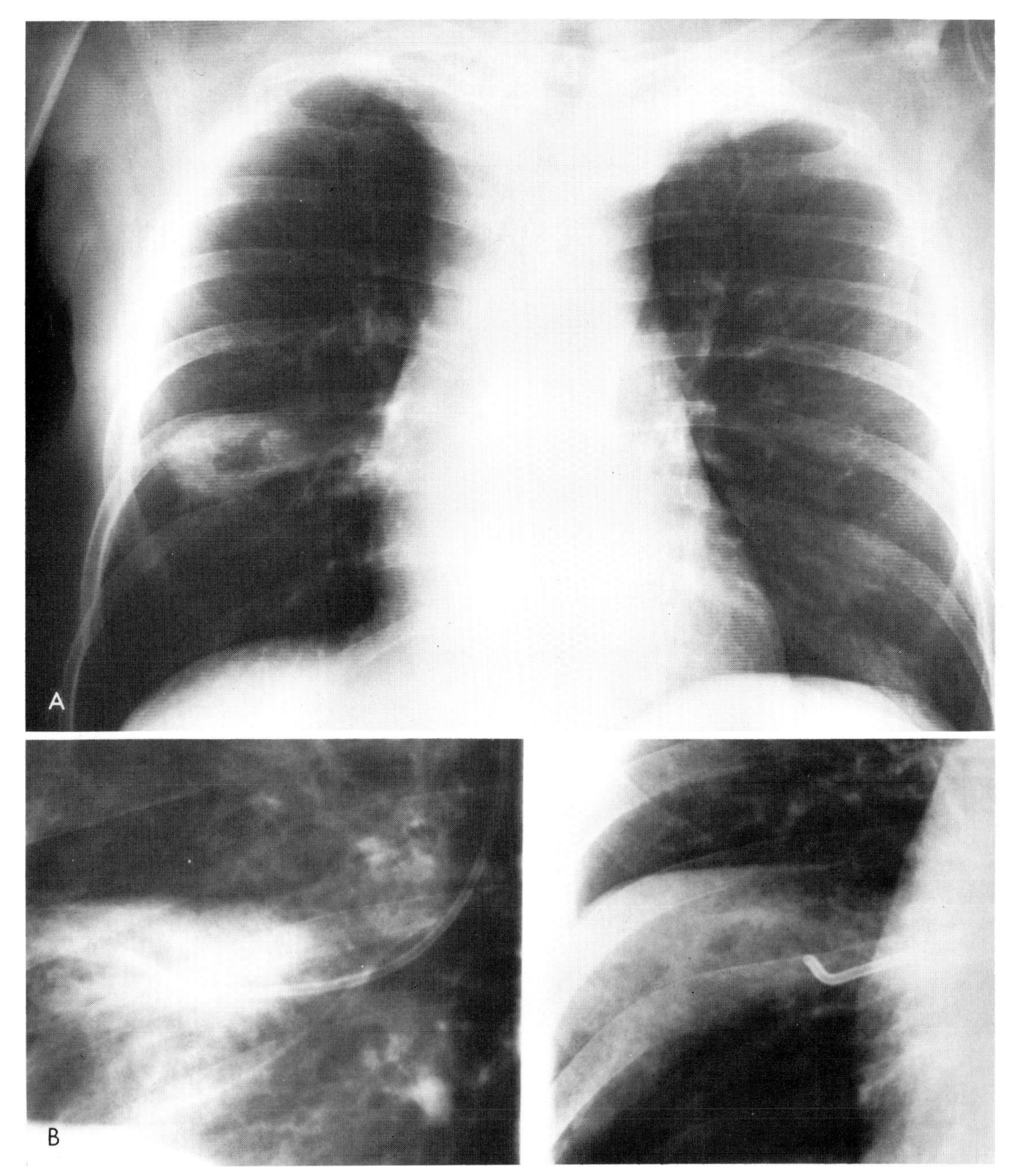

Figure 2–24. A 37 year old man on long term, high dose corticosteroid therapy, with cough and low grade fever. *A.* Anteroposterior chest radiograph demonstrates a cavitary infiltrate within the lateral segment of the middle lobe. (Mediastinal widening due to fat deposition is incidentally noted.) Sputum examination and transtracheal aspiration were negative. *B.* Fluoroscopic spot films in lateral and frontal projections confirming correct position of the catheter tip within the middle lobe infiltrate before brushing. Culture of the brush specimens revealed *Cryptococcus neoformans.*

sufficiently small to enter even a partially occluded bronchus. The catheter is advanced until it is as close to the lesion as possible. In dealing with cavitary lesions, the stiff end of the guide wire may be used in an endeavor to puncture the cavity wall if there is difficulty in entering the cavity. Correct positioning of the catheter should

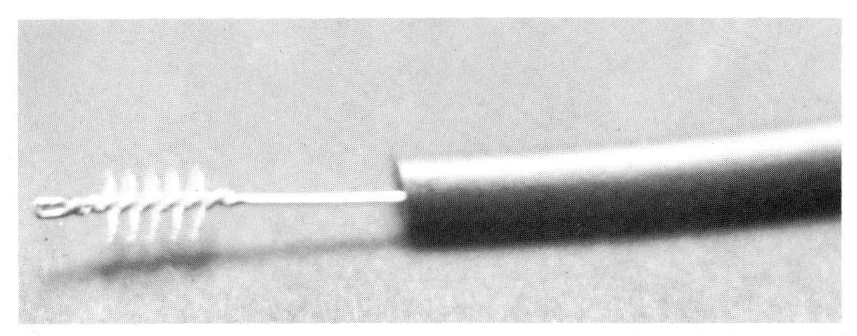

Figure 2–25. Close-up view of nylon-bristled brush protruding through the tip of the catheter.

be verified by spot films in at least two projections (Fig. 2–24). (One should not despair if, after several attempts, the lesion cannot be reached with the catheter, as brushings and washings from a nearby position may be positive, although obviously the yield is not as high as when the brush is within the lesion.)

When optimal positioning of the catheter is achieved, a small, disposable, controllable nylon-bristled brush (Fig. 2–25) is passed through the positioned catheter and advanced toward and, if possible, into the substance of the lesion. The region is vigorously scrubbed by forward and backward movements of the brush in an attempt to tear off and catch pieces of tissue on the bristles. The brush may be removed and replaced as many times as necessary to obtain material for study. Generally, following a slight repositioning of the catheter, brushings from a number of other small bronchi closely associated with the lesion are obtained. (A biopsy instrument[14,15] has not been used with the transcatheter technique at our hospital, generally being reserved for use through the fiberoptic bronchoscope.)

The brush scrapings are manually agitated in test tubes containing a balanced electrolyte solution (Polysal) to remove pieces of tissue. Depending upon the clinical situation, smears and cultures are subsequently prepared for routine bacteriologic studies and for testing for mycobacteria, fungi, and so on. If anaerobic infection is suspected, the brush scrapings are inoculated into a "nitrogen-gassed" tube. For cytologic study, the brushings in the balanced electrolyte solution are prepared as with the needle aspiration biopsy specimens. Some brush scrapings are smeared directly on frosted glass slides, which are fixed immediately in 95% ethyl alcohol, and subsequently stained by the Papanicolaou technique or the appropriate microorganism stain.

The catheter is then pulled back proximally from the wedged position within the small bronchus, and 5 cc. of sterile saline solution is injected and vigorously aspirated. This material is divided for the suitable diagnostic studies mentioned previously.

In patients with a solitary indeterminate lung lesion, a localized selective bronchogram is usually done. The finding of localized bronchiectasis proximal to or within the lesion is an ancillary substantiation that the lesion is not neoplastic if cytologic examination of the brush scrapings is negative[31] (Fig. 2–8). Patent bronchi without "pruning" of peripheral branches extending through an area of infiltration also strongly suggest non-neoplastic disease[13,35] (Fig. 2–26), although bronchoalveolar cell carcinoma or lymphoma could not be entirely excluded. Bronchography should be performed after the brushings have been obtained, since contaminating Dionosil makes cytologic diagnosis more difficult. Rarely, when difficulty in reaching a lesion is encountered, bronchography is performed first, in an endeavor to use it as a road map in guiding the catheter to a lesion.

Following removal of the catheter, the skin and subcutaneous tissues over the puncture site are massaged and a small adhesive bandage is placed over the area. The patient is instructed to hold his thumb over the cricothyroid membrane puncture site whenever he coughs during the next

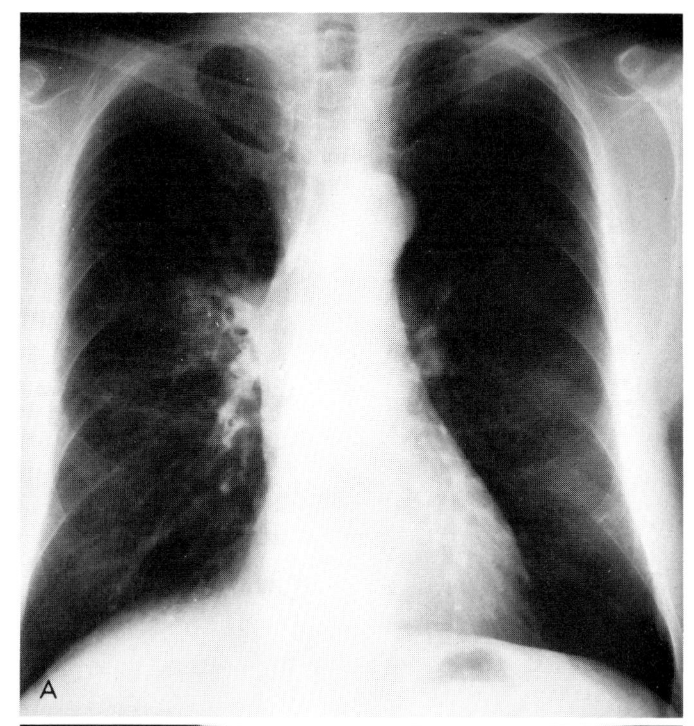

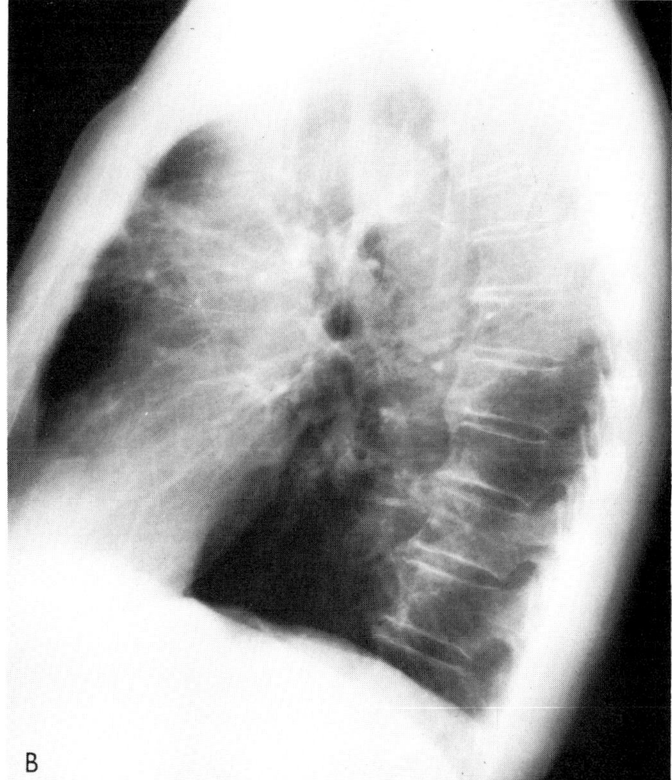

Figure 2–26. An asymptomatic 64 year old man. *A* and *B*. Posteroanterior and lateral chest radiographs demonstrate an infiltrate in the anterior segment of the right upper lobe. Sputum examination and bronchoscopy were negative.

Illustration and legend continued on the following page

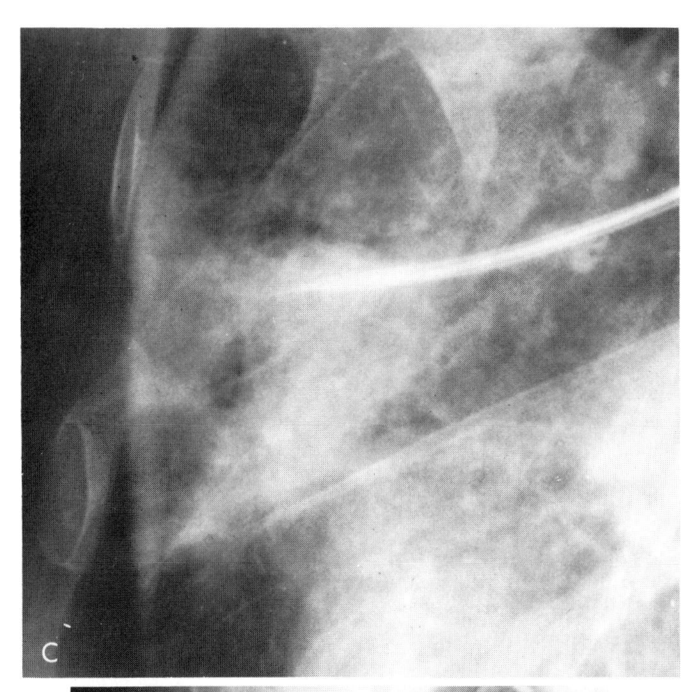

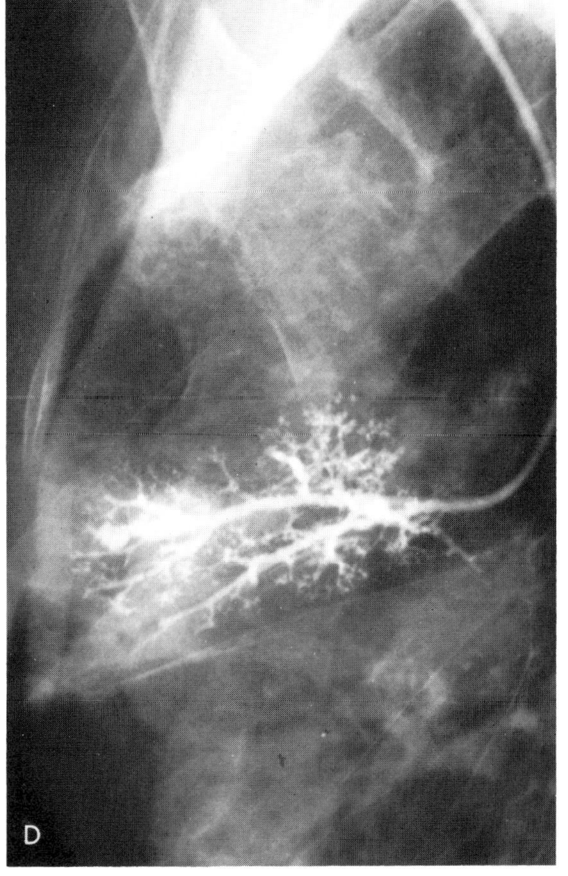

Figure 2–26 Continued. C. Fluoroscopic spot film demonstrating tip of brush and catheter within the infiltrate. Cytologic preparations and cultures were negative. *D.* Localized bronchogram showing absence of an endobronchial lesion and normal peripheral filling. The patient has remained asymptomatic with an unchanging chest roentgenogram in the subsequent two years, and the lesion is presumed to be a chronic organized pneumonia.

24 hours to prevent air from leaking into surrounding tissues. If a bronchogram was performed, the patient is placed face down on the fluoroscopy table and encouraged to cough out the contrast material. The patient is returned to his room, where he is allowed nothing by mouth for an additional 2 hours and no I.P.P.B. for 24 hours. Sputum is collected for the 24 hour period following brushing and is processed if the brushing cytology is negative. Occasionally, these sputa have been positive despite negative results from the brushing. Probably the trauma caused by the brush and the coughing that occurs when the local anesthetic wears off account for this beneficial effect.

Complications

In an experience with more than 600 bronchial brushings, this procedure has proven to be virtually free of significant complications.

There is an approximately 10 per cent incidence of subcutaneous air in the neck or upper mediastinum following transcricothyroid membrane puncture, which usually resolves spontaneously in 48 to 72 hours.

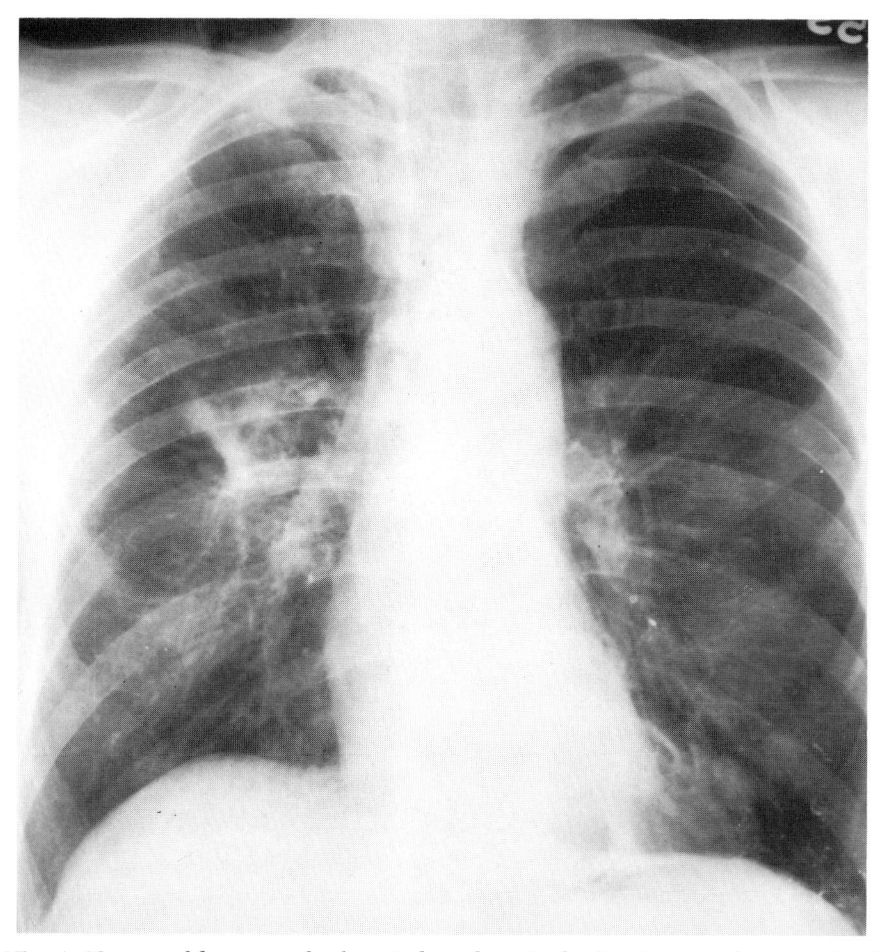

Figure 2–27. A 68 year old man with chronic lymphocytic leukemia, complaining of mild anterior chest pain, one day after bronchial brushing of right upper lobe and lingular infiltrates. Posteroanterior chest radiograph demonstrates air in the soft tissues of the neck, a pneumomediastinum, and a small left pneumothorax. The pneumothorax probably was due to dissection of air from the mediastinum into the pleural space. The symptoms and radiographic changes resolved without treatment.

Pneumothorax has occurred in five patients. Three of these were caused by inexperienced residents apparently brushing a peripheral lesion so vigorously that they perforated the lining of the pleural space with the brush. The other two were the results of mediastinal air that dissected into the pleural space (Fig. 2–27).

Minor transient blood streaking of the sputum not uncommonly occurs; this is usually an indication that the brush was in the proper spot in the abnormal tissues. While it has not occurred in our experience, severe (and even fatal) intrapulmonary hemorrhage has been reported in patients who had thrombocytopenia or hemoptysis prior to brushing.[15] It is certainly agreed that uncorrectable severe thrombocytopenia, recent severe hemoptysis, or suspected vascular lesion contraindicate bronchial brushing. A single case of septicemia following brushing of a lung abscess and two brushes that had broken off have also been reported.[15]

One case of implantation of tumor cells from a carcinoma of the lung to the site of the transcricothyroid membrane puncture has been described.[9] This is undoubtedly a rare complication, never having occurred in our experience with over 300 cases of bronchogenic carcinoma that have been brushed. In fact, one could debate whether the case that was reported was really a complication or just a fortuitous occurrence (Fig. 2–28). At present a potentially resectable lesion is not considered a contraindication to bronchial brushing, as it probably won't result in any more likelihood of tumor spread than would bronchoscopic biopsy, brushing, or washings.

Results

Fluoroscopically controlled bronchial brushing, whether through a catheter or a fiberoptic bronchoscope, produces speci-

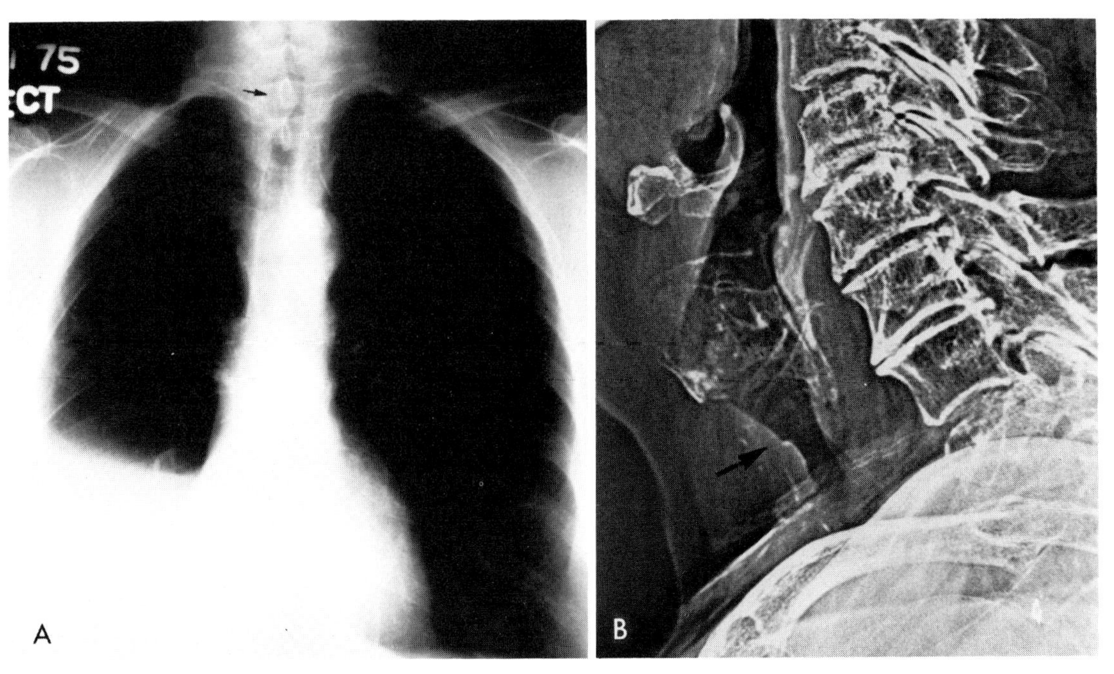

Figure 2–28. A 64 year old woman with dyspnea, who two years previously had a right middle and lower lobectomy for adenocarcinoma of the lung. Prior to surgery only rigid bronchoscopy had been performed, as sputum examination was positive. *A.* Posteroanterior chest radiograph demonstrates post-operative changes in the right hemithorax, as well as a mass impinging upon and narrowing (arrow) the right side of the proximal trachea. *B.* Lateral xeroradiograph of the neck shows a mass narrowing the anterior subglottic portion of the trachea (arrow). Biopsy revealed recurrent adenocarcinoma. This case demonstrates that subglottic seeding of lung carcinoma can occur in the absence of prior cricothyroid membrane puncture for bronchial brushing.

mens that yield a positive cytologic diagnosis in approximately 80 per cent of patients with peripherally located bronchogenic carcinoma.[15, 41, 52, 53] This is a considerable improvement over the accuracy obtained from sputum samples or rigid bronchoscopic washings in peripheral carcinomas. Bronchial brushing is much less

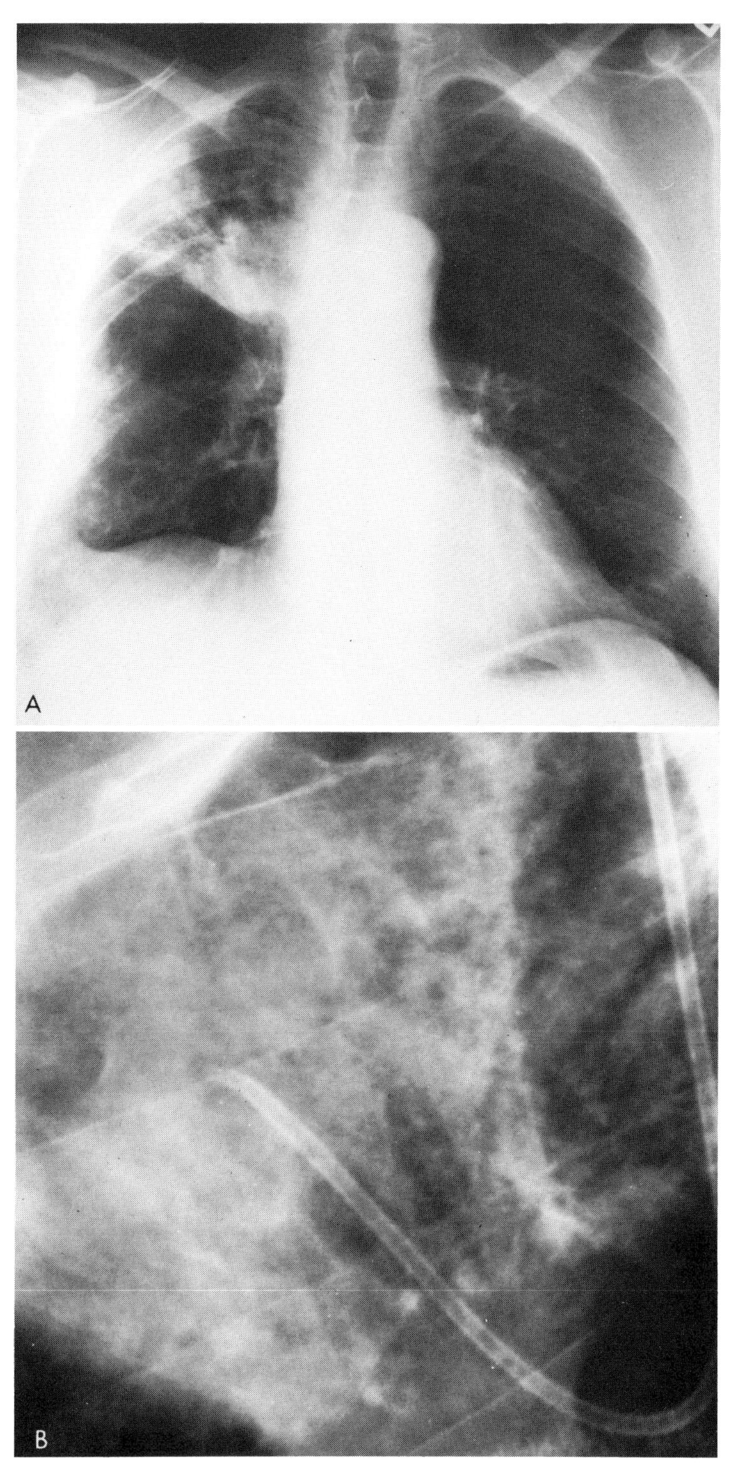

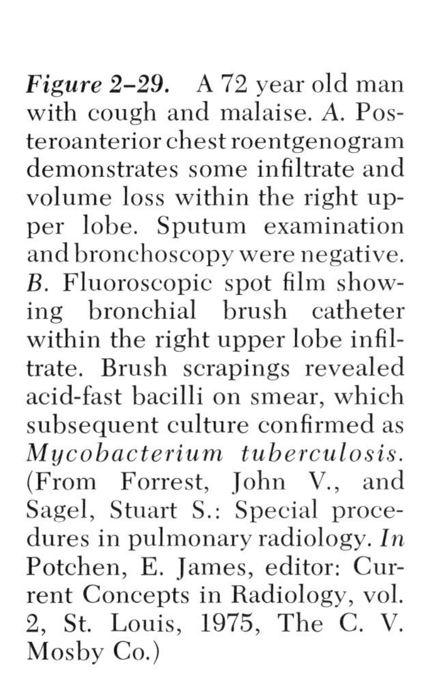
Figure 2–29. A 72 year old man with cough and malaise. *A.* Posteroanterior chest roentgenogram demonstrates some infiltrate and volume loss within the right upper lobe. Sputum examination and bronchoscopy were negative. *B.* Fluoroscopic spot film showing bronchial brush catheter within the right upper lobe infiltrate. Brush scrapings revealed acid-fast bacilli on smear, which subsequent culture confirmed as *Mycobacterium tuberculosis.* (From Forrest, John V., and Sagel, Stuart S.: Special procedures in pulmonary radiology. *In* Potchen, E. James, editor: Current Concepts in Radiology, vol. 2, St. Louis, 1975, The C. V. Mosby Co.)

accurate in the diagnosis of metastatic lesions, which are frequently extrabronchial and thus are not directly brushed. Needle aspiration biopsy is the greatly preferred diagnostic modality when metastatic disease is suspected and with nodular lesions less than 2 cm. in diameter.

Positive results from smears and cultures (about 70 per cent overall accuracy) have been obtained from brushing in a myriad of infectious conditions,[15,16,18,22] including mycobacteriosis, nocardiosis, aspergillosis, and viruses (Figs. 2–24, 2–29 to 2–31). Utilization of the transcricothyroid membrane approach greatly reduces or eliminates the problem of false-positive culture results, as there is no confusion with possible pathogens obtained from contamination by the upper respiratory tract as when an oral or nasal approach is used. While successful retrieval of organisms from *Pneumocystis carinii* pneumonia has been reported with brushing[16,35] our results have been much less favorable, with less than 10 per cent recovery. Forceps biopsy through the fiberoptic bronchoscope[40] or by bronchopulmonary lavage[12] may prove to be the most successful diagnostic procedure short of thoracotomy for this organism.

Differentiation of opportunistic infection from localized neoplastic pulmonary infiltration, such as that due to Hodgkin's disease, is often possible[20](Figs. 2–3 and 2–4).

The rate of definitive diagnosis following brushing of cavitary lesions has increased to about 90 per cent after an initial report[17] (Figs. 2–3 and 2–4, 2–31 to 2–33). A negative result if the brush has entered the cavity strongly implies that the etiology of the cavity is neither neoplastic nor infectious, but rather due to an arteritis such as Wegener's granulomatosis.

Catheterization of a large, fluid-filled abscess may have therapeutic as well as diagnostic value.[19] Purulent material may be aspirated because widening of the bronchial communication via the catheter facilitates drainage (Fig. 2–34).

While some authors have claimed a high degree of accuracy in distinguishing neoplastic from infectious infiltrates by bronchography alone,[32] the diagnosis is always inferential. Pneumonias, sarcoidosis, and asthma can produce similar roentgenographic changes.[36] The only definitive diagnosis possible by bronchography is bronchiectasis. In contradistinction, bronchial brushing can achieve a precise tissue diagnosis, permitting the direct institution of appropriate treatment—such as radiotherapy or the suitable antibiotic.

DISCUSSION

Percutaneous aspiration needle biopsy and bronchial brushing are inexpensive, relatively safe, and highly accurate diagnostic modalities that should be part of the armamentarium of every radiologist involved with the definitive diagnosis of pulmonary disease. That these examinations are comparatively easy to perform can be attested to by the fact that virtually all of the biopsy procedures performed at our hospital are done by the radiology residents after having observed several examinations. These procedures can be done in any hospital where image intensification fluoroscopy is available.

Aspiration needle biopsy and bronchial brushing not only are efficacious in providing a definitive diagnosis in patients with suspected lung neoplasm, but can also usually provide the definitive etiology of a pneumonic infiltrate when routine methods (examination and culture of sputum samples or transtracheal aspirates, serological studies) fail. Direct and often immediate evidence of the pathologic agent can be provided, uncontaminated by the upper respiratory tract flora.

No other presently available diagnostic procedure short of thoracotomy, including fiberoptic bronchoscopy, yields results as accurate as aspiration needle biopsy.[4,11,21] The simplicity and speed of performing this diagnostic test cannot be overemphasized. The diagnostic work-up of a patient must take into account the overall economics of time, staff, and apparatus required for different methods. Aspiration needle biopsy often should be considered the initial diagnostic procedure in patients with peripheral and mid lung lesions when the history, physical examination, laboratory studies, and sputum examination fail to provide a conclusive diagnosis. Patients are

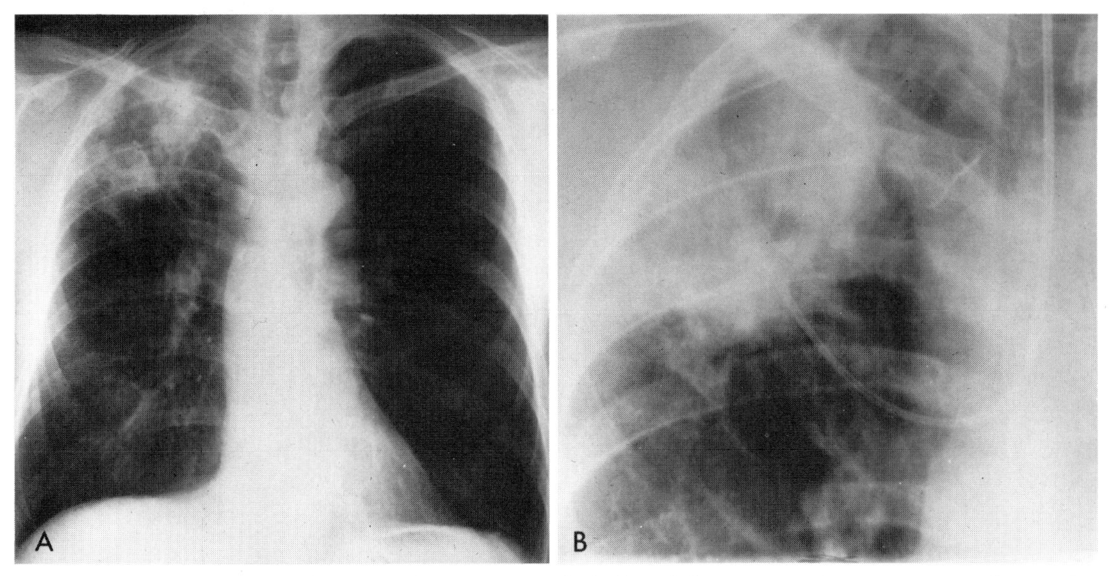

Figure 2–30. A 57 year old man with cough, weight loss and dyspnea. *A.* Posteroanterior chest radiograph demonstrates chronic obstructive pulmonary disease and a right upper lobe infiltrate. Sputum examination and culture were negative. *B.* Fluoroscopic spot film showing tip of bronchial catheter within right upper lobe infiltrate. Acid-fast bacilli were demonstrated on smear from the brush scrapings,which subsequent culture revealed to be *Mycobacterium kansasii.* (From Forrest, John V., and Sagel, Stuart S.: Special procedures in pulmonary radiology. *In* Potchen, E. James, editor: Current Concepts in Radiology, vol. 2, St. Louis, 1975, The C. V. Mosby Co.)

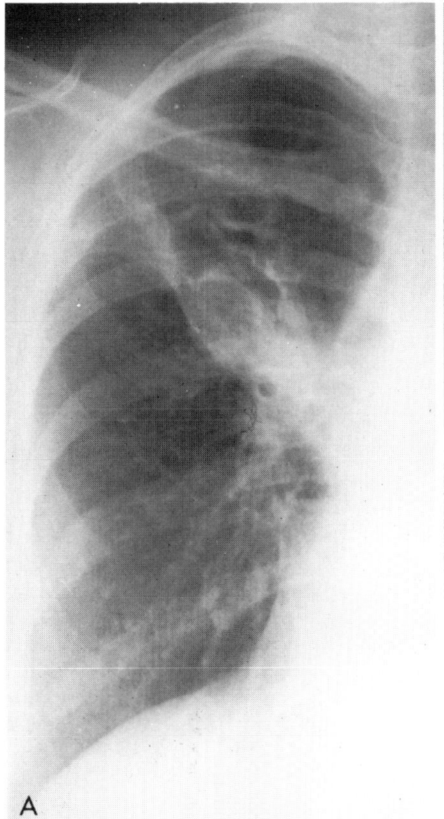

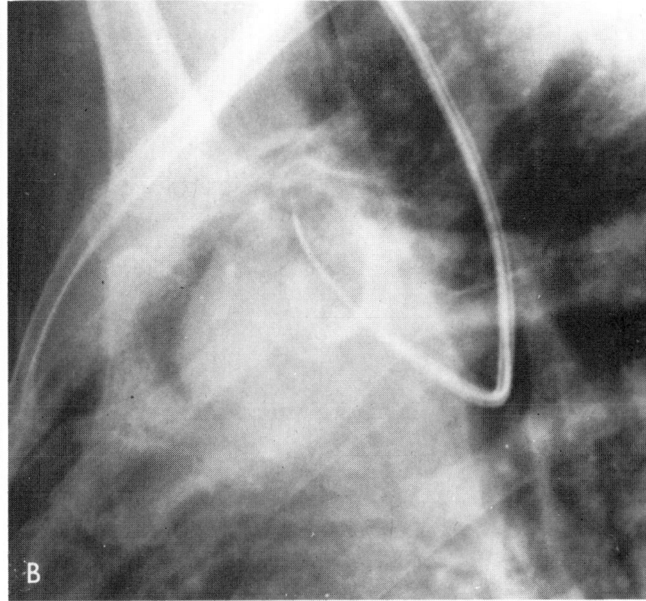

Figure 2–31. A 44 year old woman with a productive cough of 2 weeks duration and one episode of hemoptysis. *A.* Detail view of right lung, posteroanterior roentgenogram, demonstrates a 3 cm. mass (noted to be mobile on decubitus radiographs) within an irregular thin-walled cavity. Sputum examination and bronchoscopy were negative. *B.* Oblique fluoroscopic spot film showing tip of brush and catheter within the cavity. Culture of the brush scrapings yielded *Aspergillus fumigatus* and *Hemophilus influenzae.*

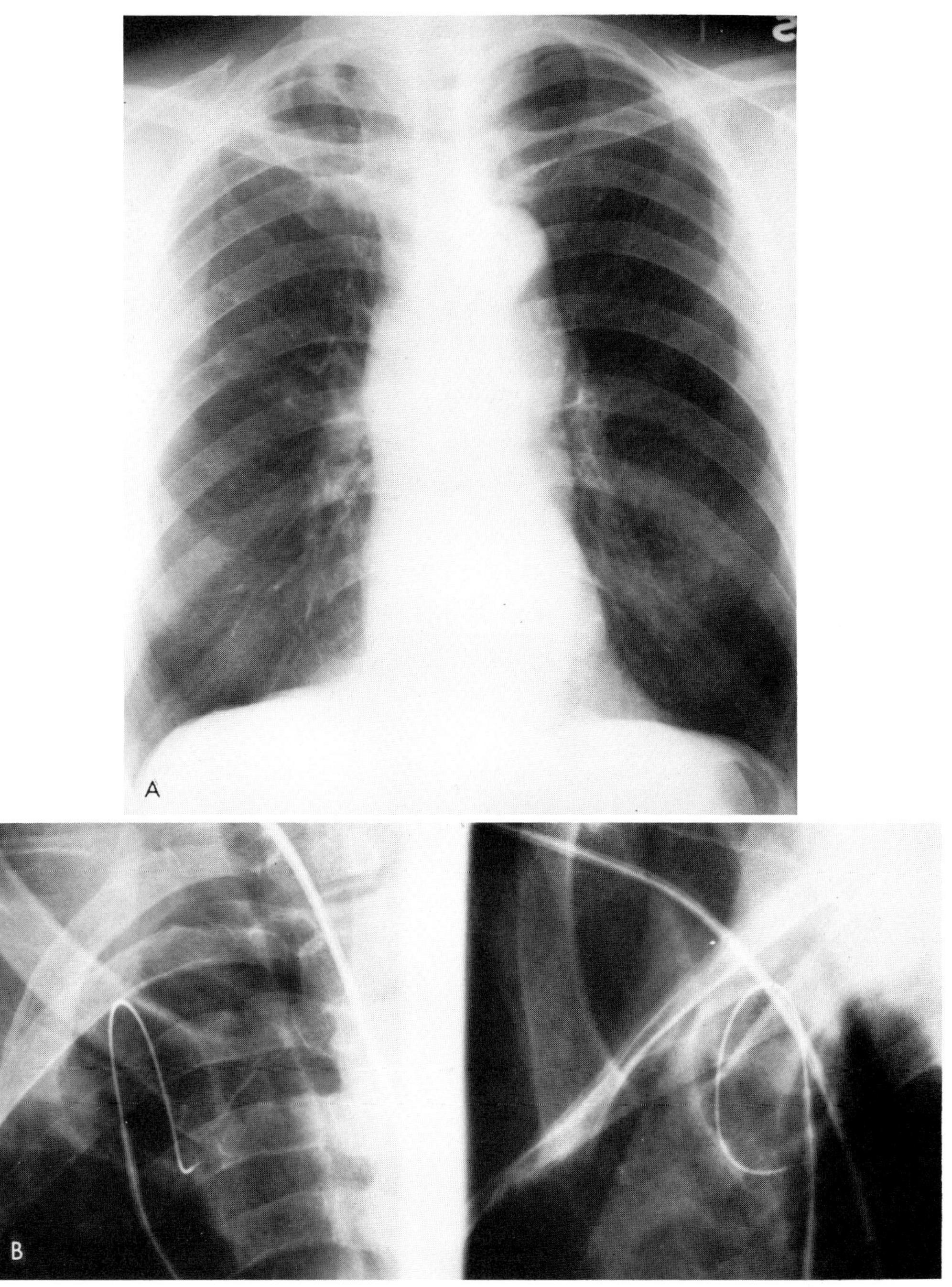

Figure 2–32. A 70 year old alcoholic man admitted for delirium tremens. No chest symptoms. *A*. Posteroanterior chest roentgenogram demonstrates a thin-walled cavitary lesion containing a small amount of fluid within the apical segment of the right upper lobe. An infected bulla was considered the most likely etiology of the lesion. Sputum examination and bronchoscopy were negative. *B*. Fluoroscopic spot films showing bronchial brush in proper location, coiled within the cavity. Cytologic preparation of the brush scrapings revealed squamous cell carcinoma cells. Surgical resection confirmed a primary cavitating lung carcinoma, which had presented with an atypical radiographic appearance. (From Forrest, John V., and Sagel, Stuart S.: Special procedures in pulmonary radiology. *In* Potchen, E. James, editor: Current Concepts in Radiology, vol. 2, St. Louis, 1975, The C. V. Mosby Co.)

only slightly discomforted, certainly much less so than by bronchoscopy, scalene node biopsy, or mediastinoscopy. Endobronchial brushing techniques are useful, but their accuracy rate is much less than that of aspiration biopsy, and the procedure is more complicated and time consuming.

Even though sputum cytology is quick and easy, the cells obtained by aspiration biopsy are much better preserved than those in sputum.[11,21] Because the accuracy of the aspiration technique (95%) is so much greater than with sputum cytology in mid and peripheral lesions,[11] and there is no difficulty collecting specimens, at times we proceed with aspiration biopsy without waiting for three negative sputum samples. This is especially true when dealing with out-patients, on whom aspiration needle biopsy can be easily performed (Fig. 2–35), followed by a 2 hour observation period, with the realization that a small percentage of patients will require a short hospitalization for treatment of a pneumothorax.

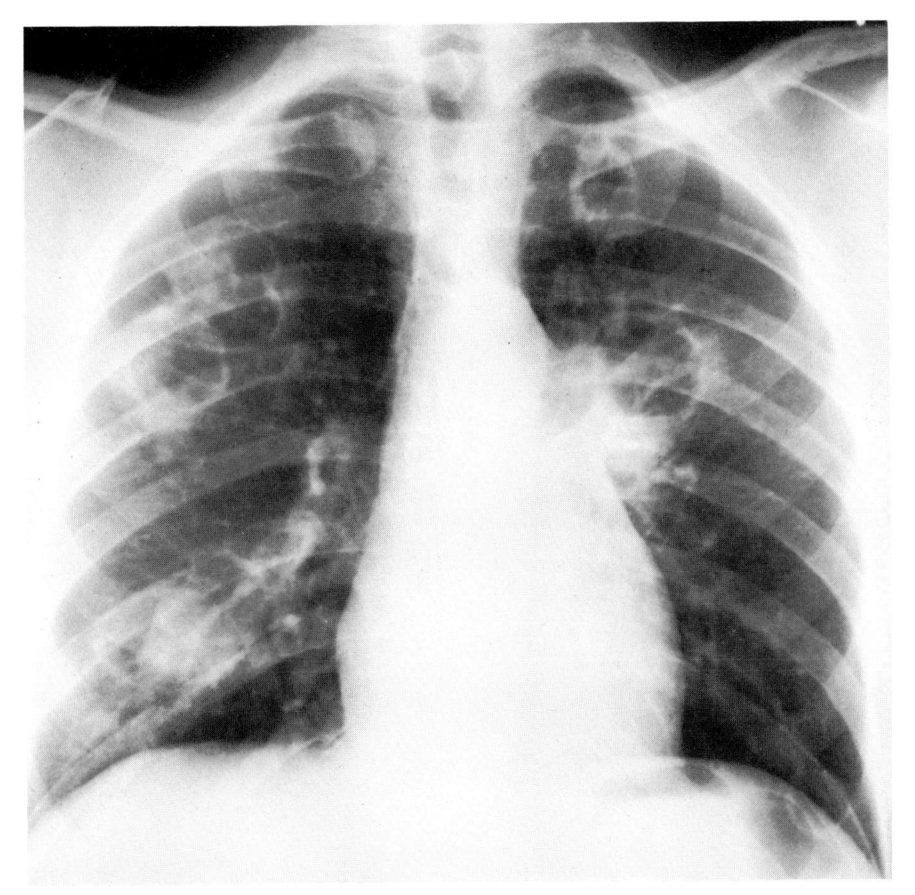

Figure 2–33. A 47 year old man, two years after supraglottic laryngectomy for carcinoma of the false cord, with cough and fever. Posteroanterior chest radiograph demonstrates multiple cavitary lesions throughout both lungs. Sputum examination and bronchoscopic washings were negative. Specimens obtained from brush biopsy of several cavities yielded squamous cell carcinoma cells; no microorganisms were cultured.

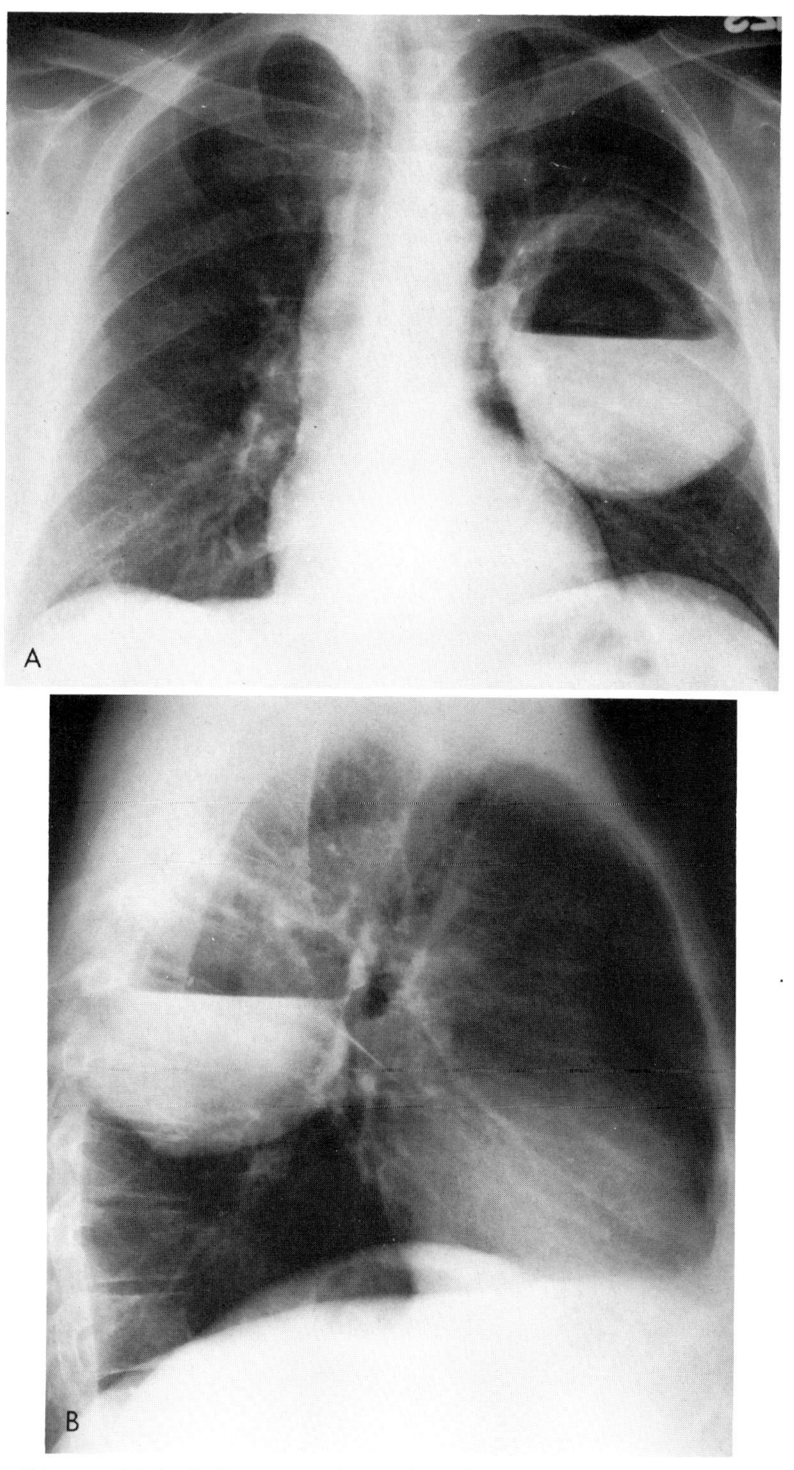

Figure 2–34. A 54 year old alcoholic man with cough and fever. *A* and *B*. Posteroanterior and lateral chest radiographs demonstrate a large, partially fluid-filled cavitary lesion within the superior segment of the left lower lobe. Antibiotic therapy and two fiberoptic bronchoscopies failed to improve the patient's clinical condition or affect drainage.

Legend continued on the opposite page

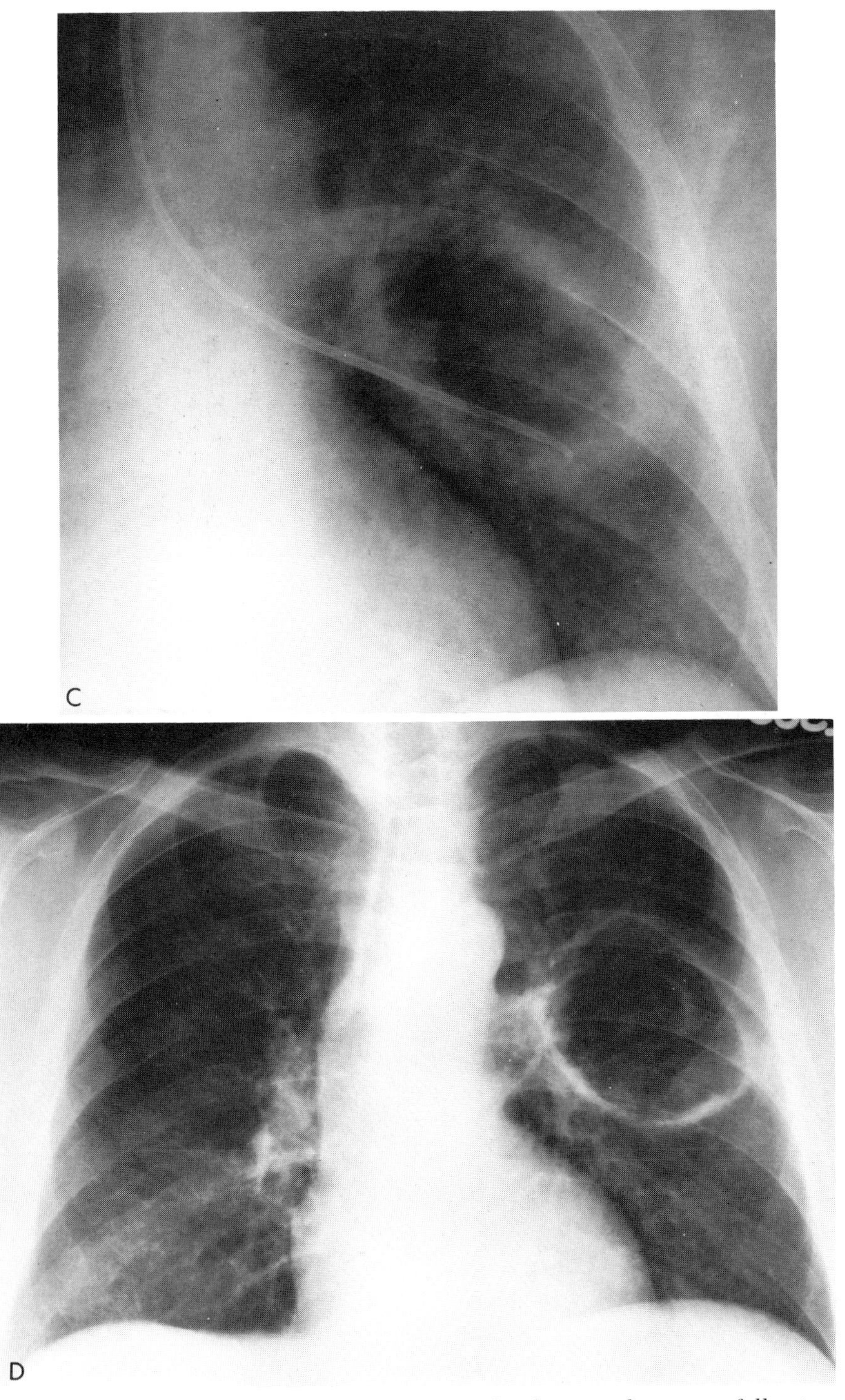

Figure 2–34 *Continued.* *C.* Fluoroscopic spot film of tip of catheter within cavity following aspiration of contents. Culture of catheter drainage revealed *Enterobacter. D.* One week later, following the catheter drainage and institution of new antibiotic therapy, the patient was virtually asymptomatic. A posteroanterior chest radiograph demonstrates a well-drained residual cavity, which subsequently closed spontaneously.

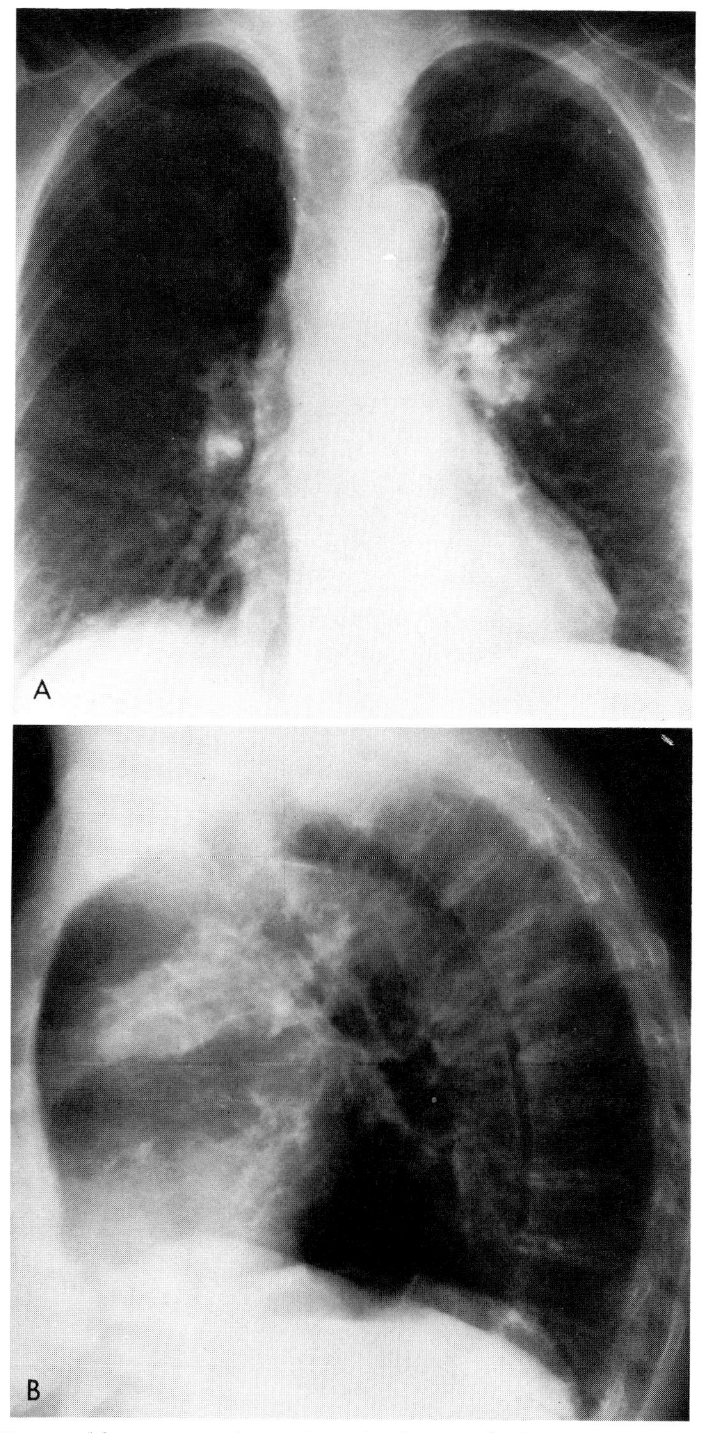

Figure 2–35. A 76 year old woman with cough and a low grade fever. *A* and *B*. Posteroanterior and lateral chest radiographs demonstrate an irregular infiltrate in the anterior segment of the left upper lobe. Treatment as an outpatient with various antibiotics was without effect. Aspiration needle biopsy of the infiltrate disclosed adenocarcinoma cells.

BIBLIOGRAPHY

1. Bandt, P. D., Blank, N., and Castellino, R. A.: Needle diagnosis of pneumonitis: Value in high risk patients. JAMA, *220*:1578-1580, 1972.
2. Berger, R. L., Dargan, E. L., and Huang, B. L.: Dissemination of cancer cells by needle biopsy of the lung. J. Thor. Card. Surg., *63*:430-432, 1972.
3. Bernstein, A., Wagaruddin, M., and Shah, M.: Management of spontaneous pneumothorax using a Heimlich flutter valve. Thorax, *28*:386-389, 1973.
4. Borgeskov, S., and Francis, D.: A comparison between fine needle biopsy and fiberoptic bronchoscopy in patients with lung lesions. Thorax, *29*:352-354, 1974.
5. Boucot, K. R., and Weiss, W.: Is curable lung cancer detected by semiannual screening? JAMA, *224*:1361-1365, 1973.
6. Boylen, C. T., Johnson, N. R., Richters, V., and Balchum, O. J.: High speed trephine lung biopsy: Methods and results. Chest, *63*:59-62, 1973.
7. Chamorro, H., Bruno, H. C., and Wholey, M. H.: Tracheobronchial studies via transcricothyroid approach. JAMA, *227*:631-633, 1974.
8. Comstock, G. W., Vaughan, R. H., and Montgomery, G.: Outcome of solitary pulmonary nodules discovered in an X-ray screening program. N. Engl. J. Med., *254*:1018-1022, 1956.
9. Curry, J. L., Regalado, R. D., Heimbach, G. Z., Stabile, J. G., and Gaulin, J. C.: Implantation transfer of pulmonary carcinoma to the trachea: A complication of percutaneous catheter brush biopsy. Chest, *65*:163-165, 1974.
10. Dahlgren, S. E., and Nordenström, B.: Transthoracic Needle Biopsy. Chicago, Year Book Medical Publishers, Inc., 1966.
11. Dahlgren, S. E., and Lind, B.: Comparison between diagnostic results obtained by transthoracic needle biopsy and by sputum cytology. Acta Cytologica, *16*:53-58, 1972.
12. Drew, W. L., Finley, T. N., Mintz, L., and Klein, H. Z.: Diagnosis of *Pneumocystis carinii* pneumonia by bronchopulmonary lavage. JAMA, *230*:713-715, 1974.
13. Felson, B.: Fundamentals of Chest Roentgenology. Philadelphia, W. B. Saunders Company, 1960.
14. Fennessy, J. J.: Bronchial brushing and transbronchial forceps biopsy in the diagnosis of pulmonary lesions. Dis. Chest, *53*:377-389, 1968.
15. Fennessy, J. J., Lu, C., Variakojis, D., Straus, F. H., and Bibbo, M.: Transcatheter biopsy in the diagnosis of diseases of the respiratory tract. Radiology, *110*:555-561, 1974.
16. Finley, R., Kieff, E., Thomsen, S., Fennessy, J., Beem, M., Lerner, S., and Morello, J.: Bronchial brushing in the diagnosis of pulmonary disease in patients at risk for opportunistic infection. Amer. Rev. Resp. Dis., *109*:379-387, 1974.
17. Forrest, J. V.: Bronchial brush biopsy in lung cavities. Radiology, *106*:69-72, 1973.
18. Genoe, G. A., Morello, J. A., and Fennessy, J. J.: The diagnosis of pulmonary aspergillosis by the bronchial brushing technique. Radiology, *102*:51-55, 1972.
19. Groff, D. B., and Marquis, J.: Treatment of lung abscess by transbronchial catheter drainage. Radiology, *107*:61-72, 1973.
20. Harlan, J. M., Fennessy, J. J., and Gross, N. J.: Bronchial brush biopsy in Hodgkin's disease. Chest, *66*:136-138, 1974.
21. Hayata, Y., Oho, K., Ichiba, M., Goya, V., and Hayashi, T.: Percutaneous pulmonary puncture for cytologic diagnosis. Its diagnostic value for small peripheral pulmonary carcinoma. Acta Cytol., *17*(6):469-475, 1973.
22. Klein, J. O.: Diagnostic lung puncture in the pneumonias of infants and children. Pediatr cs, *44*:486-492, 1969.
23. Lalli, A. F.: The direct fluoroscopically guided approach to renal thoracic and skeletal lesions. Curr. Probl. Radiol., *2*:30-41, 1972.
24. Lalli, A. F.: Roentgen-Guided Aspiration Biopsies of Thoracic, Renal, and Skeletal Lesions in Complications and Legal Implications of Radiologic Special Procedures. St. Louis, C. V. Mosby Co., 1973, p. 83-91.
25. Lauby, V. W., Burnett, W. E., Rosemond, G. P., and Tyson, R. R.: Value and risk of biopsy of pulmonary lesions by needle aspiration: Twenty-one years experience. J. Thor. Card. Surg., *49*:159-172, 1965.
26. Linsk, J. A., and Salzman, A. J.: Diagnosis of intrathoracic tumors by thin needle cytologic aspiration. Amer. J. Med. Science, *263*:181-195, 1972.
27. McCartney, R., Tait, D., Stilson, M., and Seidel, G. F.: A technique for the prevention of pneumothorax in pulmonary aspiration biopsy. Am. J. Roentgen., *120*:872-875, 1974.
28. McCartney, R. L.: Hemorrhage following percutaneous lung biopsy. Radiology, *112*:305-307, 1974.
29. McClure, C., Boucot, K., Ship, G., et al.: The solitary pulmonary nodule and pr mary lung malignancy. Arch. Environ. Health, *3*:127-139, 1961.
30. Mimica, I., Donoso, E., Howard, J. E., and Ledermann, G. W.: Lung puncture in the etiological diagnosis of pneumonia. Amer. J. Dis. Child., *122*:278-282, 1971.
31. Mintzer, R. S., Anderson, T. M., Chiles, J. T., et al.: The significance of localized bronchiectasis adjacent to pulmonary coin lesions. Chest, *64*:155-157, 1973.
32. Nelson, S. W., and Christoforidis, A. J.: Bronchography in diseases of the adult chest. Radiol. Clinics of North Amer., *11*:125-152, 1973.
33. Nordenström, B.: Needle Biopsy. Fleischner Society Course In Chest Radiology, London, 1974.
34. Norenberg, R., Claxton, C. P., Jr., and Takaro, T.: Percutaneous needle biopsy of the lung: Report of two fatal complications. Chest, *66*:216-218, 1974.
35. Repsher, L. H., Schröter, G., and Hammond, W. S.: Diagnosis of *Pneumocystis carinii* pneumonitis by means of endobronchial brush biopsy. New Engl. J. Med., *287*:340-341, 1972.

36. Rowlands, J. B., and Hare, W. S. C.: The significance of a blocked bronchus in the assessment of bronchogenic carcinoma. Australasian Radiol., *18*:27-36, 1974.
37. Sagel, S. S., and Forrest, J. V.: Fluoroscopically assisted biopsy for mid and peripheral lung lesions. JAMA, *228*:1136-1137, 1974.
38. Sanders, D. E., Thompson, D. W., and Pudden, B. J. E.: Percutaneous aspiration lung biopsy. Canad. Med. Assoc. J., *104*:139-142, 1971.
39. Sargent, E. N., and Turner, A. F.: Emergency treatment of pneumothorax. A simple catheter technique for use in the radiology department. Am. J. Roentgen., *109*:531-535, 1970.
40. Scheinhorn, D. J., Joyner, L. R., and Whitcomb, M. E.: Transbronchial forceps lung biopsy through the fiberoptic bronchoscope in *Pneumocystis carinii* pneumonia. Chest, *66*:294-295, 1974.
41. Schoenbaum, S. W., Pinsker, K. L., Rakoff, S. J., et al.: Fiberoptic bronchoscopy. Complete evaluation of the tracheobronchial tree in the radiology department. Radiology, *109*:571-575, 1973.
42. Sinner, W. N.: Transthoracic needle biopsy of small peripheral malignant lung lesions. Invest. Radiol., *8*:305-314, 1973.
43. Spjut, H. J., Hendrix, V. J., Ramirez, G. A., and Roper, C. L.: Carcinoma cells in pleural cavity washings. Cancer, *11*:1222, 1958.
44. Stevens, G. M., Weigen, J. F., and Lillington, G. A.: Needle aspiration biopsy of localized pulmonary lesions with amplified fluoroscopic guidance. Am. J. Roentgen., *103*:561-571, 1968.
45. Turner, A. F., and Sargent, E. N.: Percutaneous pulmonary needle biopsy: An improved needle for a simple direct method of diagnosis. Am. J. Roentgen., *104*:846-850, 1968.
46. Vitums, V. C.: Percutaneous needle biopsy of the lung with a new disposable needle. Chest, *62*:717-719, 1972.
47. Walls, W. J., Thornbury, J. R., and Naylor, B.: Pulmonary needle aspiration biopsy in the diagnosis of Pancoast tumors. Radiology, *111*:99-102, 1974.
48. Westcott, J. L.: Air embolism complicating percutaneous needle biopsy of the lung. Chest, *63*:108-110, 1973.
49. Willson, J. K. V., and Eskridge, M.: Bronchial brush biopsy with a controllable brush. Am. J. Roentgen., *109*:471-477, 1970.
50. Wolinsky, H., and Lischner, M. W.: Needle track implantation of tumor after percutaneous lung biopsy. Ann. Int. Med., *71*:359-362, 1969.
51. Zavala, D. C., and Bedell, G. N.: Percutaneous lung biopsy with a cutting needle. Amer. Rev. Resp. Dis., *106*:186-193, 1972.
52. Zavala, D. C., Richardson, R. H., Mukerjee, P. K., Rossi, N. P., and Bedell, G. N.: Use of bronchofiberscope for bronchial brush biopsy. Chest, *63*:889-892, 1973.
53. Zavala, D. C., Rossi, N. P., and Bedell, G. N.: Bronchial brush biopsy. Ann. Thor. Surg., *13*:519-528, 1972.
54. Zelch, J. V., and Lalli, A. F.: Diagnostic percutaneous opacification of benign pulmonary lesions. Radiology, *108*:559-561, 1973.
55. Zelch, J. V., Lalli, A. F., McCormack, L. J., and Belovich, D. M.: Aspiration biopsy in diagnosis of pulmonary nodule. Chest, *63*:149-152, 1973.

Chapter 3

BRONCHOGRAPHY

by John V. Forrest, M.D., and Stuart S. Sagel, M.D.

INTRODUCTION

Bronchography is a relatively safe, easy to perform procedure. Perusal of recent articles will reveal a wide discrepancy in opinion regarding the uses for bronchography. Some authorities rarely use the study,[8] whereas others use it frequently to evaluate many sorts of chest disease.[17] We are in agreement with those who believe that it presently has limited clinical use. Advances in cytologic and biopsy procedures have largely reduced its usefulness, especially in the diagnosis of lung cancer.

INDICATIONS

1. **BRONCHIECTASIS.** Bronchography is the definitive diagnostic method for evaluating the presence, severity, and extent of bronchiectasis. Persistent productive cough or a history of repeated pneumonias (especially when the same lobe or lobes are involved) may be clinical indications for bronchography. The plain chest radiograph is unreliable in determining the presence and anatomic distribution of bronchiectasis,[9] and surgical correction for bronchiectasis is feasible only when the disease is localized.

There is usually good correlation between clinical severity of disease and the extent and radiographic type of bronchiectasis. Cystic (saccular) bronchiectasis (Fig. 3–1) is the most severe form, and fusiform (tubular) (Fig. 3–2) is the least severe. An intermediate stage between cystic and fusiform has been termed varicose[21] since the abnormal bronchi resemble varicose veins (Fig. 3–2). Mild forms of fusiform dilatation of the bronchi are often seen with pneumonia or atelectasis and may be reversible[18] (Fig. 3–3).

If decortication of a fibrothorax is considered, bronchography will determine the extent of underlying bronchiectasis. Extensive bronchiectatic changes imply that little or no improvement in pulmonary function will result from the decortication.

2. **BRONCHO-OCCLUSIVE DISEASE.** Bronchography is helpful in determining the presence or absence of bronchial occlusion distal to the reach of the fiberoptic bronchoscope (Figs. 2–8, 2–26, and 3–4). It is often of value in the diagnosis of broncholithiasis (Fig. 3–5) and the right middle lobe syndrome and its variants (Fig. 3–6).

While some authors rely heavily on bronchography to distinguish lung cancer from benign forms of broncho-occlusive disease,[4, 17] we have found this diagnostic test alone to be almost fruitless in the definitive diagnosis of neoplastic disease (Fig. 3–7). As emphasized in the previous chapter, many benign conditions can produce bronchographic changes indistinguishable from those of neoplasm. The diagnosis of malignancy by bronchography alone always remains inferential, whereas biopsy techniques such as bronchial brushing often can achieve a definitive diagnosis, permitting the direct institution of appropriate treatment, be it surgery, radiotherapy, or a suitable antibiotic. Bronchography may be helpful in bronchial brushing as a sort of "road map" to decide which areas to brush, and to delineate the anatomy to reveal the course the brush must take to reach a peripheral lesion[5] (Fig. 3–4).

Tumors, stenosis, and dilatation of the trachea and mainstem bronchi are usually well delineated by plain films, tomography, or bronchoscopy and do not require contrast studies.

3. **HEMOPTYSIS.** Bronchography is widely used to evaluate hemoptysis of unknown etiology.[19] In our recent series of 146

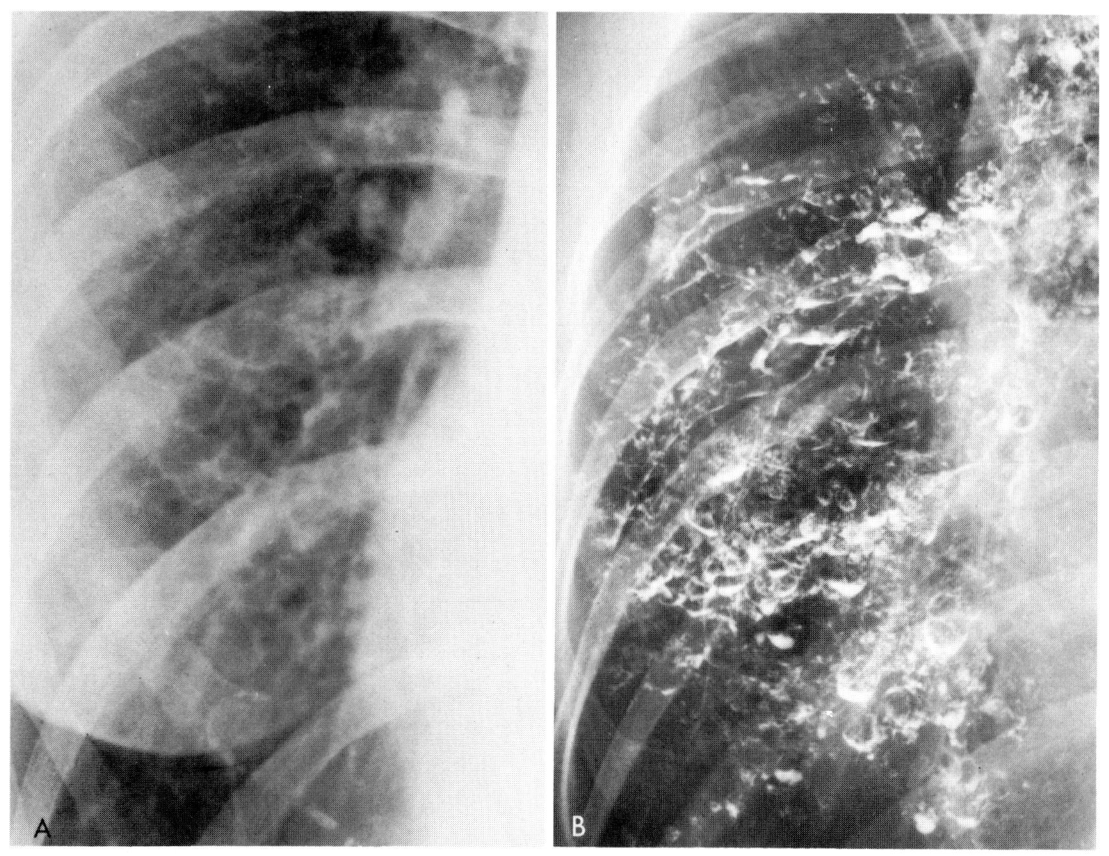

Figure 3–1. *A*. Irregular cystic densities are seen in the right mid lung field. *B*. A bronchogram confirms cystic bronchiectasis. Many of the bronchi terminate in small cysts.

patients with hemoptysis studied by bronchography, the examination was rarely of significant positive clinical help.[6] Therefore, we believe that most patients with a single episode of hemoptysis, and normal plain chest radiographic and bronchoscopic findings, do not require bronchography.

4. Obstructive airways disease. Certain bronchographic findings have been associated with chronic bronchitis and emphysema. These include irregularity of bronchial walls, slight dilatation, spasm, increased secretions (Fig. 3–8), filling of mucous glands (Fig. 3–9), and bronchiolectasis (Fig. 3–10).[11,23] The use of bronchography to evaluate these disease processes is generally unrewarding, since clinical and laboratory studies are more reliable. Most middle aged or elderly patients in the urban population have radiographic findings of chronic bronchitis on bronchography, and the severity of these findings is not well correlated with clinical status. The differentiation between severe chronic bronchitis and mild fusiform bronchiectasis is often not possible radiographically, clinically, or pathologically.

5. Fistula. Bronchography may outline fistulae between the tracheobronchial tree and pleura, esophagus, abdomen, or chest wall when the larger bronchi and trachea are involved. Most often, smaller peripheral fistulae will not be demonstrated because the viscous contrast material often will not flow into the smaller airways.[2]

TECHNIQUE

Preparation of the patient for the bronchogram requires informed consent. Most

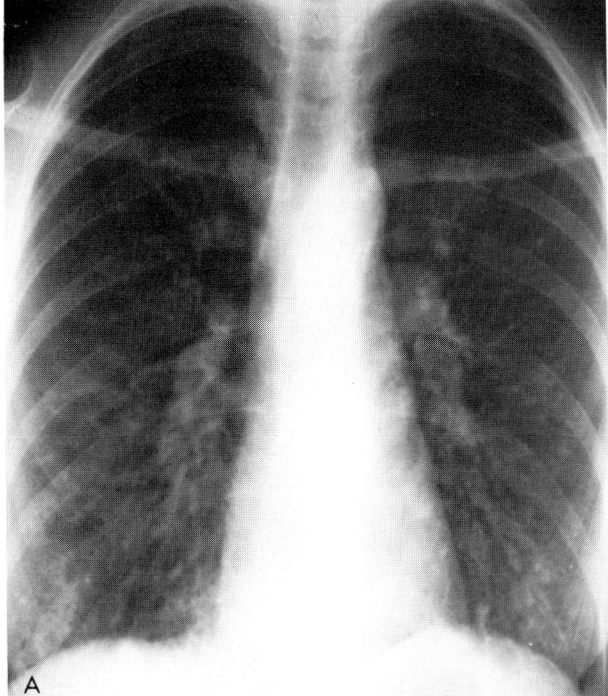

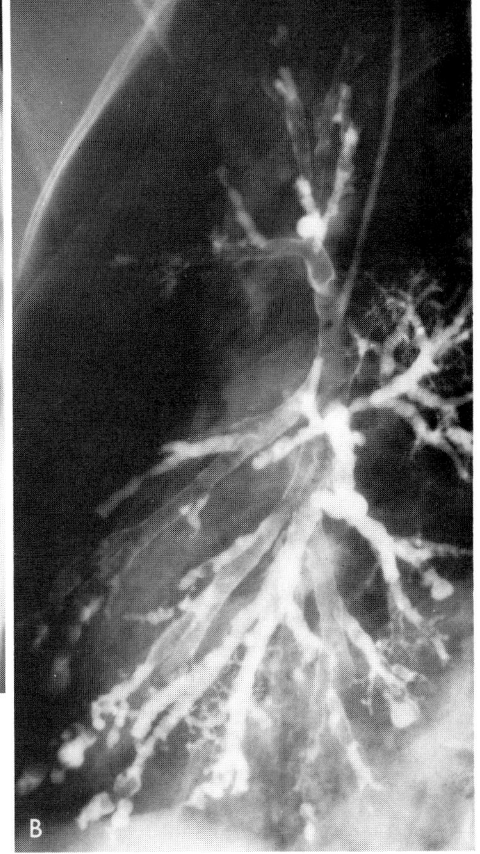

Figure 3–2. *A.* A patient with a chronic productive cough who has a diffuse increase in interstitial lung markings. *B.* Tubular and varicose bronchiectasis involves all the segments of the right lung, as demonstrated on this bronchogram. Notice how the oblique projection shows the orifices of most of the segmental bronchi well. (From Forrest, John V., and Sagel, Stuart S.: Special procedures in pulmonary radiology. *In* Potchen, E. James, editor: Current Concepts in Radiology, vol. 2, St. Louis, 1975, The C. V. Mosby Co.)

important for the success of the procedure, the patient must be well informed and relaxed because an uncooperative or anxious patient greatly increases the difficulty of the examination.

Bronchography almost always should be performed under topical anesthesia. This technique facilitates positioning for introduction of the contrast material and subsequent filming, and the coughing that is possible following the procedure results in much less retention of the viscous contrast media than if the examination is performed under general anesthesia.

Increased secretions after bronchoscopy have prompted some to recommend postponing bronchography for at least 24 hours. We have found satisfactory bronchographic detail several hours after bronchoscopy, and the patient thus can often be saved a hospital day by performing both procedures the same day.

Oily Dionosil, a solution of organically bound iodine in peanut oil, is the contrast material used generally for bronchography in the United States, and is the only one currently approved by the Federal Drug Administration.

A fine powder of the metal tantalum will coat the tracheobronchial tree when inhaled or injected through a catheter.[15] Although inhalation avoids the technical problems of catheterization, in general tantalum is an inferior agent for bronchography. Abnormal areas in the bronchial tree are often not coated, since normal areas receive the inhaled material preferentially because of relatively poor suck in the diseased segments. Even if tantalum is introduced by selective catheterization, it

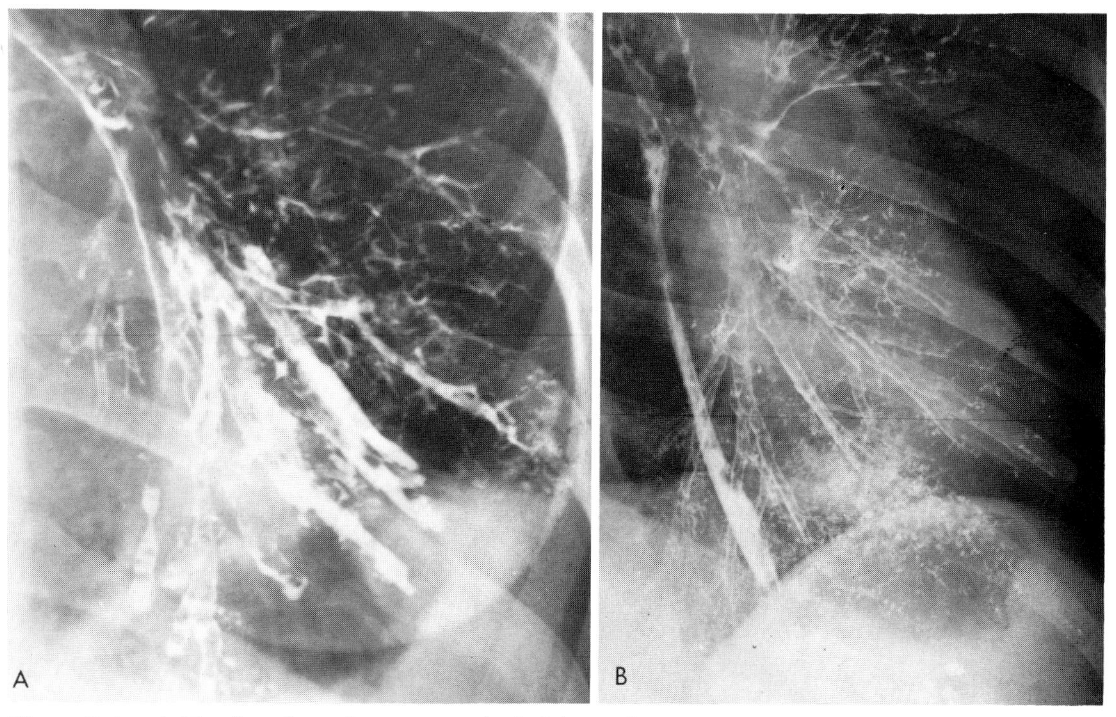

Figure 3–3. A. Fusiform bronchiectasis in the left lower lobe seen shortly after a bout of acute pneumonia. *B.* The left lower lobe bronchi are normal 8 months later.

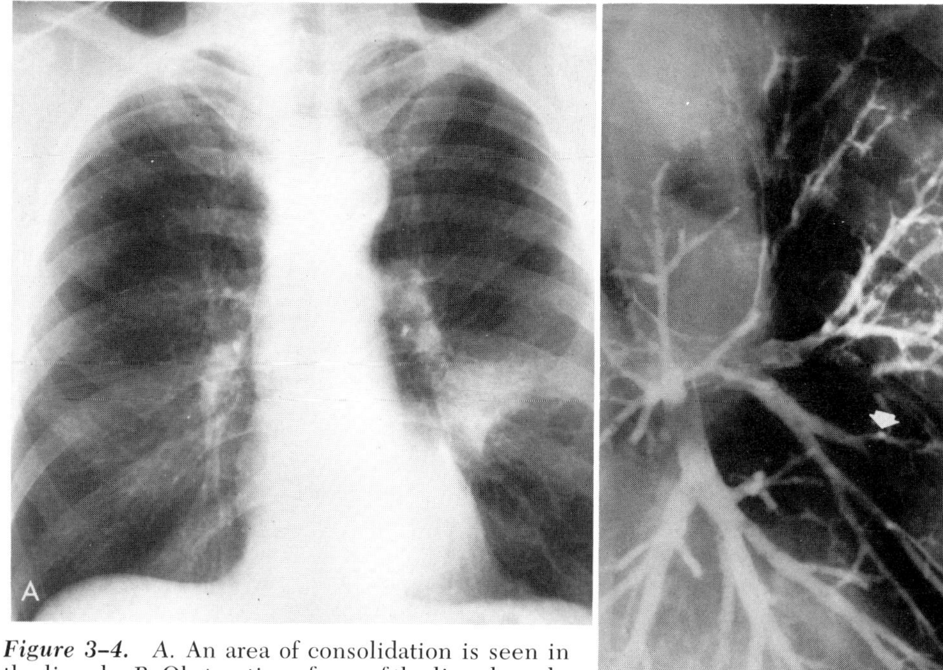

Figure 3–4. A. An area of consolidation is seen in the lingula. *B.* Obstruction of one of the lingular subsegments due to bronchogenic carcinoma (arrow) is seen on the bronchogram. This is often impossible to distinguish from benign causes of broncho-occlusive disease. Definitive diagnosis was achieved by bronchial brushing of the involved subsegment, which yielded epidermoid carcinoma cells. (From Forrest, John V., and Sagel, Stuart S.: Special procedures in pulmonary radiology. *In* Potchen, E. James, editor: Current Concepts in Radiology, vol. 2, St. Louis, 1975, The C. V. Mosby Co.)

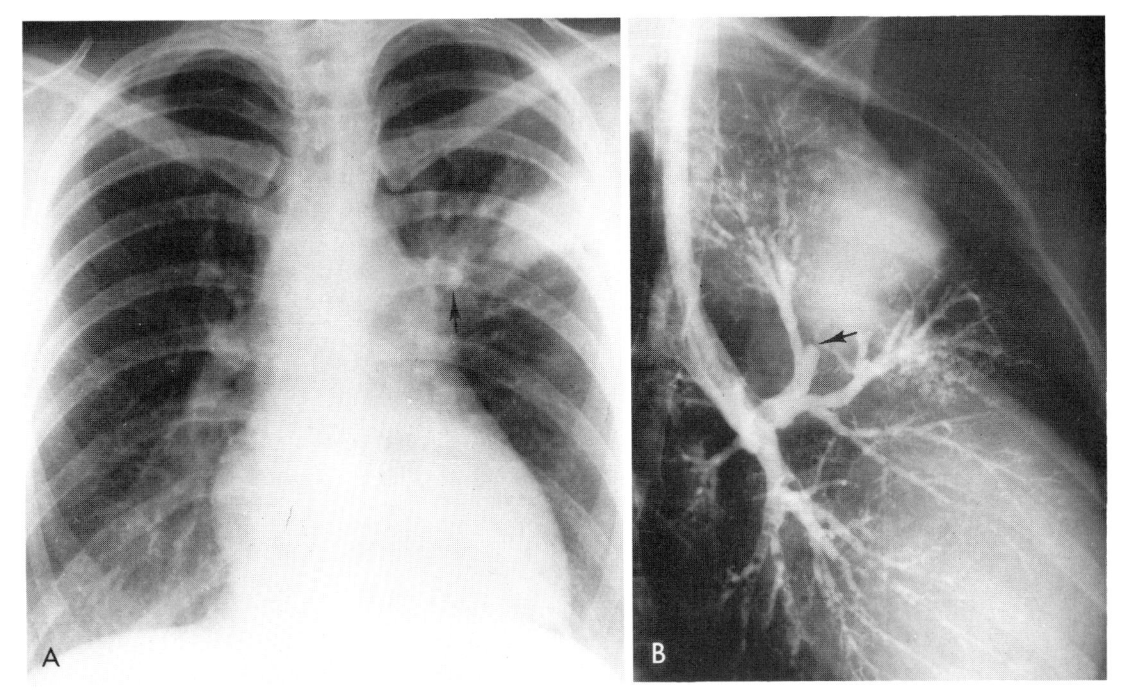

Figure 3–5. *A.* Area of consolidation is seen in the left upper lobe. A small calcification is evident centrally (arrow). *B.* A bronchogram reveals complete obstruction of the anterior segment of the left upper lobe due to a broncholith (arrow). (From Forrest, John V., and Sagel, Stuart S.: Special procedures in pulmonary radiology. *In* Potchen, E. James, editor: Current Concepts in Radiology, vol. 2, St. Louis, 1975, The C. V. Mosby Co.)

often coats mucus and secretions present in the diseased areas, thus greatly obscuring fine detail. Tantalum may remain in the peripheral airways for long periods of time after the study is completed, and it is also flammable and tends to spread throughout the radiographic room.[12] While tantalum is a very good research tool for outlining the tracheobronchial tree, at present its clinical usefulness is extremely questionable.

Contrast material may be placed into the tracheobronchial tree by many methods.[4] The use of a catheter under fluoroscopic control allows local studies to be performed, with better control of filling and selective refilling of poorly visualized areas[24] (Fig. 3–11). We personally favor the use of the cricothyroid membrane approach for greater patient comfort, reduction in the amount of local anesthetic needed, and better control of the catheter for selective studies.[22] The procedure is often combined with bronchial brushing when material is needed for cytologic or bacteriologic examination (Figs. 2–8, 2–26, and 3–4). Premedication and the technique of catheter introduction are identical to those described for bronchial brushing in Chapter 2.

Under fluoroscopic control, the catheter is advanced to the area to be studied. After the patient is moved into the lateral position, lying on the side to be studied, contrast medium is instilled. The contrast medium thus flows equally into all the lobar bronchial orifices being studied, and spillover to the other lung is prevented. Slight changes in position are easily accomplished, such as moving the patient to a somewhat more prone position to favor filling of the middle lobe. If both sides are to be studied, the right side is usually done first in order to better visualize the middle lobe orifice in the lateral projection. When sufficient coating is achieved, spot films are obtained in various projections. These films are taken in mid-inspiration, since very deep inspiration may spread contrast material to unanesthetized peripheral bronchi and induce coughing. Lateral and oblique films usually show the major bron-

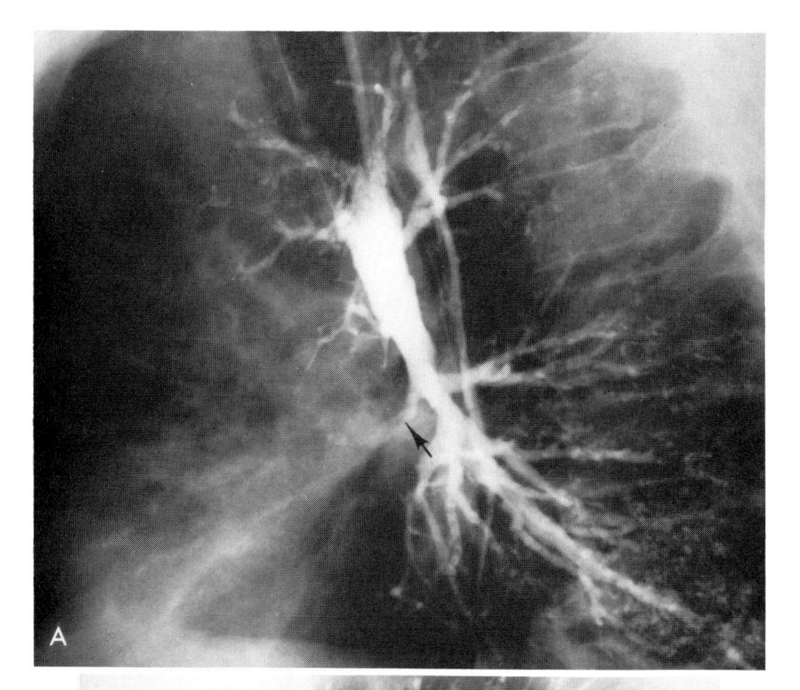

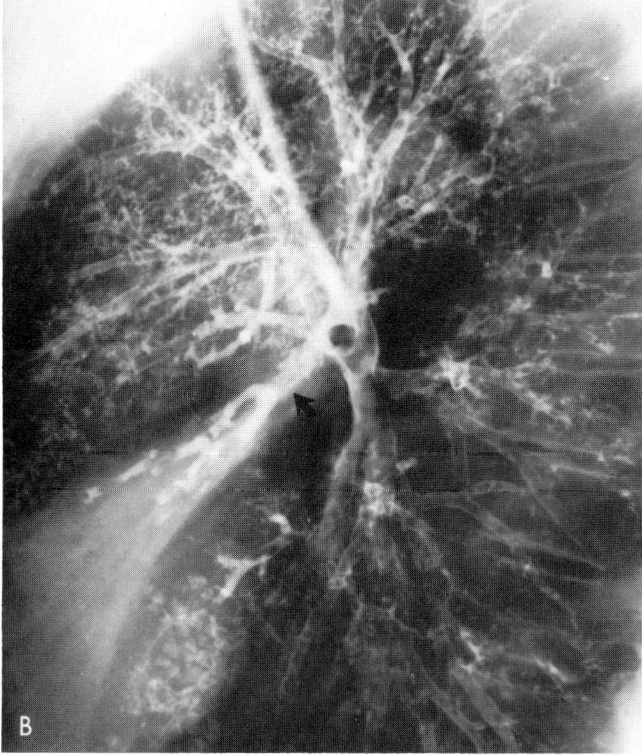

Figure 3–6. *A.* Right middle lobe syndrome with chronic pneumonia and atelectasis. The right middle lobe bronchus is occluded on the bronchogram (arrow). *B.* Another example of a right middle lobe syndrome with chronic atelectasis and consolidation. In this instance the right middle lobe bronchus is patent (arrow). (From Forrest, John V., and Sagel, Stuart S.: Special procedures in pulmonary radiology. *In* Potchen, E. James, editor: Current Concepts in Radiology, vol. 2, St. Louis, 1975, The C. V. Mosby Co.)

Figure 3–7. *A* and *B.* Posteroanterior and lateral chest radiographs in an asymptomatic man demonstrate an elliptical density in the anterior segment of the right upper lobe. *C.* Bronchogram, right posterior oblique projection, demonstrates complete occlusion of the anterior segment of the right upper lobe by a "mass" (arrow). The apical bronchi are displaced inferiorly and the middle lobe bronchi superiorly about the atelectatic segment. Classic bronchographic criteria would regard this as a typical case of obstructing carcinoma. However, histologic examination of the resected right upper lobe disclosed a fibrotic contracted anterior segment secondary to old granulomatous disease with some inspissated mucus in the segmental bronchial orifice.

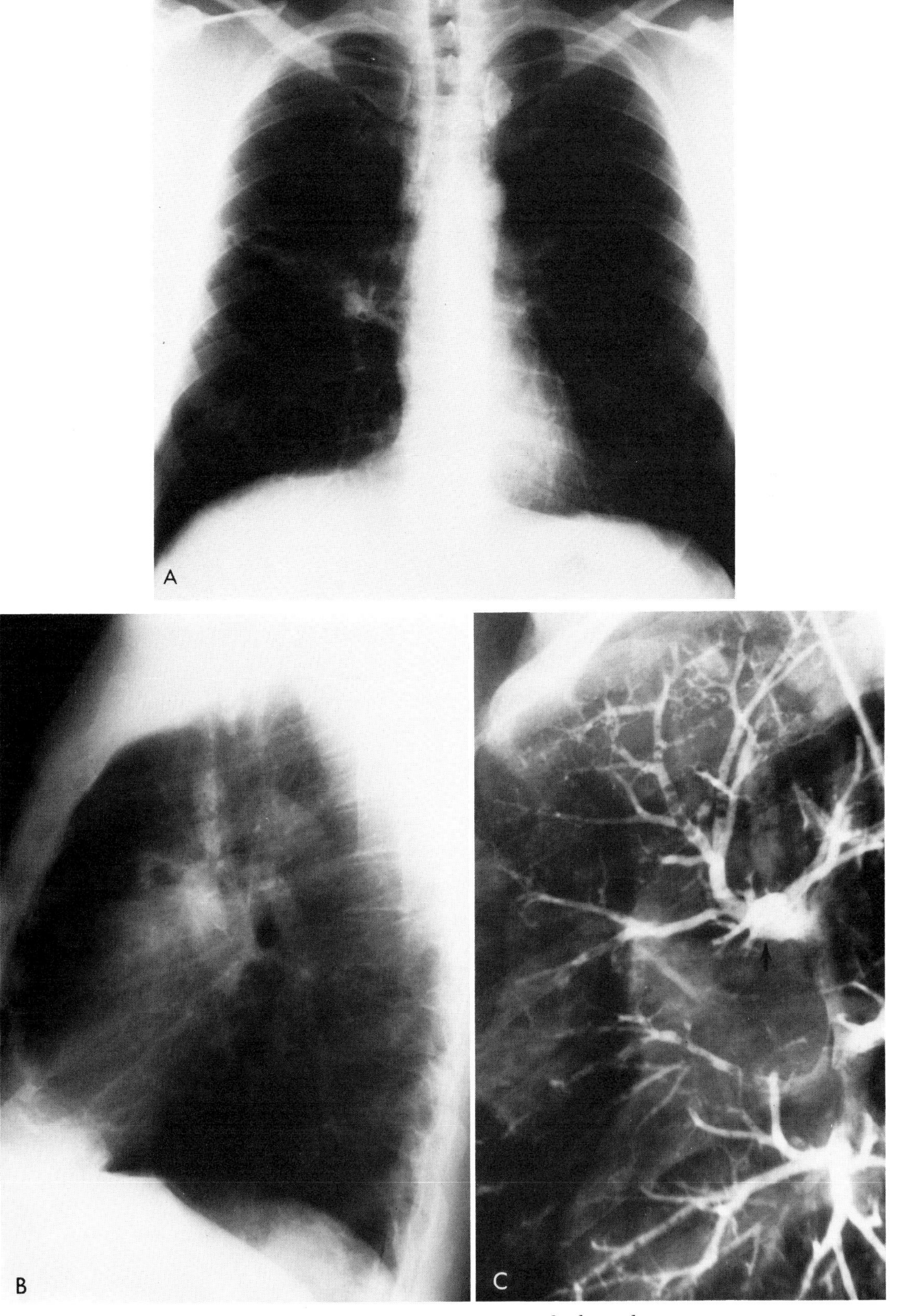

Figure 3–7. *See opposite page for legend.*

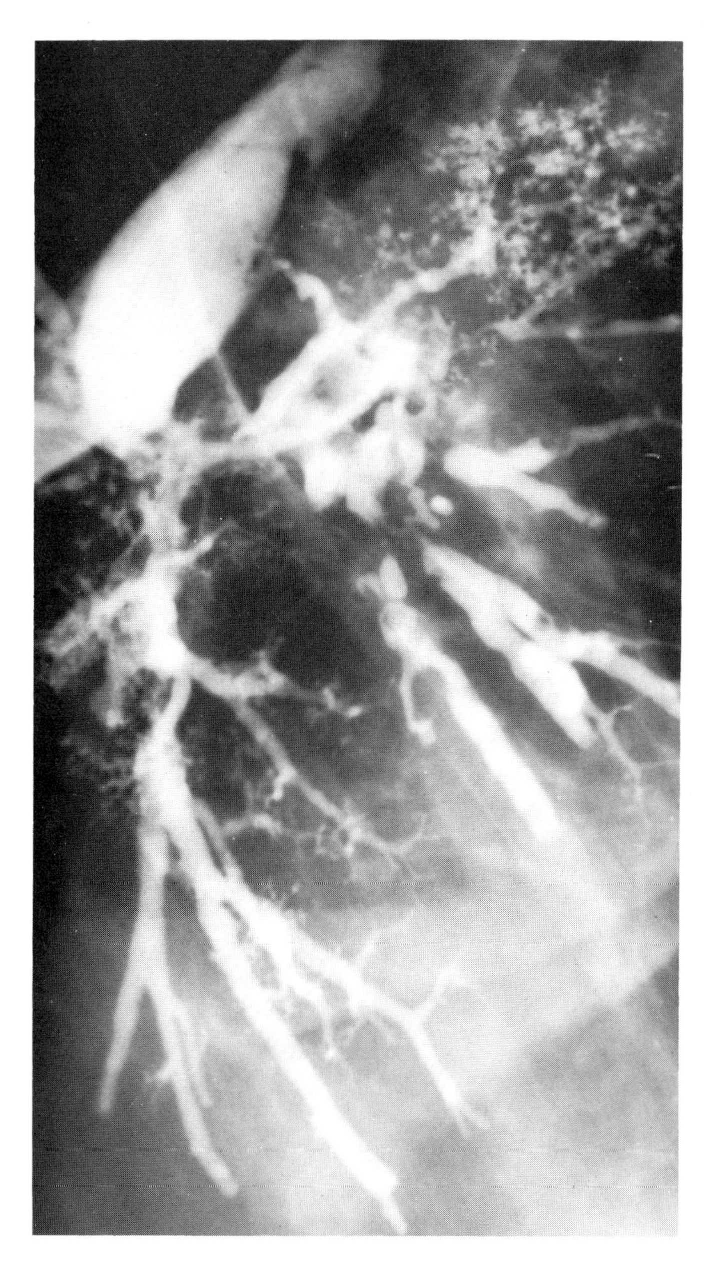

Figure 3–8. A bronchogram of a patient with severe, chronic bronchitis shows slight dilatation and irregularity of the bronchi, with incomplete filling and lucent defects due to spasm and increased secretions. (From Forrest, John V., and Sagel, Stuart S.: Special procedures in pulmonary radiology. *In* Potchen, E. James, editor: Current Concepts in Radiology, vol. 2, St. Louis, 1975, The C. V. Mosby Co.)

chial orifices better than do frontal films[4, 14] (Fig. 3–2B). With good quality fluoroscopic spot films, standard 14 × 17 inch radiographs are rarely if ever necessary. A post-cough film has been advocated to evaluate more peripheral airways, particularly in order to see bronchiectasis involving only smaller bronchi.[1] In our personal experience, this film has been of doubtful value.

Cinebronchography may be used to record fluoroscopic observations of bronchial spasm, collapse, and stenosis. This technique has been helpful in studying the pathophysiology of the bronchial tree but rarely is necessary for clinical evaluation.[7]

CONTRAINDICATIONS AND COMPLICATIONS

While rare, allergic reactions or overdose of local anesthetic are potentially fatal.[3, 20]

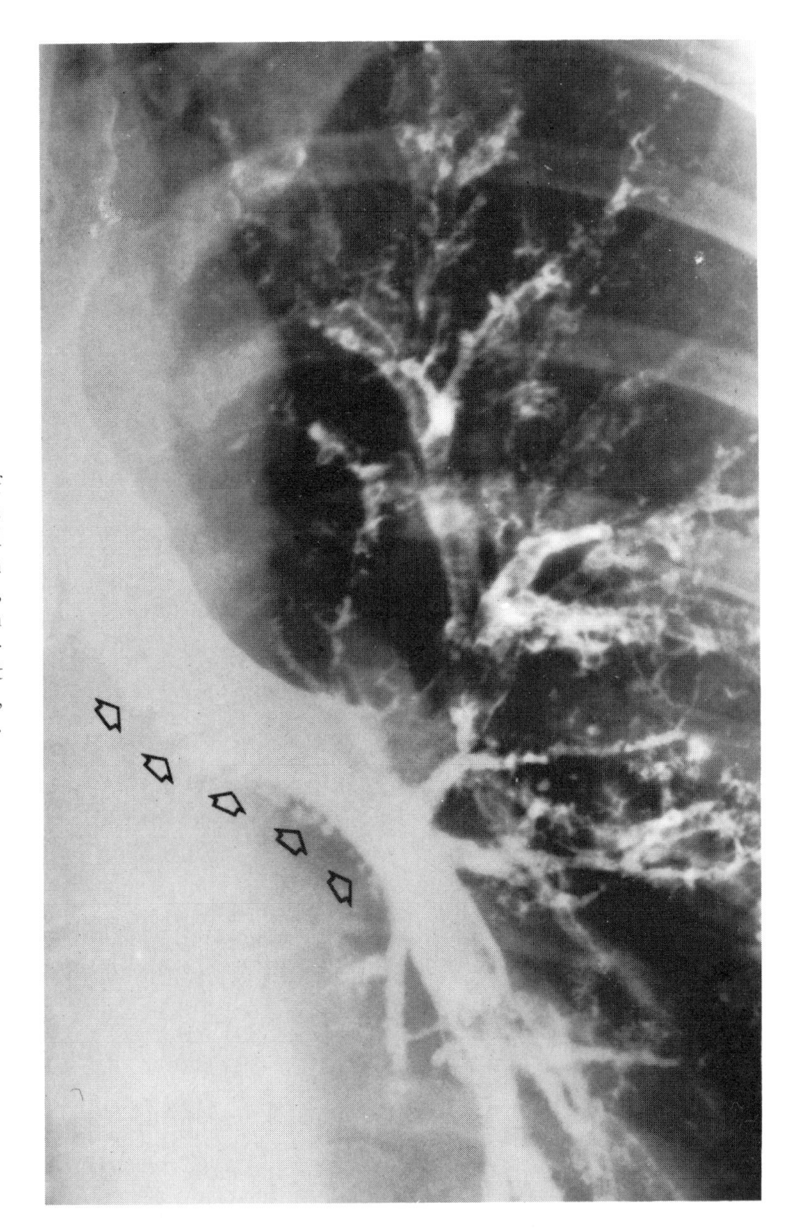

Figure 3–9. Bronchogram of patient with chronic bronchitis shows filling of many dilated mucous glands (arrows). (From Forrest, John V., and Sagel, Stuart S.: Special procedures in pulmonary radiology. *In* Potchen, E. James, editor: Current Concepts in Radiology, vol. 2, St. Louis, 1975, The C. V. Mosby Co.)

If a study is necessary in a patient who is allergic to local anesthetic material, general anesthesia must be used. True allergy to the oily Dionosil is rare, but when present it is certainly a contraindication to the examination.[17] Alternate contrast material with different chemical properties, such as barium sulfate[16] or tantalum powder, might be indicated in this situation.

A patient with a very labile medical condition, such as cardiac arrhythmia, would not be a candidate for bronchography.

Dyspnea precipitated by the introduction of the viscous contrast medium is the most common complication of bronchography. Unilateral bronchography results in an approximate 20% reduction in pulmonary function, whereas bilateral bronchography reduces it by approximately 30%.[3] Thus, severe respiratory insufficiency would be an absolute contraindication for bronchography, since the contrast medium will occlude or partially occlude some airways during the course of the examination, fur-

Text continued on page 82

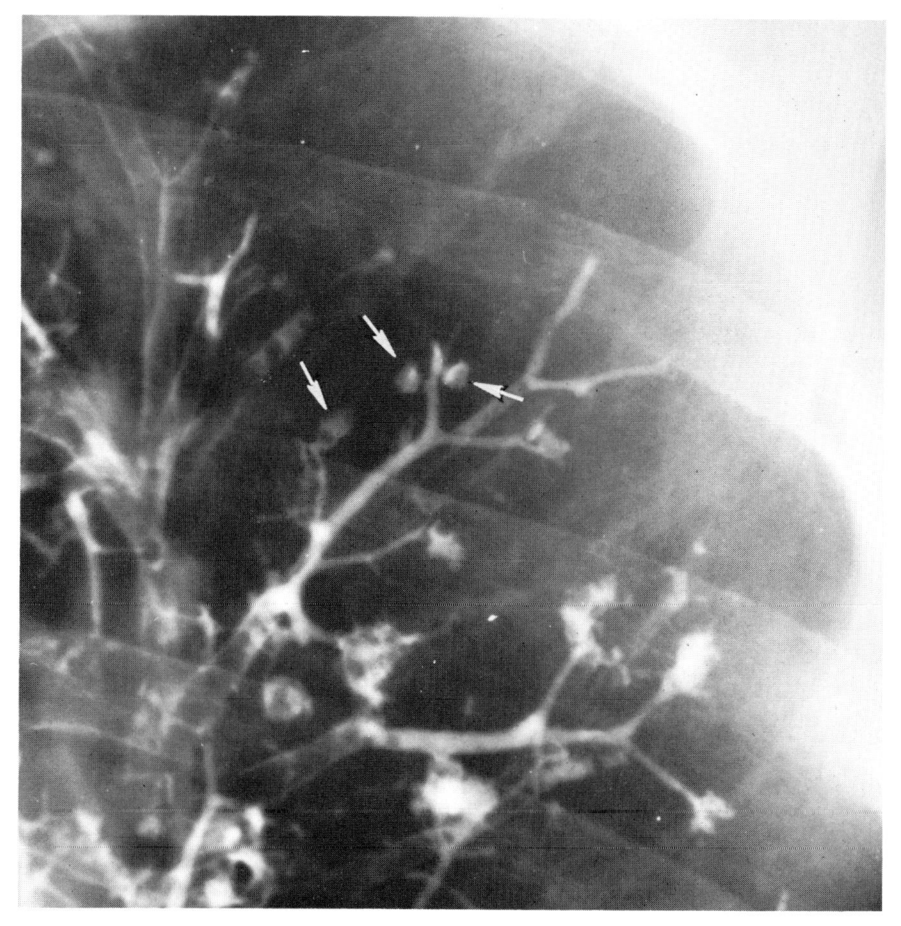

Figure 3–10. Bronchogram of a patient with emphysema shows sparse peripheral filling of bronchi (the pruned tree appearance) and bronchiolectasis (arrows). (From Forrest, John V., and Sagel, Stuart S.: Special procedures in pulmonary radiology. *In* Potchen, E. James, editor: Current Concepts in Radiology, vol. 2, St. Louis, 1975, The C. V. Mosby Co.)

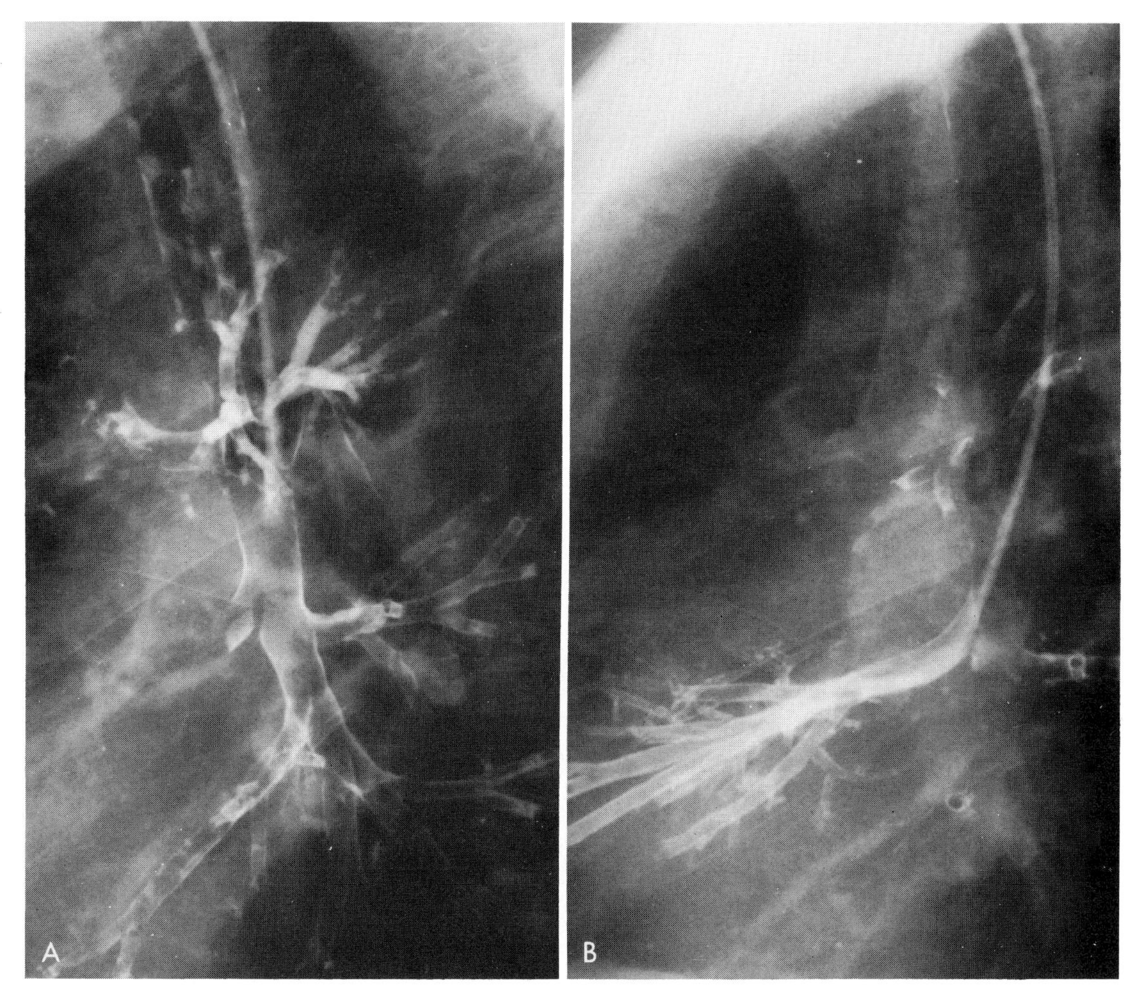

Figure 3–11. *A.* Right middle lobe bronchi are not filled (even after injecting contrast media with patient prone), suggesting possibility of broncho-occlusive disease. *B.* Selective catheterization of the right middle lobe bronchus allows filling and excludes bronchial occlusion. (From Forrest, John V., and Sagel, Stuart S.: Special procedures in pulmonary radiology. *In* Potchen, E. James, editor: Current Concepts in Radiology, vol. 2, St. Louis, 1975, The C. V. Mosby Co.)

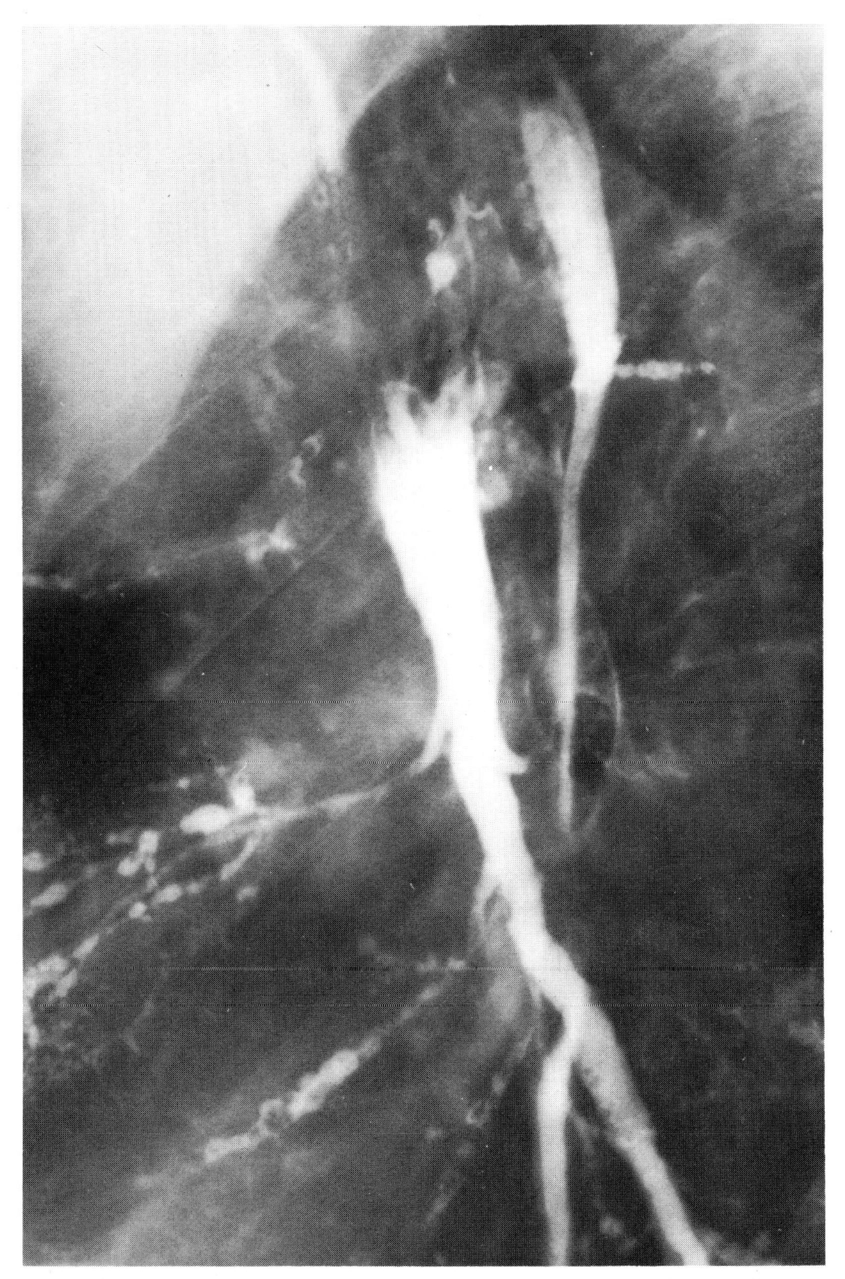

Figure 3–12. Lateral view of a right-sided bronchogram shows poor filling and narrowing of many bronchi due to spasm in an asthmatic.

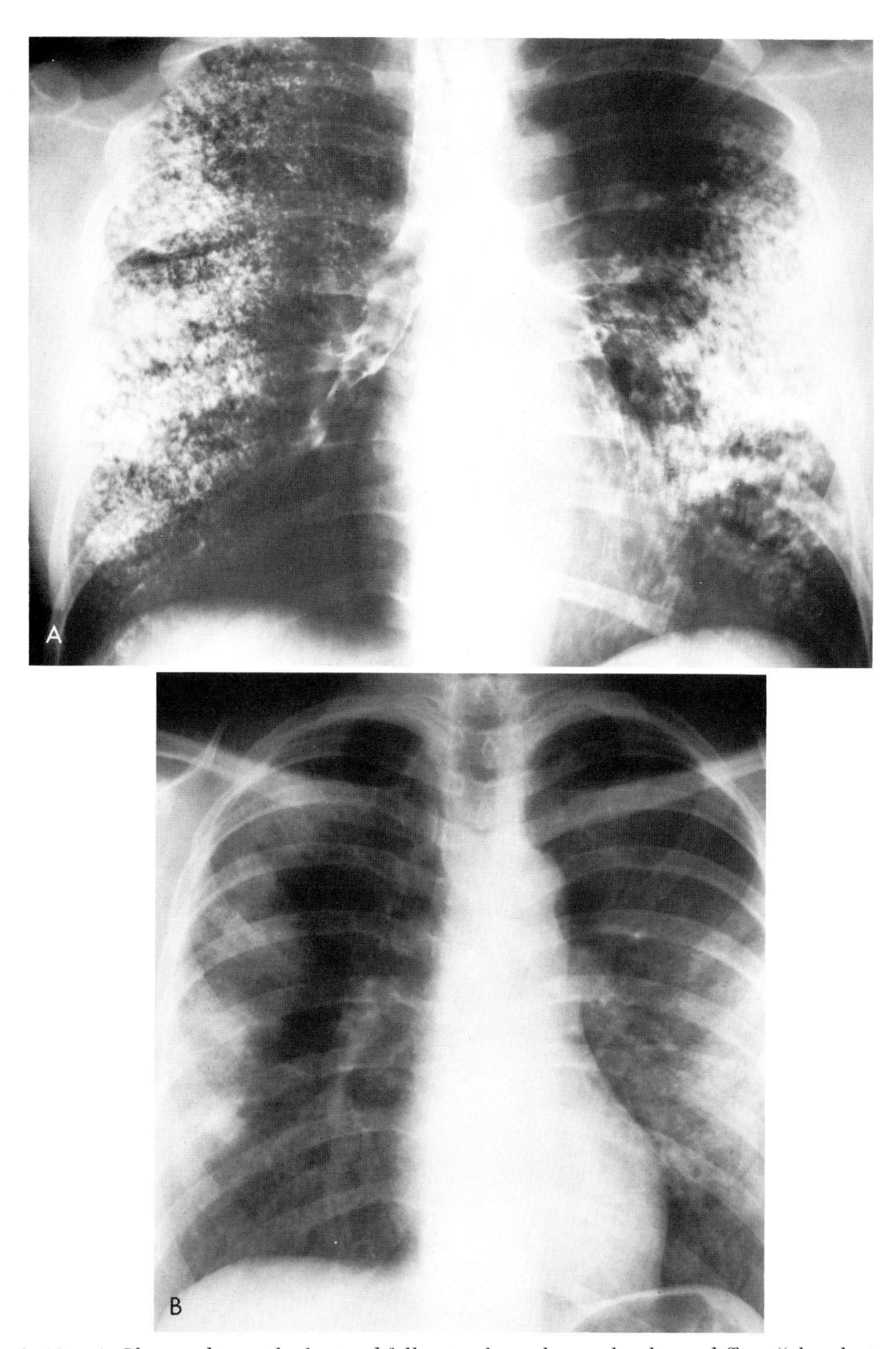

Figure 3–13. A. Chest radiograph obtained following bronchography shows diffuse "alveolarization." B. Four days later there was extensive peripheral consolidation and the patient was febrile with symptoms of pneumonia. Chemical and superimposed bacterial pneumonia have been caused by filling of the peripheral bronchioles by oily Dionosil. (From Forrest, John V., and Sagel, Stuart S.: Special procedures in pulmonary radiology. *In* Potchen, E. James, editor: Current Concepts in Radiology, vol. 2, St. Louis, 1975, The C. V. Mosby Co.)

ther diminishing already compromised pulmonary function.[3,4] Selective filling of a localized segment with a small amount of contrast medium may be permissible.

The tolerance of asthmatics to bronchography is difficult to predict.[10] Occasionally, severe bronchospasm will occur (Fig. 3–12), but other patients with severe asthma tolerate the procedure well. The study should not be performed during an acute attack.

If a large amount of oily Dionosil is coughed or aspirated into the most peripheral airways, the characteristic appearance of "alveolarization" is seen (Fig. 3–13A). This contrast may cause no effect on the patient, but secondary chemical or superimposed bacterial pneumonia may ensue (Fig. 3–13B). Coughing during the procedure or overfilling with contrast medium increases the risk of this complication. Decanting half the oil from the unmixed bottle of oily Dionosil will increase the viscosity of the contrast agent and decrease filling of the peripheral bronchioles.[17]

Localized or segmental areas of atelectasis may occur following bronchography, particularly when coughing is ineffective in expectorating the viscous contrast medium, such as when the examination is performed under general anesthesia.

Laryngeal spasm and edema due to mechanical irritation from the catheter may occur occasionally. The transcricothyroid membrane approach can result in neck infection which could spread to the mediastinum.[13] Contrast material left in the soft tissue of the neck after such a study may

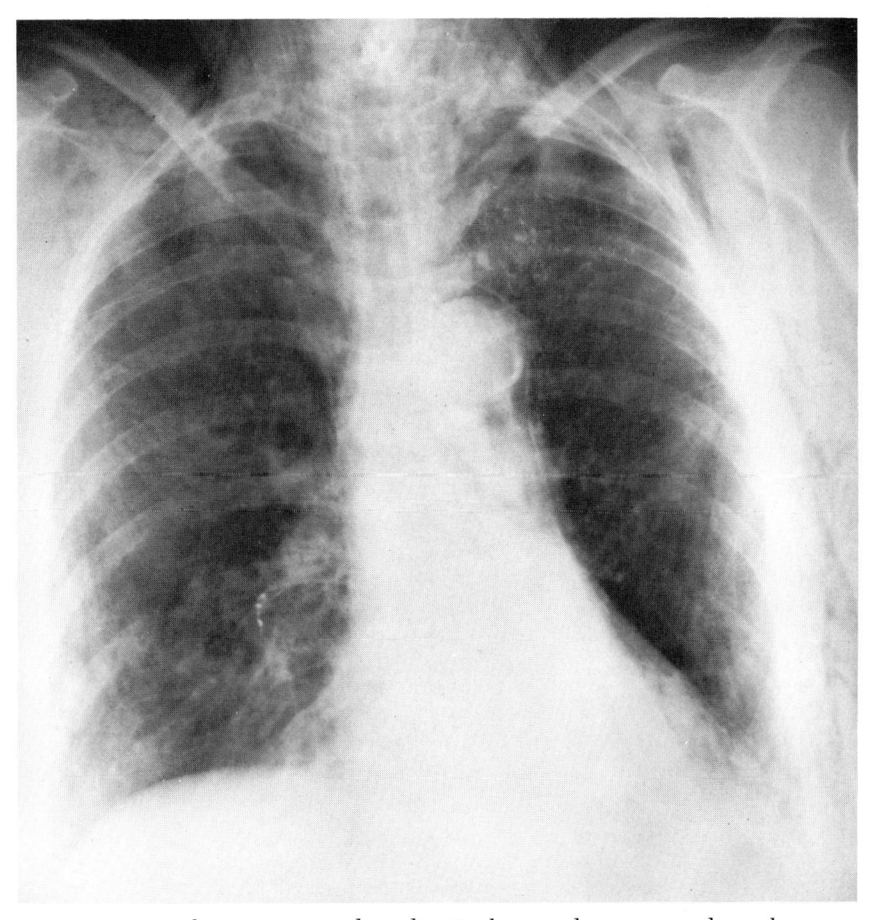

Figure 3–14. Extensive subcutaneous and mediastinal air is demonstrated on chest roentgenogram obtained 24 hours after a bronchogram was performed using the transcricothyroid membrane technique. (From Forrest, John V., and Sagel, Stuart S.: Special procedures in pulmonary radiology. *In* Potchen, E. James, editor: Current Concepts in Radiology, vol. 2, St. Louis, 1975, The C. V. Mosby Co.)

cause a small sterile abscess.[25] Subcutaneous air due to leakage at the wound site is a frequent complication of this approach but usually is of no significance. Occasionally, large amounts of air will collect subcutaneously and dissect into the mediastinum (Fig. 3–14), rarely perforating into the pleural space and causing a pneumothorax. Massaging the neck wound for 5 minutes after the procedure and instructing the patient to cover the wound with the finger for the next day whenever he has to cough will greatly reduce the incidence of air leakage into the surrounding tissues.

BIBLIOGRAPHY

1. Abrams, H. L., Hencky, G., and Kaplan, H. S.: Delayed films in bronchography. Calif. Med., *78*:104–107, 1953.
2. Burford, T.: Lack of bronchographic filling of peripheral fistulae. Personal communication.
3. Christoforidis, A. J.: Bronchography. *In* Meaney, T. F., et al.: Complications and Legal Implications of Radiologic Special Procedures. St. Louis, C. V. Mosby Co., 1973, pp. 102–116.
4. Christoforidis, A. J., and Johnson, J. C.: Bronchography. *In* Current Problems in Radiology. Chicago, Year Book Medical Publishers, Inc., July-August, 1973, pp. 1–48.
5. Fennessy, J. J.: Transbronchial biopsy of peripheral lung lesions. Radiology, *88*:878–882, 1967.
6. Forrest, J. V., Sagel, S. S., and Omell, G. H.: The use of bronchography in hemoptysis. (Submitted for publication.)
7. Fraser, R. G., Macklem, P. T., and Brown, W. G.: Airway dynamics in bronchiectasis. A combined cinefluorographic-manometric study. Amer. J. Roentgen., *93*:821–835, April 1965.
8. Fraser, R.: Bronchography 1972. J. Canad. Assoc. Radiol., *23*:236–237, 1972.
9. Fraser, R. G., and Paré, J. A. P.: Diagnosis of Diseases of the Chest. Philadelphia, W. B. Saunders Co., 1970, p. 1048.
10. Ibid., p. 119.
11. Freimanis, A. K., and Molnar, W.: Chronic bronchitis and emphysema at bronchography. Radiology, *74*:194–205, 1960.
12. Friedman, P. J., and Tisi, G. M.: Alveolarization of tantalum powder in experimental bronchography and the clearance of inhaled particles from the lung. Radiology, *104*:523–535, 1972.
13. Hemley, S. D., and Kanick, V.: Some observations on transcricothyroid bronchography. Amer. J. Roentgen., *92*:578–583, Sept. 1964.
14. Leuenberger, P., and DeBrito-Paiva, E.: Atlas of Segmental Bronchography. Paris, Kodak-Pathe Medical Division, 1973.
15. Nadel, J. A., Wolfe, W. G., and Graf, P. D.: Powdered tantalum as a medium for bronchography in canine and human lungs. Invest. Radiol., *3*:229–238, 1968.
16. Nelson, S. W., Christoforidis, A. J., and Pratt, P. C.: Further experience with barium sulfate as a bronchographic contrast medium. Amer. J. Roentgen., *92*:595–614, 1964.
17. Nelson, S. W., and Christoforidis, A. J.: Bronchography in diseases of the adult chest. Radiol. Clinics of North Amer., *11*:125–152, 1973.
18. Nelson, S. W., and Christoforidis, A. J.: Reversible bronchiectasis. Radiology, *71*:375–382, 1958.
19. Olsen, A. M., and O'Neil, J. J.: Bronchography. A report of the Committee on Brochoesophagraphy. Dis. Chest, *51*:663–668, 1967.
20. Proctor, D. F.: Anesthesia for peroral endoscopy and bronchography. A review. Anesthesiology, *29*:(5)1025–1036, 1968.
21. Reid, L.: Reduction in bronchial subdivision in bronchiectasis. Thorax, *5*:233–247, 1950.
22. Sargent, E. N., and Turner, A. F.: Percutaneous transcricothyroid membrane selective bronchography. Amer. J. Roentgen., *104*:(4)792–801, 1968.
23. Simon, G., and Galbraith, H. J. B.: Radiology of chronic bronchitis. Lancet, *2*:850–852, Oct. 1953.
24. Steckel, R. J., and Grillo, H. C.: Catheterization of the trachea and bronchi by a modified Seldinger technic: A new approach to bronchography. Radiology, *83*:1035–1038, 1964.
25. Zuckerman, S. D., and Jacobson, F.: Transtracheal bronchography. Amer. J. Roentgen., *87*:(5)840–843, 1962.

Chapter 4

PULMONARY ANGIOGRAPHY

by Allan L. Simon, M.D., and Stuart S. Sagel, M.D.

INTRODUCTION

Pulmonary angiography is a helpful method of identifying alterations in the pulmonary vessels caused by intrinsic vascular or pulmonary parenchymal disease. The earliest method of opacifying the pulmonary vessels was by injection of contrast medium into a peripheral vein or the right atrium. Although this method provides both visualization of the pulmonary circulation and assessment of the size and function of the right heart chambers, there is significant loss of detail of the pulmonary vessels due to dilution of the contrast medium by unopacified blood. Also, both arm vein and right atrial injection may obscure the right pulmonary artery and its branches by the presence of contrast medium in the superior vena cava and right atrium. Therefore, this chapter will deal primarily with injections into the main pulmonary artery and distally. While right atrial injection theoretically might demonstrate a rare thrombus in the right atrium, right ventricle, or right ventricular outflow tract as the cause of pulmonary embolism, we have personally seen only one such case.

INDICATIONS

As with any other radiologic technique, each case should be individualized and the decision as to performance of angiography made on the basis of available clinical and radiographic information. The general criteria for selection of patients for pulmonary angiography have one common denominator: the addition of meaningful information from careful inspection of the pulmonary vessels. Presenting signs and symptoms may include dysphagia, dyspnea, hemoptysis, positive radiographs, or laboratory tests.

PULMONARY EMBOLISM. The most common application of pulmonary angiography is in the diagnosis of pulmonary embolism. Angiography is the most specific test available for establishing the diagnosis of embolism,[4, 11, 20] but should be reserved for cases in which the usual screening test findings (chest radiograph, radioisotopic perfusion and ventilation scans, and blood gases) are equivocal or inconsistent.[16] It is not necessary to perform an angiogram in a patient who has a normal chest radiograph, classic radioisotopic studies for embolism, and a good clinical history. Pulmonary angiography is indicated to differentiate pulmonary embolism from other antecedent or intercurrent pulmonary disease which may be causing abnormal chest radiographic or radioisotopic ventilation-perfusion abnormalities. Also, pulmonary angiography is recommended to establish a definitive diagnosis of pulmonary embolism whenever caval interruption is contemplated, and should be mandatory to assess the size, location, and extent of the emboli before embolectomy is performed. Additionally, it may be of value in patients at high risk from anticoagulant therapy (e.g., gastrointestinal bleeding, stroke, post-operative).

VASCULAR ANOMALIES. Angiography should be performed in patients who are suspected of having pulmonary vascular slings, abnormalities in pulmonary venous drainage, arteriovenous malformations, pulmonary venous varices, and so forth. These diagnoses are usually suggested on the basis of chest radiographic abnormalities. The value of angiography in pulmonary arteriovenous malformation, in addition to establishing the diagnosis, is to visualize smaller lesions which may not be seen on routine chest films or laminography.

Bronchogenic carcinoma. In the past, pulmonary angiography was used in preoperative evaluation to determine the extent of involvement of mediastinal structures by carcinoma. With the development of mediastinoscopy, this technique is seldom necessary. A rare indication for pulmonary angiography may be to determine whether the proximal left pulmonary artery is invaded by a carcinoma near the left hilum.[10]

CONTRAINDICATIONS

Recent myocardial infarction. This problem most frequently is encountered in patients being considered for angiography in the diagnosis of pulmonary embolism. The presence of ischemic or necrotic myocardium is potentially a lethal problem. The passage of a catheter through the heart may initiate an irreversible arrhythmia, and the consequences of contrast injection on ventricular function may seriously compromise the patient's cardiac status. It is imperative that this diagnosis be excluded by serial enzyme analyses or electrocardiograms. If necessary, the start of the examination should be delayed until this diagnosis is excluded.

History of contrast material reaction. This contraindication needs no explanation. If the study is mandatory, it is recommended that the procedure be done with steroid and antihistamine premedication.

TECHNIQUE

This procedure should be undertaken only in a radiographic room equipped with physiologic and electrocardiographic monitoring equipment, a DC defibrillator, image intensified fluoroscopy, rapid serial film changer, and high capacity modern x-ray equipment.

A complete pulmonary angiographic examination should include a brief hemodynamic assessment of right heart function. The catheter will necessarily traverse the right atrium and right ventricle in order to inject contrast medium into the main pulmonary artery, and the simple expedient of measuring intracardiac pressures may reveal valuable information.

The individual performing the pulmonary angiogram should be completely conversant with all the potential complications of right heart catheterization and their treatment. The overall risk (morbidity and mortality) from pulmonary angiography should be negligible, as shown in a recent cooperative study.[25] Right heart catheterization and pulmonary angiography were performed 310 times in the Urokinase-Pulmonary Embolism Trial in a number of institutions without mortality. There were five episodes of ventricular arrhythmias requiring treatment and one case of cardiac perforation.

Preparation. The angiographer should be thoroughly familiar with the patient's clinical status and should visit the patient, explain the procedure, and obtain informed consent. Whenever possible, the patient should have been fasting for at least four hours prior to the examination (although this may not be possible because of the urgent nature of the examination). Some form of preoperative medication should be given intramuscularly as the patient leaves the floor on the way to the radiology department. Our preference is Demerol, 2/3 to 1 mg. per kg. (50 to 75 mg.) and Vistaril, 1 mg. per kg. (75 mg.). If the angiogram must be done within two hours after the patient has eaten, substitute 10 mg. of Compazine for the Vistaril.

Catheterization site. Our preferred site for introduction of the catheter is the antecubital fossa. In thin patients with well visualized veins, the procedure can be done percutaneously using a sheath system. However, many patients are obese or have had numerous venipunctures and therefore require an incision to reach either a medial or medially directed antecubital vein or the basilic vein. Alternatives such as the percutaneous jugular approach and the percutaneous femoral route have their proponents.[14, 23] The authors prefer the arm rather than the leg, since it is easier to advance the catheter through the right heart chambers and into the pulmonary artery, and to position the catheter for any necessary selective injection. Another objection to the use of the femoral route is the possible dislodgement of a clot in the femoral vein or inferior vena cava. However, inferior venacavography with the catheter well down in the femoral vein certainly can minimize the risk.

CATHETERS. Closed end, side-hole catheters are preferred for pulmonary angiography to minimize recoil into the right ventricle during injection. This greatly reduces the incidence of arrhythmias attendant with contrast angiography. The woven Dacron standard angiographic catheters (NIH or Eppendorf type) are the most commonly used. However, the recent enthusiasm for disposable catheters has resulted in a number of other plastic materials used in catheter construction. These newer catheters are preferable if they conform to the physical characteristics of woven Dacron (i.e., rigidity, malleability, shape retention).

A "pigtail" catheter is quite suitable for main pulmonary artery injection.[23] The catheter may be introduced percutaneously, although use of a sheath in the arm or the femoral position makes it possible to introduce closed end catheters percutaneously. The curved end of the catheter contacting the right ventricular wall is less likely to cause rhythm disturbances than is the tip of the angiographic catheter. Similarly, the blunt curve leading edge of the catheter is much less likely to perforate the cardiac chamber than is the tip of even a soft Eppendorf catheter.

The introduction several years ago of a balloon-tipped flow guided catheter system promises to be quite helpful to the pulmonary angiographer. The balloon-tipped catheter greatly facilitates entry into the pulmonary artery and passes through the right ventricle without extrasystoles. The original angiographic catheters suffered from too few side-holes and a too small lumen (a No. 7 or 8 French catheter is necessary for flow rate adequate to visualize vessels well). However, newer versions of the flow-guided system have a more suitable lumen and side-holes, allowing for better injection. The balloon catheter is easy to advance into segmental vessels for selective injections and therefore may become the method of choice for catheterization of the pulmonary artery.

CATHETERIZATION. The catheter is advanced into the right atrium and then attached to a manometer for recording pressures in the right atrium, especially the mean pressure. The catheter is then introduced into the right ventricle under pressure and electrocardiographic monitoring, and ventricular systolic and diastolic pressures are recorded. After the catheter is advanced into the pulmonary artery, systolic, diastolic, and mean pressures should be obtained. Simultaneously with the measurement of the pulmonary artery pressure, systemic blood pressure should be determined. The pulmonary artery pressure should always be related to systemic pressure, because pressure which is normal under ordinary hemodynamic circumstances can be grossly abnormal in a patient with shock. If pulmonary artery diastolic pressure is elevated, the pulmonary wedge pressure should be determined by means of an end-hole catheter. This information concerning the left-sided cardiac pressure is required to explain the elevated pulmonary arterial pressure. This pressure is best determined before angiography. However, if the positioning of the catheter has been unduly difficult, the wedge pressure can be obtained after angiography and the return of right-sided pressures to the preangiographic levels. This expedient eliminates replacing the angiographic catheter with an end-hole catheter, recording pressures, and reintroducing the angiographic catheter.

SITE OF INJECTION. The main pulmonary artery is preferred for the first injection. Optimal catheter position is checked by use of a small test injection of contrast medium. This should result in flow through both pulmonary arteries without recoil of the catheter to the right ventricle.

A contraindication to injection in the main pulmonary artery is severe pulmonary hypertension. The more closely the pulmonary artery systolic pressure approximates the systemic arterial systolic pressure, the more poorly tolerated is pulmonary angiography. Injection of contrast medium into the pulmonary artery normally results in transient pulmonary hypertension. If pulmonary artery systolic pressure is greater than 60 mm. of Hg, the risk of arrhythmia and even fatality with pulmonary angiography is greatly increased.[22] Main pulmonary artery injection is best avoided with these patients. Two possible alternative methods can be employed. The safest course of action in this case is to withdraw the catheter to the right atrium for injection. This site of injection will avoid the acute increase in the right ventricular afterload but has the disadvantage of poor visualization of the pulmonary vessels. The preferred option is to advance the catheter into the hilar pulmonary artery on either side and do selective injections, one lung at a time. Care in placing the catheter distally in the left or right pulmonary artery is extremely important (Fig. 4–1).

INJECTION. Somewhat less than 1 ml. per kilogram body weight (50 to 60 ml.) is the recommended volume. The contrast materials to be used are the mixtures of sodium and meglumine diatrozoates, metrizoates, or iothalamates, containing about 40 mg. per ml. iodine (Renografin-76, Hypaque-M 75%, Vascoray and Isopaque 440 are examples). The injection should be done by power injector in 1½ to 2 seconds. As mentioned previously, this can be accomplished only with the use of No. 7 or 8 French catheters with multiple side holes.

RADIOGRAPHY

FACTORS. Use 70 to 90 kV, the highest current, and the shortest exposure time possible (10 milliseconds should be the goal). A scout film should be taken to check quality and position. The kilovoltage should be high enough so that the spine shadow is of moderate greyness; this insures proper visualization of the main pulmonary artery.

FILMING. The anteroposterior supine projection is used for the first survey arteriogram with injection into the main pulmonary artery. This allows both an assessment of symmetrical flow through the lungs and a general look at the distribution and size of the pulmonary vessels. The sequence should be at least 2 films per second for 4 seconds, followed by 1 film per second for 6 to 8 seconds, depending on the circulation time through the lung. (Patients with low cardiac output or suspected long circulation time should have the 1 film per second prolonged up to 10 seconds.) Two films per second for the first 4 seconds is a minimal rate, and 3 per second for the first 2 to 3 seconds is optimal if the film changer will allow this sequence. The study should not be considered complete unless the left heart chambers and aorta are visualized, since occasionally pericardial effusion and dissecting aortic aneurysm may present with symptoms similar to those of pulmonary embolism.

SELECTIVE INJECTIONS. Selective injection may be performed after the survey main pulmonary artery injection to improve visualization of a branch pulmonary vessel.[3, 4, 11, 19, 20] The site of injection and study is determined by the location of the suspected pathologic condition. Selection of the appropriate site is made on the basis of the area of abnormality detected on either the initial angiogram, the plain chest radiograph, or the radioisotopic scan. In this case the catheter is placed far enough into the origin of the vessel selected to preclude any recoil, and the reduction in the amount of contrast material is proportional. Injections into the right or left pulmonary artery should have about 60 per cent (30 to 40 ml.) of the volume of the main pulmonary artery injection and should be injected in 1 to 1½ seconds. Injections into the lobar vessels should be about 20 to 30 ml., and injections into the segmental vessels should be about 10 to 15 ml. The injection time should be about 1 second. The filming sequence need not visualize the left heart chambers in the selective injections if they were demonstrated previously on the main pulmonary artery injection. Generally, 2 to 3 frames per second for 4 seconds suffices.

PROJECTIONS. Selective injections are most advantageous when combined with a change in the projection of the patient.[12] The proximal right pulmonary artery and most of the right lung are best demonstrated by slight elevation of the patient's right side (10° to 15° LPO). The best differentiation between lesions in the right middle and lower lobes is performed by steep right posterior oblique or right lateral projection. The proximal left pulmonary artery and proximal left lung are best demonstrated by moderate elevation of the patient's left side (30° to 45° RPO). The best differentiation into the various lobes and segments of the left lung also is done by steep left posterior oblique or left lateral projections.

SPECIAL TECHNIQUES

1. *Magnification.* Selective injection combined with direct radiographic magnification can increase the visualization of the pulmonary vessels by several orders of magnitude.[11] Ultrafine focal spot tubes and

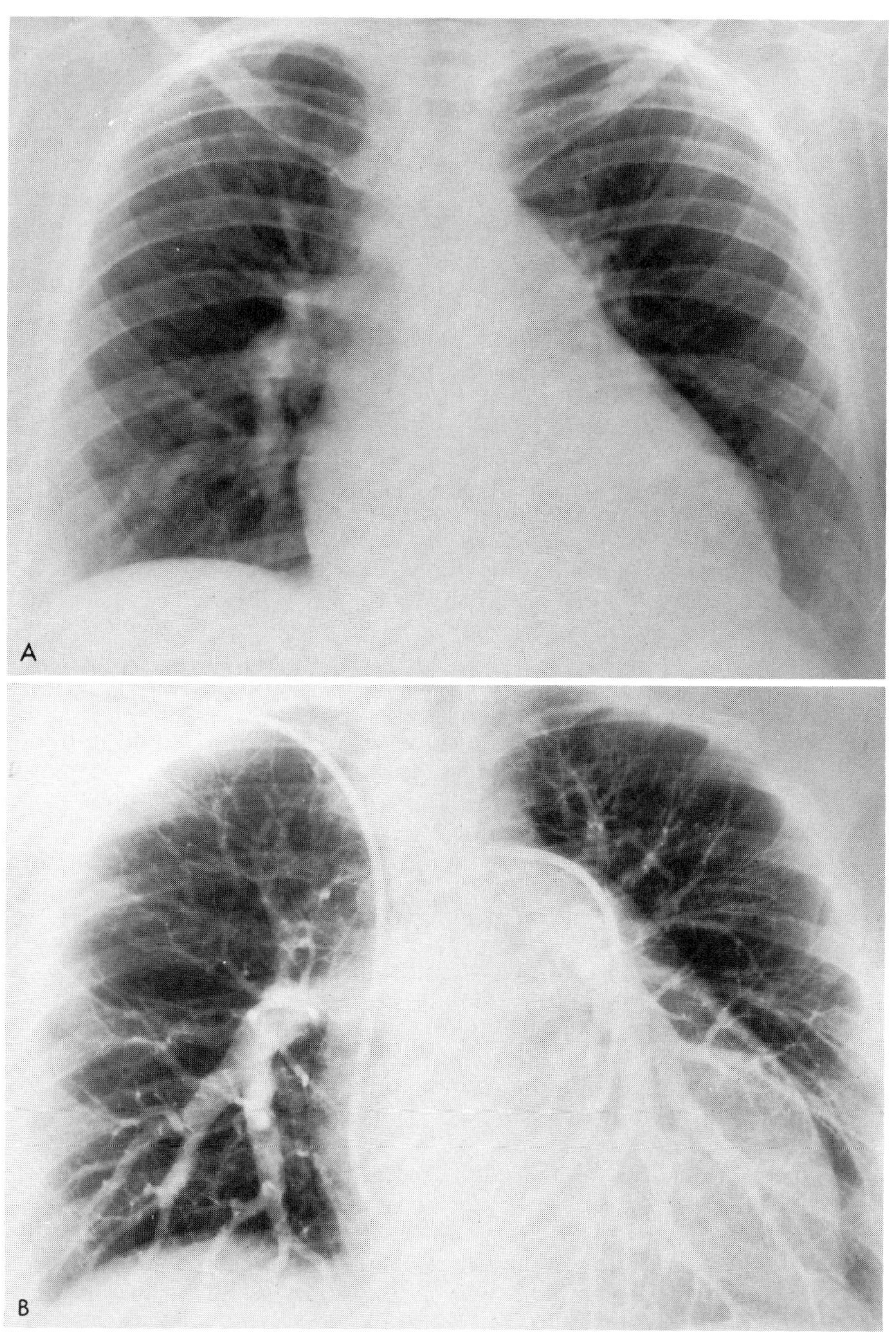

Figure 4–1. A 25 year old woman with systemic lupus erythematosus and increasing shortness of breath. *A.* Posteroanterior chest radiograph demonstrates cardiomegaly and enlarged central pulmonary arteries, consistent with pulmonary arterial hypertension. Pulmonary angiography was performed to exclude pulmonary emboli. Pressure in the main pulmonary artery was 120/60 (mean 84) mm. Hg. Because of markedly elevated pressures, catheter was placed in left pulmonary artery and 25 cc. of contrast media injected. *B.* Angiogram demonstrates that pressure injection has caused catheter to recoil proximally, opacifying the pulmonary arteries to both lungs. The patient experienced a cardiac arrest immediately after injection and could not be resuscitated. This case illustrates the danger of pulmonary angiography in patients with severe pulmonary arterial hypertension. Placement of the catheter more distal in the left pulmonary artery probably would have prevented recoil and its subsequent complication.

high resolution filming systems such as vacuum cassettes enable the demonstration of lesions in the smaller pulmonary vessels, below the segmental level. Ordinary pulmonary angiography allows fairly accurate demonstration of disease in the lobar and segmental vessels. Visualization of the subsegmental vessels is difficult, but the use of magnification angiography extends the limits.

2. *Cinearteriography.* Cinearteriography has been used in analysis of pulmonary circulatory dynamics;[17] with the improving resolution of image intensifiers, cine systems may ultimately replace large film angiography.

Image intensified rapid serial spot film angiography (70, 90, 100 mm., and larger) has a potential similar to cineangiography. The resolving power of present systems is rapidly approaching that of large film changers. In the near future angiography may be performed more conveniently using these techniques and at a much lower radiation dose rate.

COMPLICATIONS

Arrhythmia is the most serious complication encountered. This commonly occurs during passage of the catheter through the right ventricle, with one or more extrasystoles resulting from contact of the catheter with the right ventricular wall. This can be minimized by careful catheter technique or the use of balloon-tipped catheters. It is not uncommon to have up to 4 or 5 extrasystoles during passage of the catheter through the right ventricle; however, the number of these premature beats should be kept to a minimum. Ventricular tachycardia may occur if the extrasystoles are not terminated by removal of the catheter from the chamber immediately. Ventricular fibrillation may occur if the ventricular tachycardia is allowed to persist. Fibrillation should be treated by immediate institution of cardiopulmonary resuscitation including oxygen therapy, closed chest massage, and electric defibrillation.

Severe bradycardia or arrest may occur during the catheterization. This is most frequently encountered as the catheter enters the right atrium and is thought to be caused by vasovagal reaction. The bradycardia, if severe, should be treated by injection of atropine; asystole requires more vigorous resuscitation measures.

Cardiac perforation may occur in the right ventricular outflow tract or as the result of mistakenly advancing the catheter through the coronary sinus. The use of a balloon-tipped catheter minimizes this risk, as do careful catheter manipulation and soft catheters. It is imperative that this complication be recognized immediately; if tamponade or circulatory embarrassment occurs, pericardiocentesis is necessary.

Other complications, such as dislodgement of an existing clot, can occur. This can be minimized by the use of test injections prior to angiographic runs. In addition, knotting or breakage of the catheter can occur and is minimized by careful catheterization technique. Air embolism, another possible complication, can be avoided by careful attention to the details of hook-up of pressure lines and connector tubing. Thrombosis in the catheter can occur if there is infrequent flushing with heparinized solutions. In the event of thrombosis, the catheter must be replaced; absolutely no attempt must be made to flush the catheter while it is present in the body.

DATA ANALYSIS

The angiographer must carefully analyze the data as it is obtained, and make decisions as to the next step in the study. For example, the type and site of arteriography depend upon the right ventricular and pulmonary artery pressures; similarly, the need for a site of selective injection is determined from analysis of the main pulmonary artery injection.

HEMODYNAMICS. There are three important components to the right atrial pressure: A-wave height, V-wave height, and mean pressure. The normal value for the A-wave, which follows atrial contraction and the electrocardiographic P-wave, is 7 mm. Hg (range 2 to 14). Normal pressure for the V-wave, which occurs during ventricular contraction, is 4.5 mm. Hg (range 2.5 to 8). The normal value of the mean right atrial pressure (the most important component) is 4.5 mm. Hg (range minus 2 to 10).

Right ventricular pressure is measured at peak systole and at end diastole. The nor-

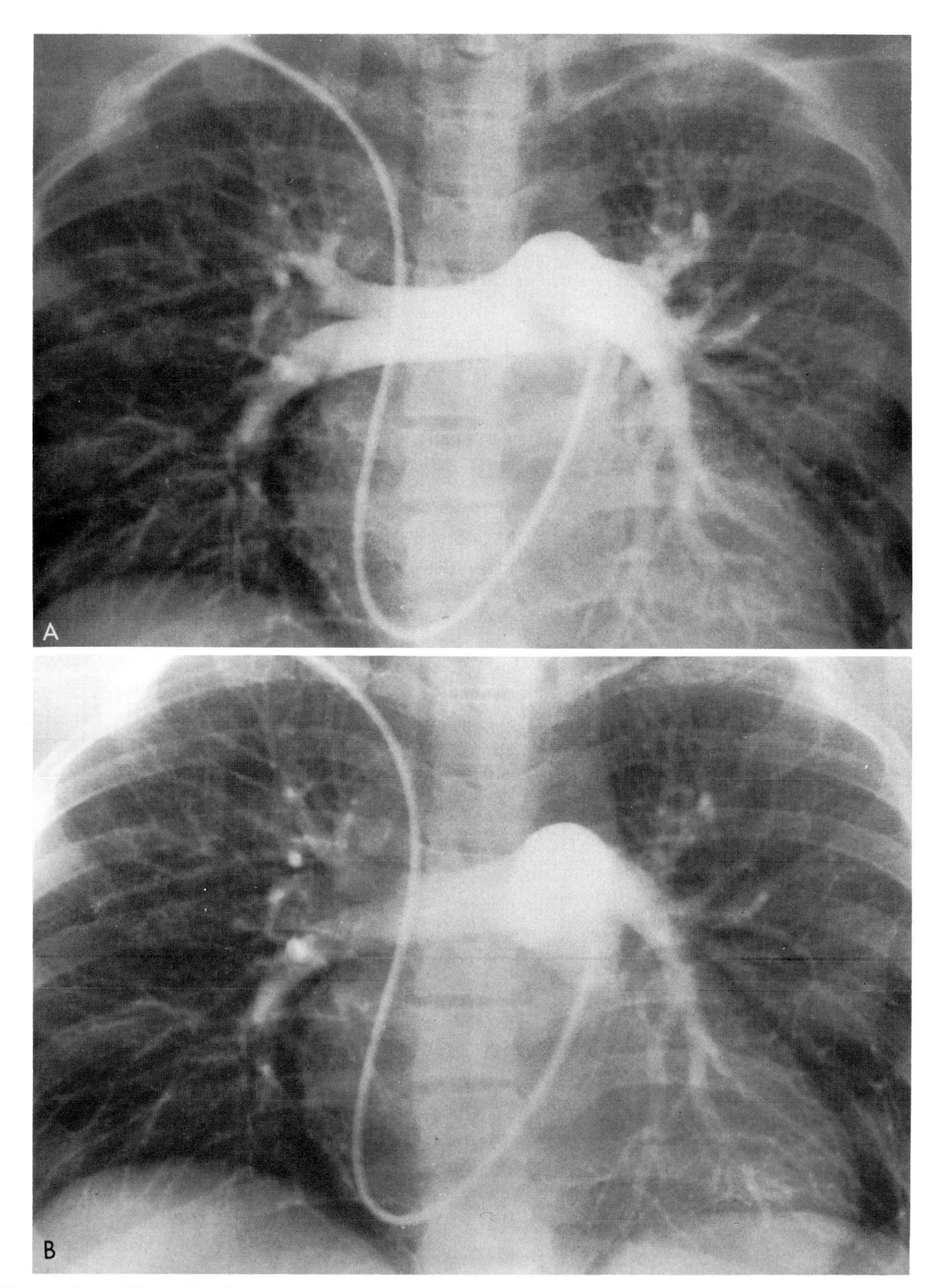

Figure 4–2. Normal pulmonary angiogram. *A.* Arterial phase, systole. Non-opacified right ventricular blood is opening the pulmonic valves and causing a normal filling defect in the supravalvular portion of the main pulmonary artery. *B.* Arterial phase, diastole. The sinuses of Valsalva are distended, and no filling defect is seen at this time. The pulmonary vessels in all the lung zones are opacified symmetrically. *C.* Levogram phase (see text).

Illustration continued on the opposite page

mal systolic pressure is 25 mm. Hg (range 15 to 35). The normal end diastolic pressure, measured 0.04 second after the onset of the QRS complex on the electrocardiogram, is 4.5 mm. Hg (range minus 5 to 14).

Pulmonary artery pressure measured at peak systole is 21 mm. Hg (range 11 to 30). The lowest pulmonary artery diastolic pressure can range from 2 to 16 mm. Hg, the average being 10. The mean pulmonary arterial pressure is 14 mm. Hg (range 8 to 22).

If pulmonary arterial pressure, especially the diastolic, is elevated, it is wise to obtain a pulmonary arterial wedge pressure. This corresponds to left atrial pressure. The normal value of the mean pulmonary wedge pressure is 9 mm. Hg (range 4 to 15). Pressures in the main pulmonary artery may be elevated because of increased postcapillary pressure, as in mitral disease or left ventricular failure. Increase in the capillary or precapillary resistance due to parenchymal disease with distortion and obliteration of vessels, or due to arterial obstructive disease (such as that caused by embolism or vasculitis), may also cause elevations in the main pulmonary artery pressure.

As mentioned in the technical section, a severely elevated pulmonary arterial pressure, specifically peak pressure measuring 60 mm. Hg or greater, should alert the angiographer to proceed cautiously. In these cases, the right ventricle may be severely compromised and the injection may cause acute right ventricular strain and failure. Selective distal main pulmonary artery injections of approximately 30 ml. of contrast material seem to be safe.

ANALYSIS OF THE ANGIOGRAM. The best method for insuring careful scrutiny of the angiogram is an anatomic and physiologic flow progression.

1. *Arterial Phase.* The injection should opacify the main pulmonary artery back to the pulmonic valves. During systole one should see a wash-in of non-opacified right ventricular blood and a non-opaque filling defect entering the main pulmonary artery through the open pulmonic valves (Fig. 4–2A). In diastole, the valves should coapt, distending the sinuses of Valsalva (Fig. 4–2B). Any filling defects which are present

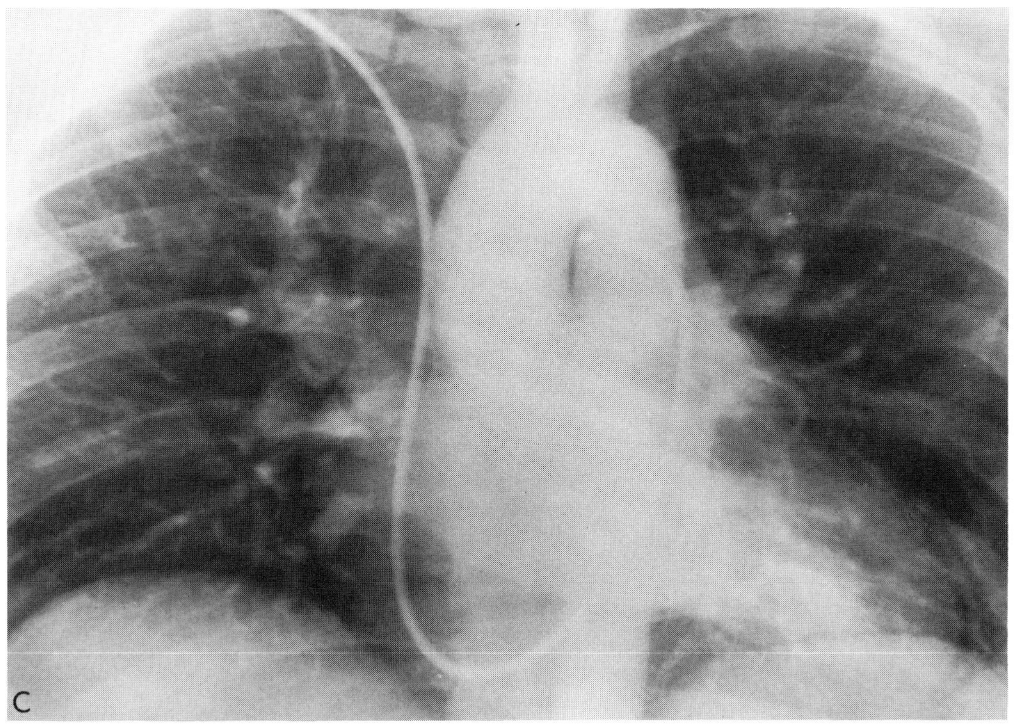

Figure 4–2 Continued.

in the main pulmonary artery in diastole should be considered pathologic. If the early films are made at 3 frames per second, there are two or three diastoles to see if the filling defects are indeed real. The presence of a catheter through the pulmonic valve may result in a small amount of pulmonary insufficiency. Occasionally, the catheter will recoil into the right ventricle and opacify the outflow tract of the right ventricle, and this should not be confused with true pulmonary insufficiency. The proximal right and left main pulmonary arteries are then examined. Flow should be symmetrical and, therefore, equal portions of the right and left pulmonary artery are opacified on each succeeding angiographic film. Asymmetries of flow may occur because of catheter position; however, any asymmetry of flow should be noted, and structural abnormalities that may be responsible for this should be excluded on subsequent films.

The right pulmonary artery branches at about the level of the hilum, giving rise to a large branch to the upper lobe (Fig.4–2A). The trunk subsequently gives off branches to each of the three segments of the right upper lobe. Occasionally, two vessels originate directly from the right pulmonary artery to supply the upper lobe.

The continuation of the main right pulmonary artery, now called the intermediate pulmonary artery (to correspond with the bronchial terminology), gives rise to a vessel which bifurcates to supply the segments of the middle lobe. The continuation of the right pulmonary artery, now called the lower lobe artery, gives rise to a small vessel which feeds the superior segment. It then divides and each division subdivides, resulting in approximately four segmental vessels to the lower lobe.

The course of the left pulmonary artery is more difficult to follow. The main left pulmonary artery is more perpendicular to the plane of the film, causing a great deal of foreshortening. The first branch from the left pulmonary artery is the artery to the left upper lobe. This vessel usually gives rise to two or three segmental branches. As on the right side, there may be two vessels arising directly from the left pulmonary artery to feed the left upper lobe.

The intermediate left pulmonary artery then gives rise to a single vessel, which bifurcates immediately to supply the lingular segments of the left upper lobe. These are quite similar to the arteries to the right middle lobe.

The anatomy of the left lower lobe pulmonary artery and its branches is roughly similar to the right lower lobe architecture. Although the bronchial anatomy is not symmetrical, the pulmonary artery anatomy is frequently symmetrical.

In evaluating the segmental vascular anatomy, one should ascertain that there are enough segmental vessels.[3] In addition, the method of branching should be carefully analyzed. The bifurcations of the vessels are quite smooth and have sharp angles. The total cross-sectional area of the branches should be slightly greater than the total cross-sectional area of the vessels which have given rise to these branches. Bookstein has arrived at this formula: the sum of the squares of the diameters of the branches should be equal to about 1.2 times the square of the diameter of the vessel proximal to the bifurcation.[2] The course of the vessels is quite straight and radiates out from the hilum to the appropriate segment.

2. *Parenchymal Phase.* The pulmonary arterial phase lasts up to about 2 seconds. This is followed by a phase in which the major vessels are not well seen. Instead, there is a diffuse increase in density of the lung fields and prominence of the reticular pattern of the lung. At this time, the contrast material resides in the smaller pulmonary vessels, although some of it has presumably diffused into the interstitial tissues as it does in other organ systems. Remnants of distal arteries, as well as fragments of proximal pulmonary veins, may be filled at this time. The structures seen in this phase of the pulmonary arteriogram are analogous to the anatomic structures usually visualized on perfusion lung scans.

The density of this phase is proportional to the amount of contrast material held in the parenchyma of the lung. This is dependent upon two major factors. It is directly proportional to the amount of contrast material perfusing an area of lung; thus, an area of lung that for any reason receives less arterial supply will have less density than its neighbors. Similarly, an area of lung that receives more blood supply will be denser than the surrounding lung. The density of this phase is also inversely proportional to the transit time of the contrast material. Therefore, any process such as vascular pooling or postcapillary obstruction will result in an increase in the density of this phase.

Filling defects in the parenchymal phase may be caused by any type of pulmonary pathology which results in a local increase in vascular resistance. The most common cause of a decrease in perfusion is vascular obstruction, as in embolism. However, localized areas of pneumonia, interstitial disease, or airway obstruction can increase the intravascular resistance and result in lack of parenchymal filling. Any lesion compressing vessels, such as large bullae, or a process destroying the parenchyma will result in a defect in this phase.[4, 20]

Increases in local density during this phase can be caused by arteriovenous malformations or localized atelectasis. A diffuse, generalized increase in density during this phase can be seen in postcapillary obstruction or in any process which slows the circulation time through the lungs.

3. *Pulmonary Venous and Levogram Phase.* The parenchymal phase is usually seen for one or two films in the middle of the study. As the parenchymal opacification slackens, the pulmonary veins opacify (Fig. 4–2C). There is usually simultaneous opacification of four groups of pulmonary veins. A pair of veins from the right upper lobe drain into the left atrium in the northwest quadrant of the atrium. A group of veins drains the right lower lobe. These usually join in a single trunk and enter the left atrium in its southwest quadrant. A pair of veins drain the left upper lobe and drain as a trunk into the mid portion of the left side of the atrium. The left lower lobe veins may drain as a separate trunk into the left atrium in the southeast quadrant, or may join the trunk draining the right upper lobe. Symmetry of circulatory flow through the veins is the normal state. Any area which does not receive arterial supply and which may have a parenchymal filling defect will result in considerably less venous opacification from that region.

The left atrium usually fills from 3 to 4

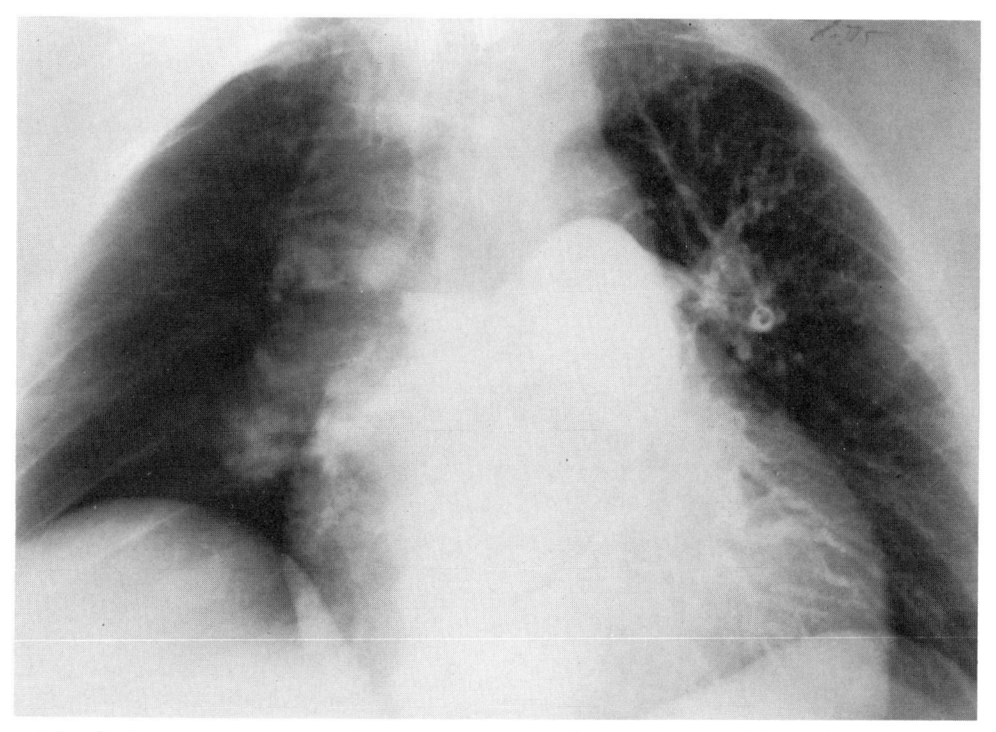

Figure 4–3. Pulmonary angiogram demonstrating complete occlusion of the right pulmonary artery. The "trailing edge" of the embolus is well seen in the occluded vessel. Multiple emboli are also present throughout the left lung.

seconds after the beginning of injection. Congestive failure or shock will prolong the circulation time and result in much later filling.

Some assessment should be made of the size of the left atrium, left ventricle, and aorta.

ANGIOGRAPHIC ABNORMALITIES

I. Alterations In Arterial Phase

NONFILLING OF A VESSEL

Pulmonary Embolism. An embolus may cause complete occlusion of a pulmonary artery, and massive pulmonary embolism may occlude the main right or left pulmonary artery (Fig. 4–3). Advancing the catheter just proximal to the unfilled vessel and performing another injection is valuable for confirmation of occlusion plus added detail[3, 4, 12] (Fig. 4–4). The appearance of a totally occluding pulmonary embolus is fairly characteristic, in that one sees the amputated stump of a vessel, often containing the trailing edge of the embolus[20] (Figs. 4–3 and 4–5), rather than a smooth, flush occlusion. Complete occlusion of a vessel leaving no stump may cause a false negative angiogram. One might overlook the absence of a segmental vessel, since the number and distribution of these vessels varies. However, a segmental vascular occlusion results in a filling defect in the parenchymal phase and should lead the angiographer to a careful study of the regional pulmonary vessels coursing to the unfilled parenchyma.

Other Causes: Malignant mediastinal or

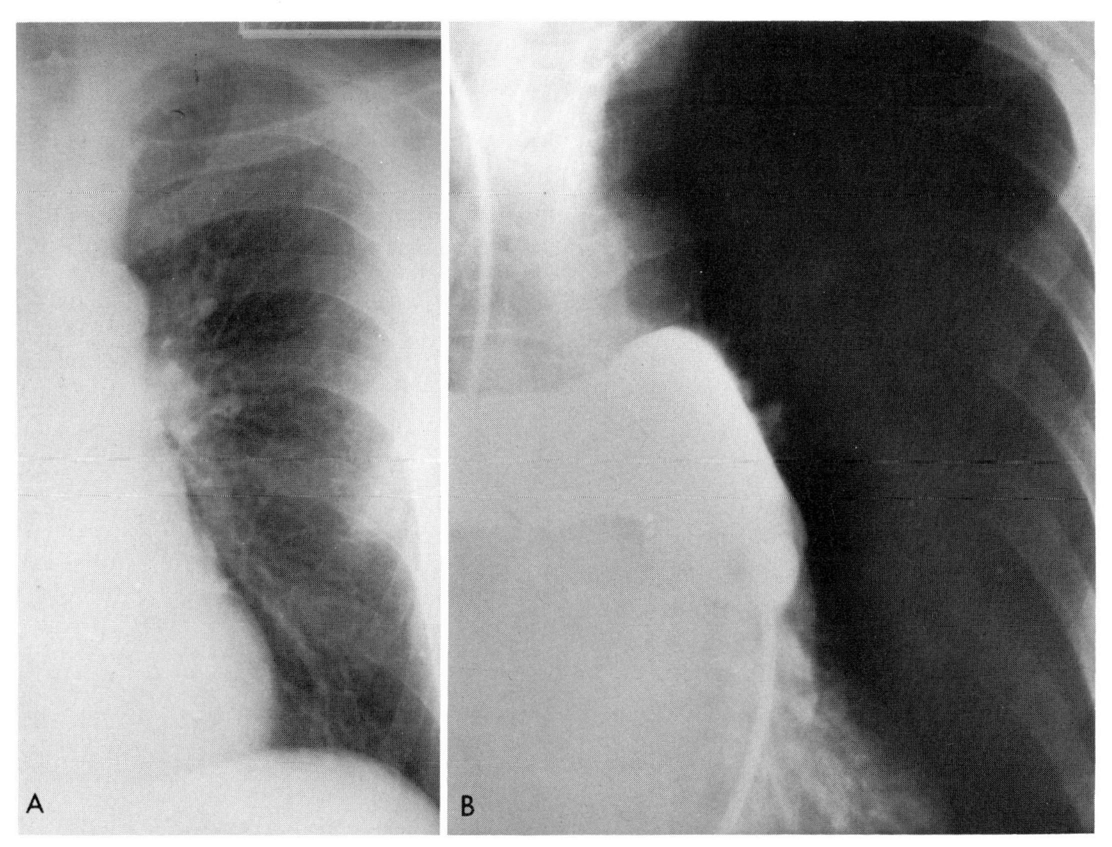

Figure 4–4. A 67 year old man with sudden onset of dyspnea, left chest pain, and hypotension. *A.* Detail of left chest, posteroanterior roentgenogram, demonstrates no abnormality. *B.* Pulmonary angiogram following main pulmonary artery injection demonstrates complete absence of filling of the left pulmonary artery. *C.* Selective left pulmonary arteriogram in the right posterior oblique projection demonstrates emboli occluding the segmental arteries of the left lung.

Illustration continued on the opposite page

hilar neoplasm or fibrosing mediastinitis may cause obstruction of a major pulmonary artery by extrinsic compression or invasion. Congenital absence of a pulmonary artery is a rare developmental defect in which complete non-filling of a pulmonary artery may occur[21] (Fig. 4–6). The diagnosis can be made by examination of the plain chest film, which shows a hypoplastic lung with a more reticular pattern, usually due to bronchial arterial collateral supply, and a tiny or absent hilum on the affected side. Localized areas of atelectasis, pneumonia, bullae, peripheral neoplasm, or fibrosis may result in segmental or subsegmental pulmonary arteries not filling from a main pulmonary arterial injection. Selective angiography will often demonstrate patent vessels in these entities (Figs. 4–7 and 4–8).

INTRALUMINAL FILLING DEFECTS

Pulmonary Embolism. This condition may present as one or more filling defects within the lumen of the pulmonary arteries, as well as cut-off of a vessel.[3, 11, 20] The filling defects have a variable appearance. The embolus may be fully intraluminal, showing a small string of contrast material on all sides between the filling defect and the vessel (Figs. 4–9 and 4–10). The filling defect may attach itself to one wall of the vessel, and thus no line of contrast material will be visible (Figs. 4–11 and 4–12).

Pulmonary embolism has the following characteristics which aid in the diagnosis.[25] The emboli tend to be multiple, so that more than one vessel is affected. The emboli are usually seen at sites of vessel bifurcation, and frequently an embolus will straddle the orifices of more than one ves-

Text continued on page 100

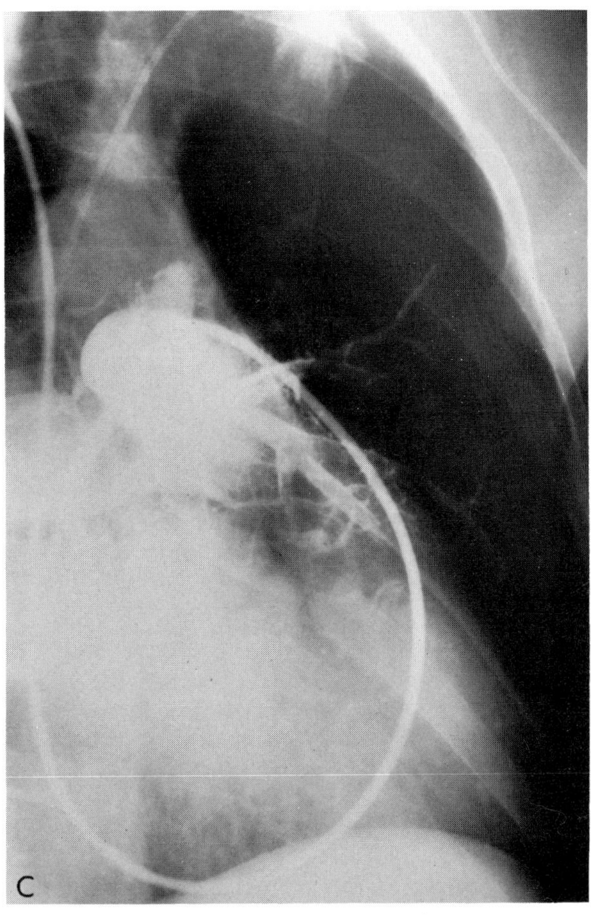

Figure 4–4 *Continued.*

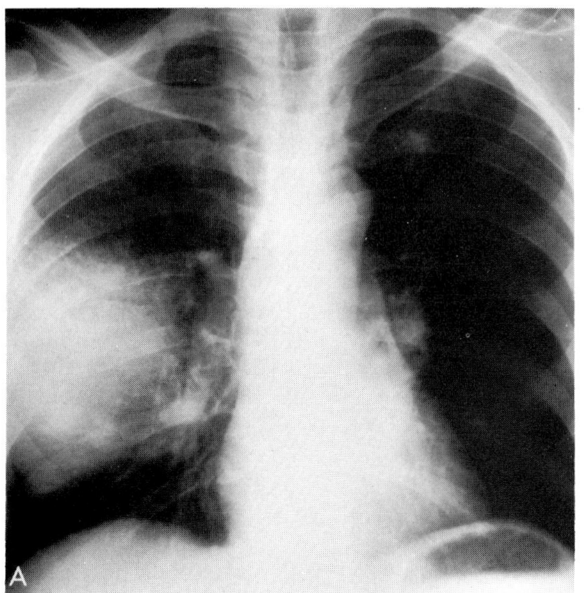

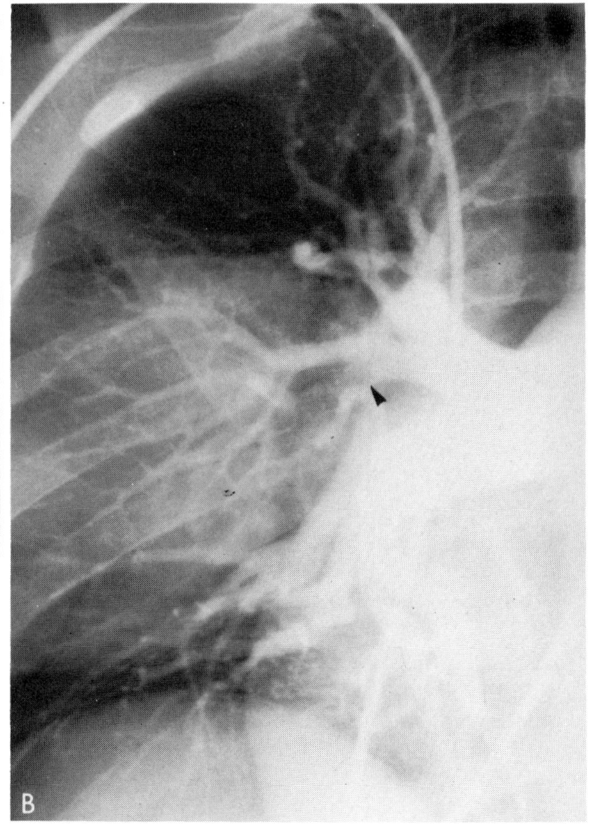

Figure 4–5. A 65 year old man, 7 days after colectomy, with right chest pain, dyspnea and fever. *A*. Posteroanterior chest roentgenogram demonstrates consolidation of right mid lung field. A radioisotopic perfusion scan showed a defect in this area only. *B*. Pulmonary angiogram, following selective right pulmonary artery injection in the right posterior oblique projection, demonstrates occlusion of the stump of the anterior segmental artery of the right upper lobe by an embolus, whose "trailing edge" is well seen (arrow).

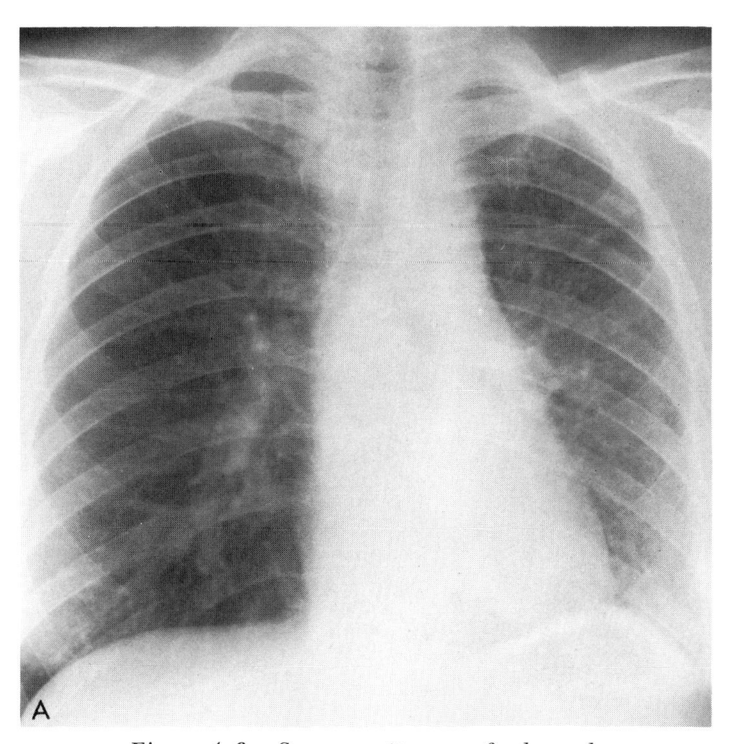

Figure 4–6. *See opposite page for legend.*

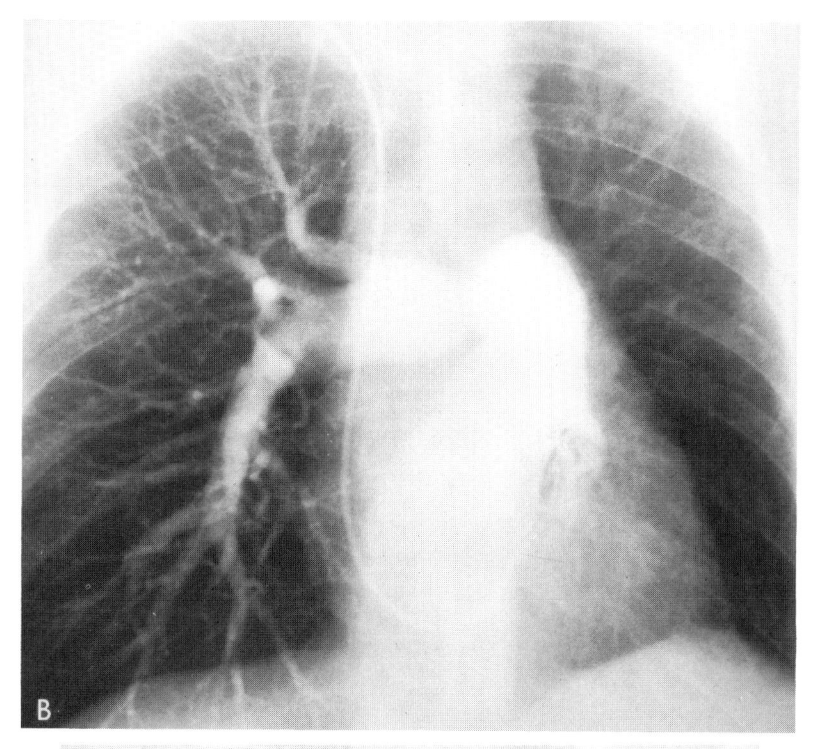

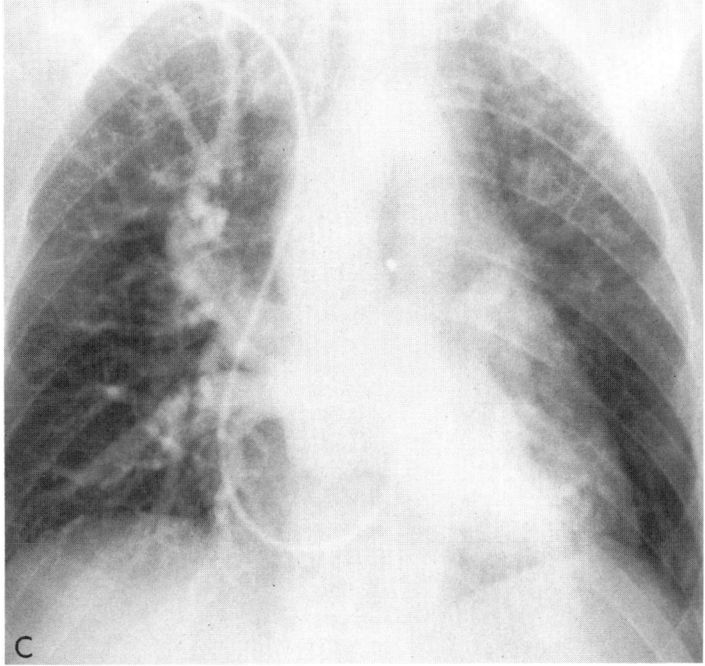

Figure 4–6. Congenital absence of the left pulmonary artery. *A*. Posteroanterior chest radiograph demonstrates a small left hemithorax, without a definite left hilar shadow, and a reticular pattern throughout the left lung. *B*. Pulmonary angiogram following injection into the main pulmonary artery shows absence of filling of the left pulmonary artery. (During injection, the catheter recoiled into the right ventricle). Constriction of the origin of the right pulmonary artery with slight post-stenotic dilatation is also present. *C*. Levogram phase of pulmonary angiogram shows neither parenchymal opacification nor venous drainage from the left lung.

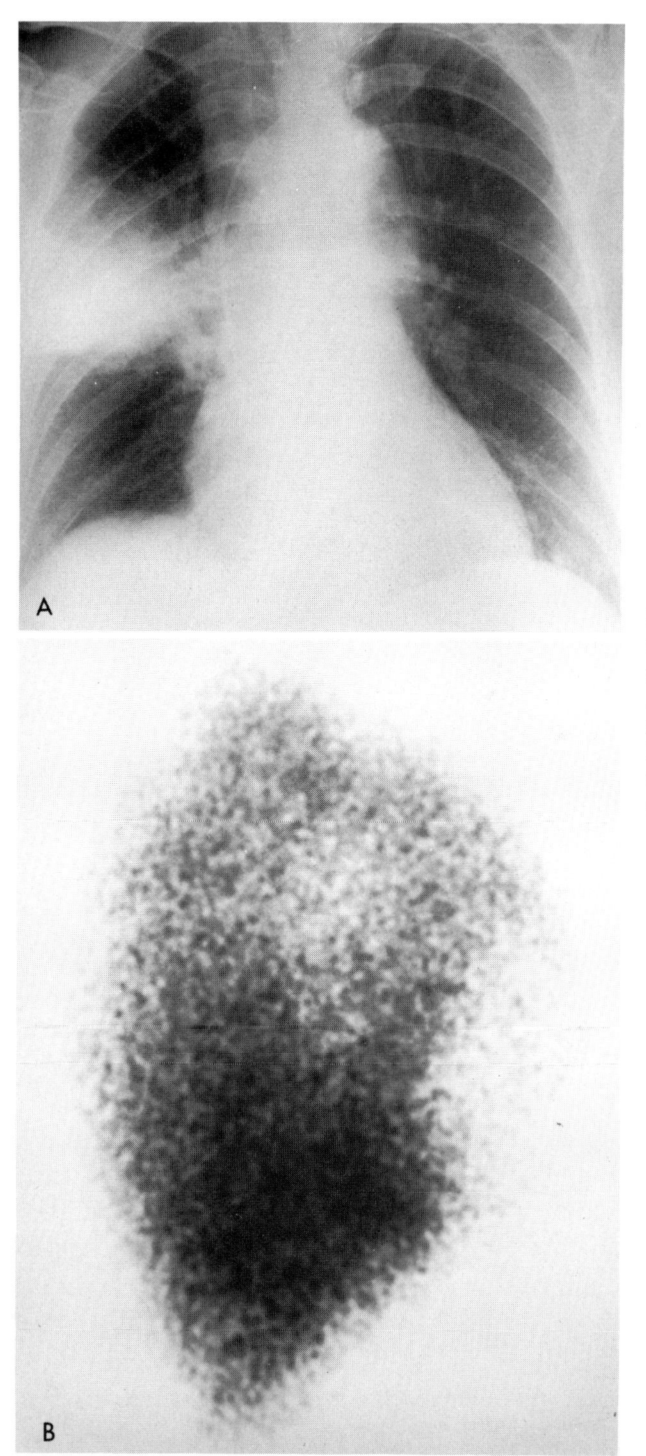

Figure 4-7. A 69 year old woman with cough, fever, chills, right chest pain, and dyspnea, 2 days after colon surgery. *A.* Anteroposterior chest roentgenogram demonstrates right upper lobe consolidation. *B.* Radioisotopic perfusion scan, right lateral view, shows right upper lobe perfusion defects.

Legend continued on the opposite page

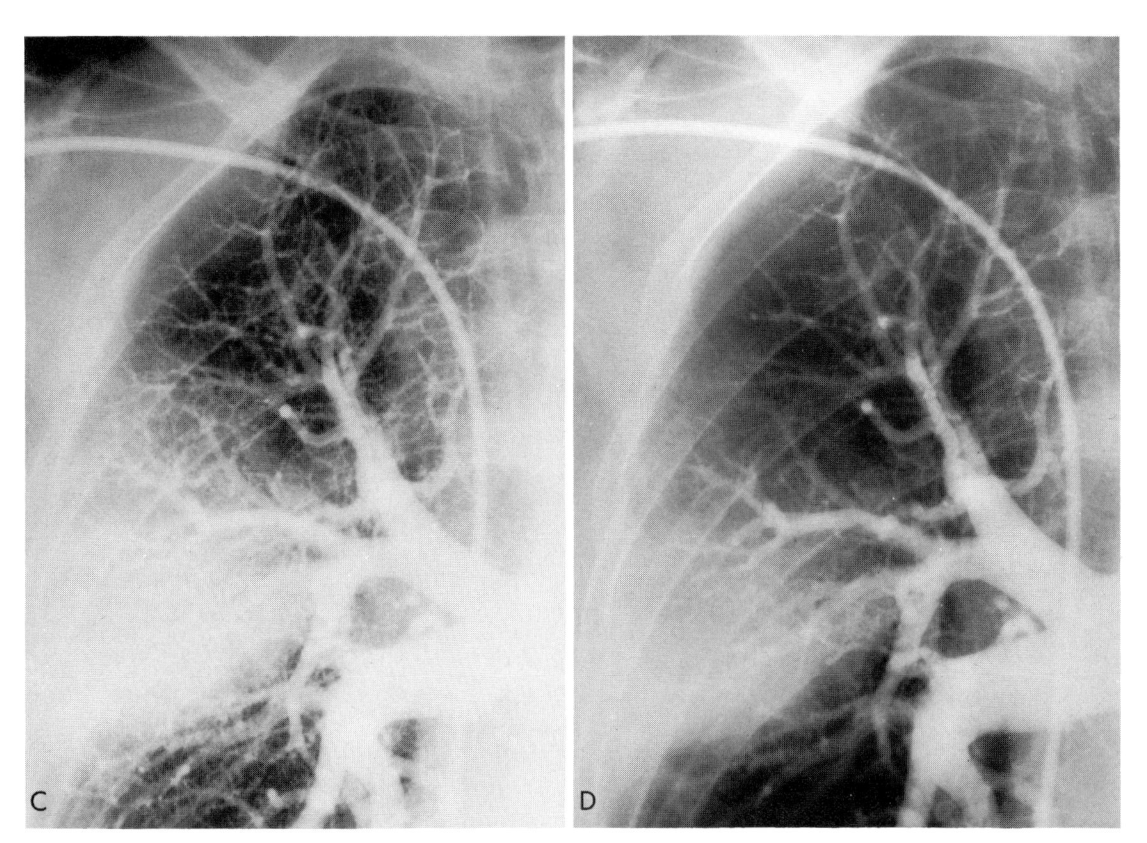

Figure 4–7 *Continued.* *C* and *D*. Early and late arterial phases from selective right pulmonary arteriogram demonstrate filling of all right upper lobe arteries, without evidence of emboli. (Compare to Fig. 4–5.) Sputum cultures one day later grew out pneumococci, and the patient made an uneventful recovery following penicillin therapy.

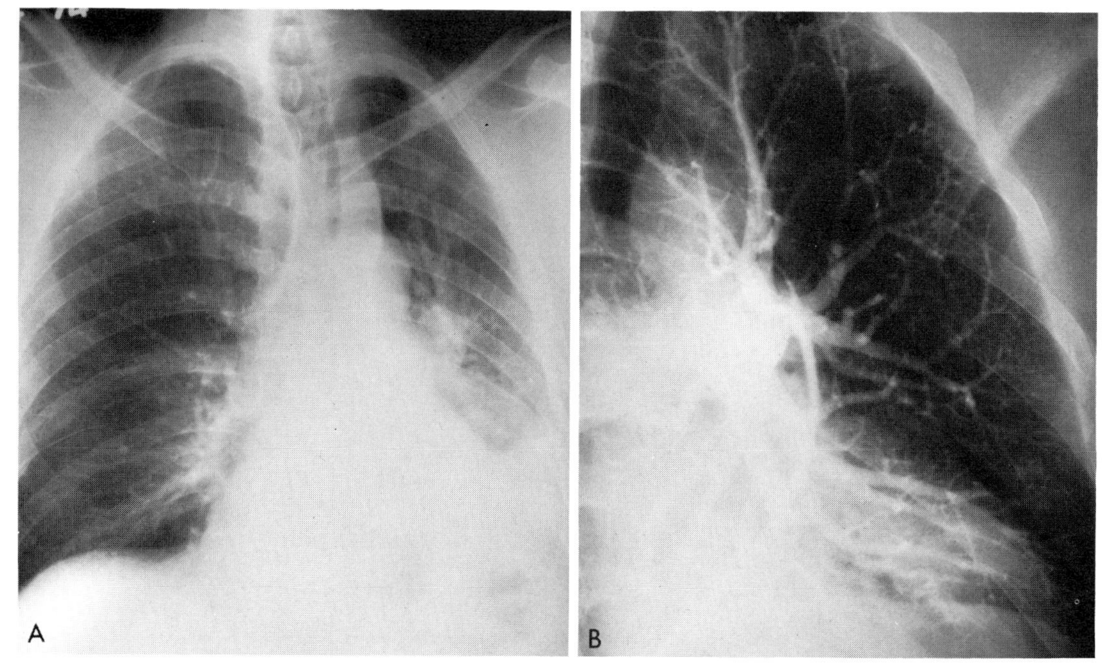

Figure 4–8. A 48 year old man with coronary artery disease and recent onset of cough, chest pain, and dyspnea. *A.* Posteroanterior chest radiograph demonstrates marked left lower lobe volume loss. Both radioisotopic perfusion lung scan and pulmonary angiogram following main pulmonary artery injection showed diminished perfusion of the left lower lobe. *B.* Selective left pulmonary arteriogram demonstrates crowding of vessels in the left lower lobe without evidence of emboli. Bronchoscopy was negative. Antibiotics given for presumed bronchitis resulted in alleviation of symptoms after several weeks, but the chest radiograph remained unchanged. The volume loss was felt to be due to chronic fibrosis.

sel. The most common site for occurrence of pulmonary embolism is in the right lower lobe, followed very closely by the left lower lobe (Table 4–1). The area of lung beyond the obstructed vessel will demonstrate decreased opacification in the parenchymal phase (Fig. 4–11) and decreased opacification of the pulmonary veins. Frequently, one can find atelectasis (Fig. 4–10) or delayed flow through the area involved.

A difficult task of the angiographer in the diagnosis of pulmonary embolism is the detection of a false-positive due to overlapping vessels. Occasionally, the summation of two vessels filled with contrast material will appear denser than do the nonoverlapped vessels, and this appearance will mimic an intraluminal filling defect. This can be recognized on close observation by tracing the overlapping vessels. Sometimes, one must resort to a selective injection with some rotation of a patient to eliminate the overlap.

The other false-positive for pulmonary embolism is nonfilling of a vessel due to other conditions.

It cannot be overemphasized that a definitive angiographic diagnosis of pulmo-

TABLE 4–1. Location of Pulmonary Emboli*

ANATOMY OR LOCATION	NUMBER OF VESSELS INVOLVED WITH EMBOLI
Main pulmonary artery	3
Proximal right pulmonary artery	45
Proximal left pulmonary artery	66
Right upper lobe arteries	186
Left upper lobe arteries	99
Right middle lobe arteries	108
Lingular arteries	108
Right lower lobe arteries	295
Left lower lobe arteries	255

*Compilation of 148 patients from Urokinase-Pulmonary Embolism Trial.

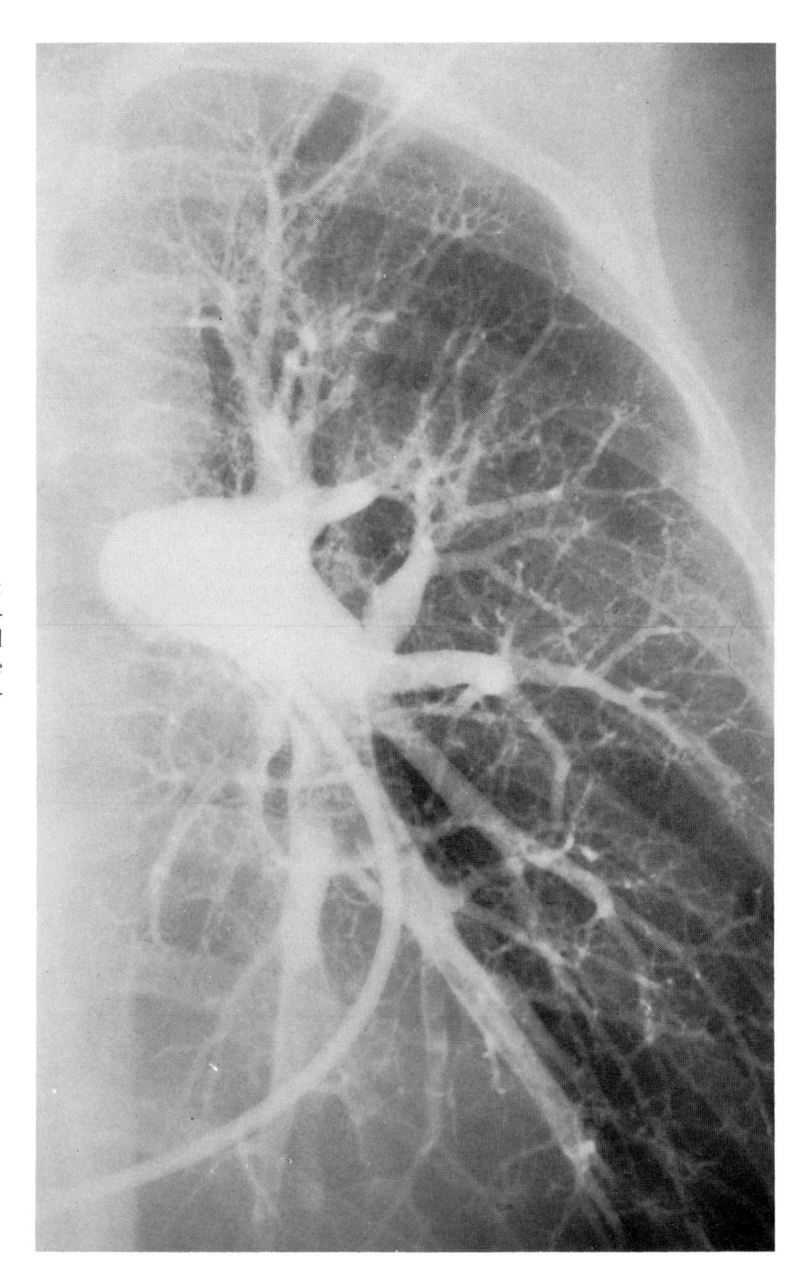

Figure 4–9. Selective left pulmonary arteriogram demonstrates a large intraluminal embolus in the lower lobe artery extending into the segmental branches.

nary embolism should be based solely on the demonstration of intraluminal filling defects or characteristic arterial occlusions.[4, 20] Pulmonary emboli involving larger branches can usually be recognized following the main pulmonary artery injection of contrast medium. However, emboli often involve only peripheral branches, and selective segmental injections, often with various degrees of obliquity, may be necessary to demonstrate the pathognomonic findings and to make a confident differential diagnosis.[4, 11, 12, 20] Vessels as small as 2 mm. in diameter can be well seen with these selective techniques.[11, 19, 24]

While pulmonary embolism can produce other angiographic changes, these may also be produced by other diseases affecting the lung. These changes assume varying levels of importance, depending upon the underlying cardiopulmonary status of the patient (Table 4–2, p. 103).

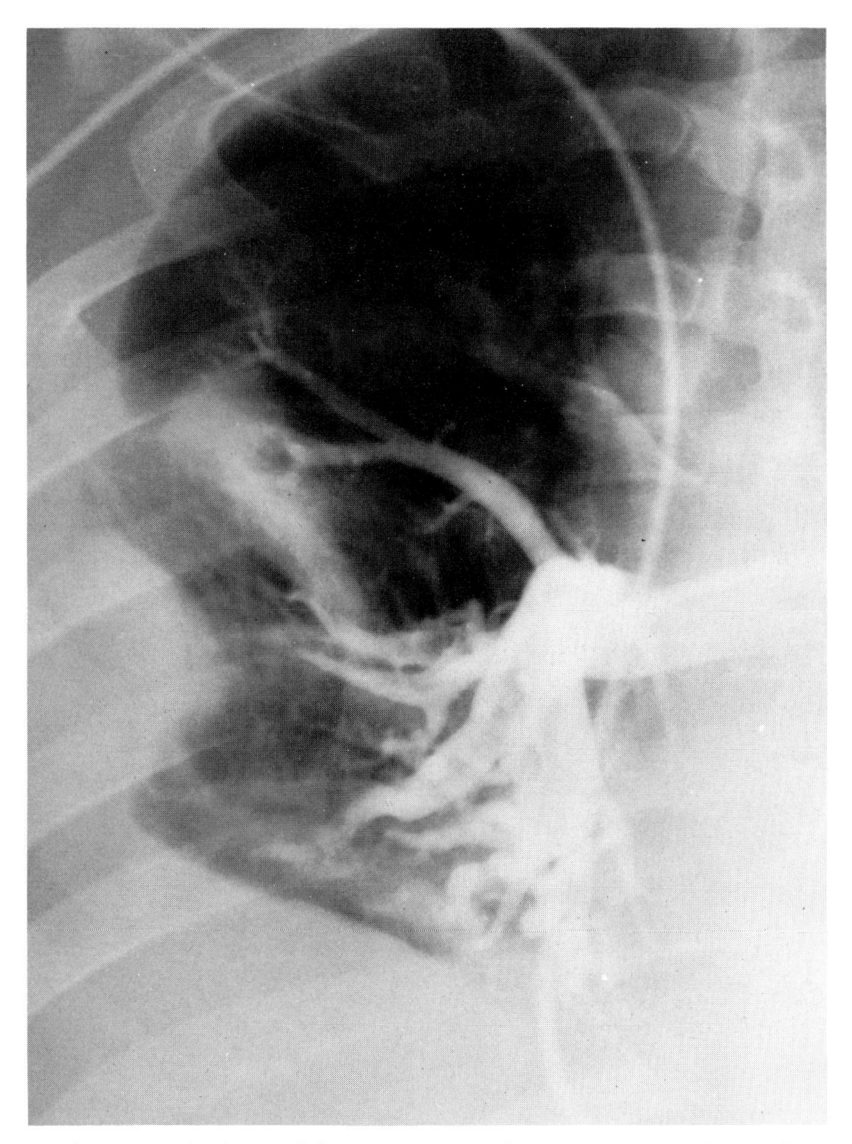

Figure 4–10. Selective right lower lobe arteriogram demonstrates intraluminal thrombi within segmental arteries. Marked volume loss within right lower lobe and a right pleural effusion are present.

Large pulmonary emboli have been overlooked because of vessel overlap. The most frequent area for this oversight is the proximal left pulmonary artery, which may be overlapped by the main pulmonary artery or the right ventricle (Figs. 4–13 and 4–14).

Large central intraluminal emboli may be overlooked if the angiographic technique results in a light film and inadequate penetration of the mediastinal portion of the pulmonary artery. Careful attention to angiographic technique should eliminate this cause for false-negative diagnosis.

Other Entities. Other pathologic conditions may rarely present as intraluminal pulmonary arterial filling defects, usually involving the most central arteries.[15] Primary mediastinal tumors and lymphomas may invade the pulmonary arterial wall and proliferate intraluminally. Helminthic infection and foreign bodies must also be considered. However, the diagnosis should be quite apparent from the history.

CONSTRICTIONS ALONG THE VESSEL WALL

Coarctation of the Pulmonary Artery. This presents as a symmetrical hour-glass constriction at the origin of a pulmonary ar-

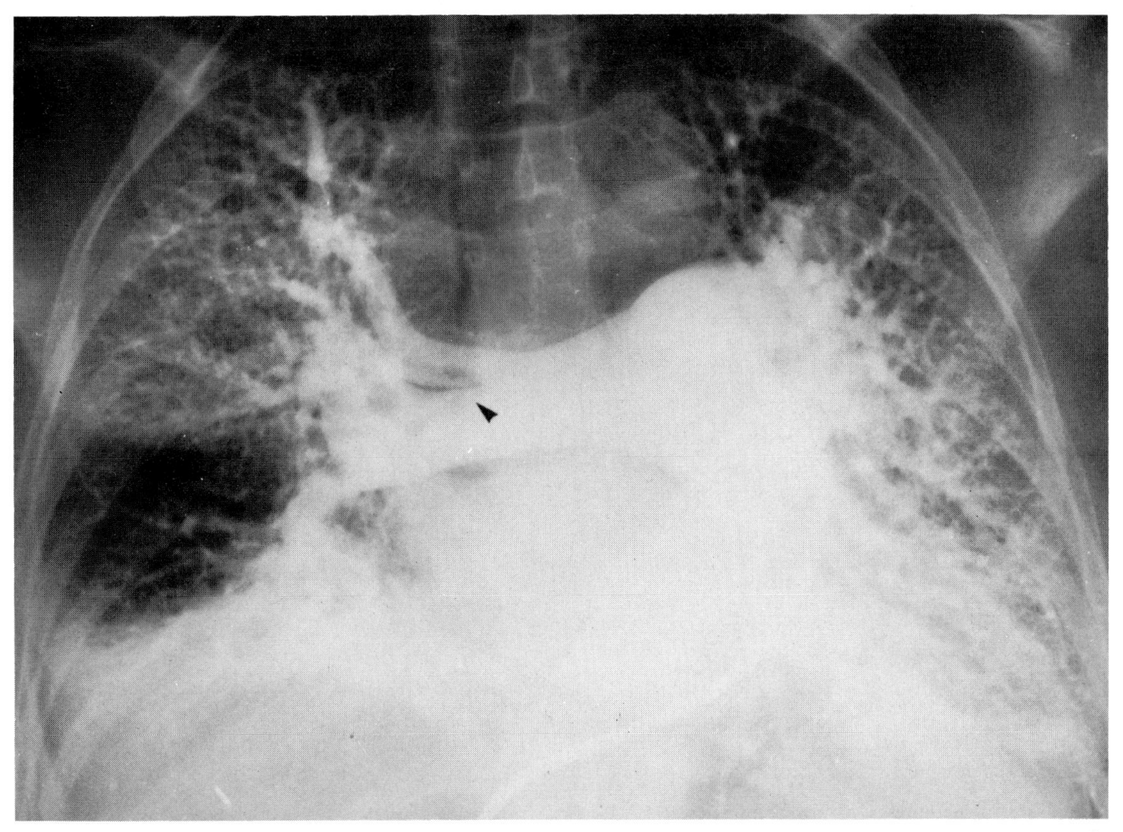

Figure 4–11. Pulmonary angiogram demonstrates embolus straddling the bifurcation of the right pulmonary artery (arrow), with a portion within the right upper lobe artery and the remainder in the intermediate artery. The embolus is applied to the wall, as no contrast medium is seen between the embolus and intima. Decreased opacification of the middle lobe is noted.

tery or branch (Figs. 4–6B and 4–15). The stenoses may be short or long, unilateral or bilateral.[8] There is generally some poststenotic dilatation of the pulmonary artery beyond the constriction. Probably congenital in origin, coarctation is an isolated lesion in 40 per cent of its occurrences. However, it is frequently seen in association with other congenital cardiac lesions, most commonly pulmonary valvular stenosis. It has been described in the postrubella syndrome and associated with supravalvar aortic stenosis in the hypercalcemia syndrome, and has been demonstrated as part of the tetralogy of Fallot complex.[8] Advancing the catheter beyond the stenosis and obtaining a pressure tracing from the catheter while withdrawing it to the main pulmonary artery determines the hemodynamic significance of the stenosis.

Pulmonary Atheroma. This appears

TABLE 4–2. Criteria for Angiographic Diagnosis of Pulmonary Embolism*

1. Definite
   Intraluminal filling defects and/or cut-off of arteries.

2. Probable
   Oligemia and/or asymmetry of blood flow in patients who do not have coexistent lung or heart disease.

3. Equivocal
   Presence of oligemia and/or asymmetry of blood flow in patients with lung disease or heart disease, or presence of uncertain abnormalities, i.e., possible filling defects or possible cut-off.

4. Negative
   No angiographic abnormality consistent with pulmonary embolism.

*Modified from Dalen, J. E., et al., Amer. Heart J., 81:175–185, 1971.

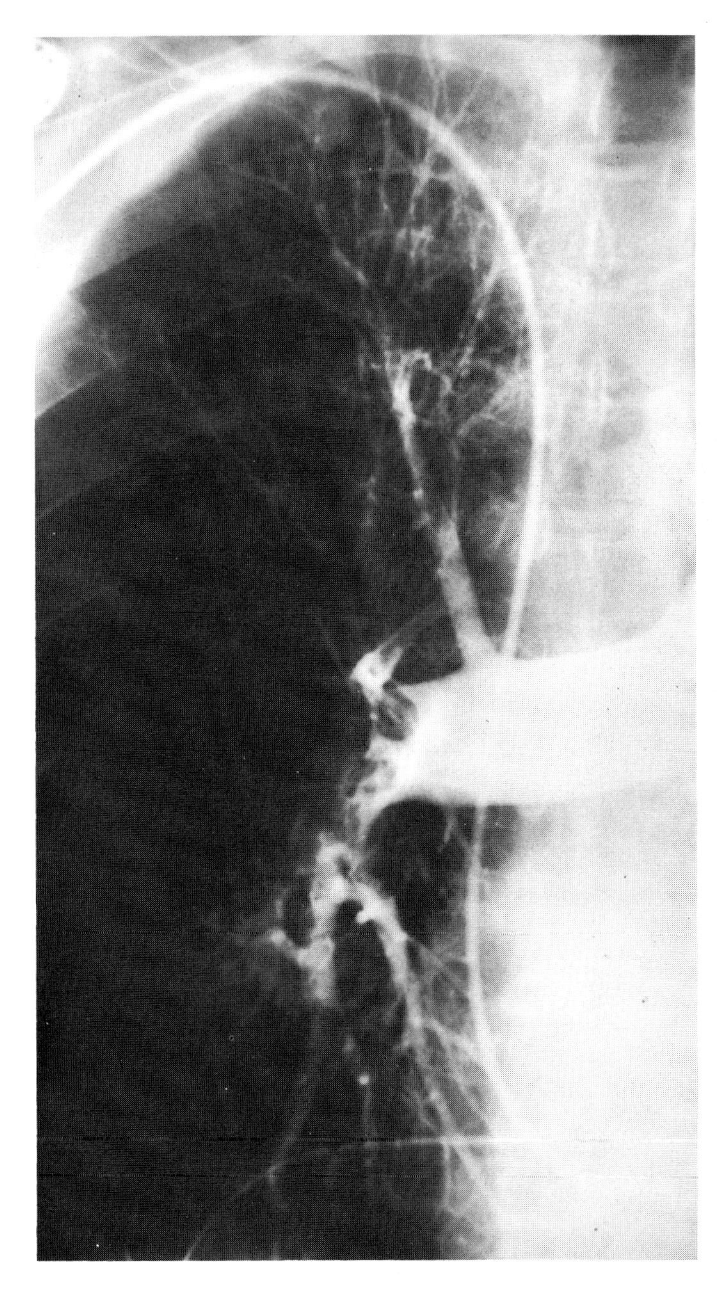

Figure 4–12. Selective right pulmonary arteriogram demonstrates a large embolus attached to the wall of the distal right pulmonary artery, occluding all but a single upper lobe and two lower lobe segmental arteries.

similar to branch stenoses, in that there are segmental constrictions in the pulmonary arterial branches. The atheromatous plaques may develop from long-standing pulmonary arterial hypertension due to any cause, or may be the remnant of an organized pulmonary embolism with plaque formation and bridging. This form of acquired stenosis differs from the congenital variety in that the constriction tends to be asymmetric (more marked on one wall). In addition, there is a rounding of the usually sharp angles which bifurcating vessels make with each other. Often, other small irregularities in the walls of vessels are present and there is no poststenotic dilatation (Fig. 4–16). Hemodynamic data help to make this diagnosis more secure by the finding of systemic pressure in the pulmonary system when these angiographic findings are present. The central pulmonary arteries are usually quite dilated, and this may be visible on the plain chest radiograph.

DILATATION OF VESSELS

Large central pulmonary arteries can be seen in a number of circumstances and are usually the result of increased flow or increased resistance in the pulmonary vascular bed.

High Flow States. In conditions such as left to right shunts, severe anemia, or arteriovenous malformations (systemic or pulmonary), there is generalized dilatation of the vessels. Macroscopic pulmonary arteriovenous malformations are visible on the angiogram. Microscopic arteriovenous shunts have been described in some patients with hepatic cirrhosis,[18] but are not usually visible on the angiograms.

High Resistance. High resistance in the pulmonary vascular bed results in dilated pulmonary arteries. Distribution of the dilatation in this case is different from that of the high flow state in that only the central pulmonary arteries are dilated. Generally the main and hilar pulmonary vessels are large; the branches beyond change to a relatively normal diameter. In addition, the undilated vessels may exhibit irregularities in the wall, including asymmetric constrictions along their course and markedly blunt and rounded bifurcation angles. The diagnosis of high resistance pulmonary hypertension is a hemodynamic diagnosis, determined by the presence of systemic pressures in the pulmonary circulation. If the presence of chronic pulmonary thromboembolism is a consideration, angiography becomes quite important.

There are multiple etiologies for the end stage of pulmonary hypertension. A common etiology is Eisenmenger's syndrome, occurring after a long-standing left to right shunt and resulting in reversal of the shunt due to severe resistance.[5]

Idiopathic Pulmonary Artery Dilatation. This is a diagnosis of exclusion. Occasionally one is presented with an abnormal radiographic finding of a large main pulmonary artery in a young or middle aged patient, generally female (Fig. 4–17). The differential diagnosis lies between silent mitral valve disease with pulmonary hypertension, thromboembolic or idiopathic pulmonary hypertension, and idiopathic pulmonary artery dilatation. Catheterization in these patients will exclude the first two possibilities. Angiography demonstrates a large pulmonary artery, leading to the exclusion diagnosis of idiopathic pulmonary artery dilatation.[6]

DISPLACEMENT OF VESSELS

Parenchymal Space-Occupying Lesions. Such lesions in the lung may be manifested by the deflection of pulmonary vessels around the lesion. Large bullae commonly cause this phenomenon (Fig. 4–18). Despite the extreme sensitivity of angiography for recognition of parenchymal bullae, this examination is rarely indicated for diagnosis or evaluation. Plain chest roentgenography, tomography, and radioisotopic perfusion and ventilation almost always suffice in detecting bullous areas and in assessing the integrity of the remaining lung tissue.

Crowding of Vessels. This condition, secondary to loss of parenchymal volume, can be seen either in bronchial obstruction or with parenchymal lung disease (Figs. 4–7 and 4–8). Main pulmonary arterial injections will frequently show nonfilling of vessels in collapsed segments. Selective injections show vascular crowding with poor visualization of the small branches (Figs. 4–8B and 4–19A). The parenchymal phase generally shows a very dense stain persisting as the veins from other sections of lung are filled (Fig. 4–19B).

Small vessels may become tortuous and have a corkscrew appearance. This is occasionally seen in the lower lobes of the normal lung if the angiogram is done in expiration. Atelectasis also causes this appearance. Presumably, vessels appear tortuous because of redundancy in a slightly compressed lung. The vessels would be normal if the lung were fully expanded. However, peripheral vascular tortuosity also occurs in patients with elevated pulmonary vascular resistance, such as large left to right shunts.

REDISTRIBUTION OF FLOW

Main pulmonary artery injections follow the general pulmonary flow patterns.

Text continued on page 110

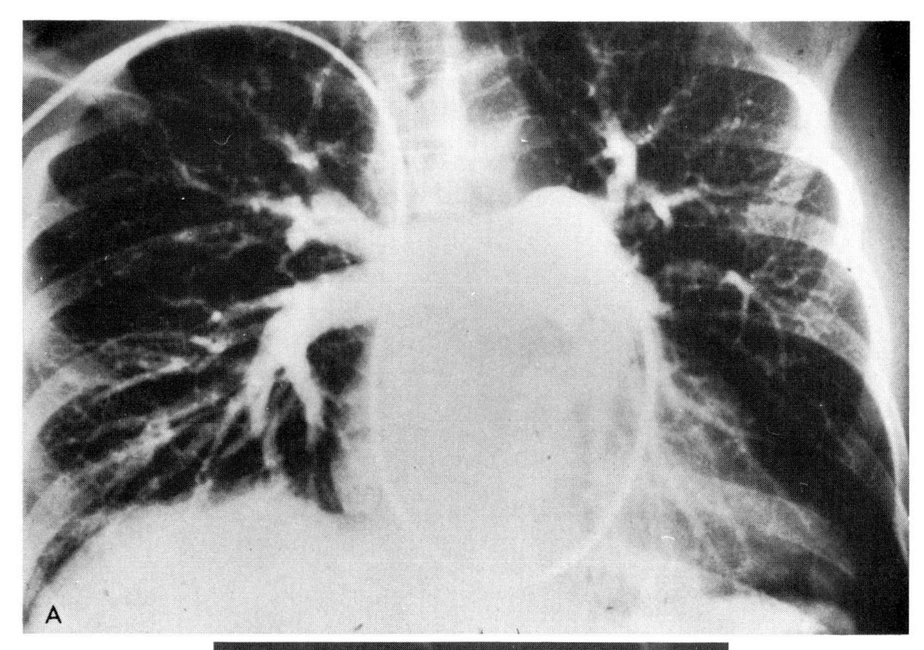

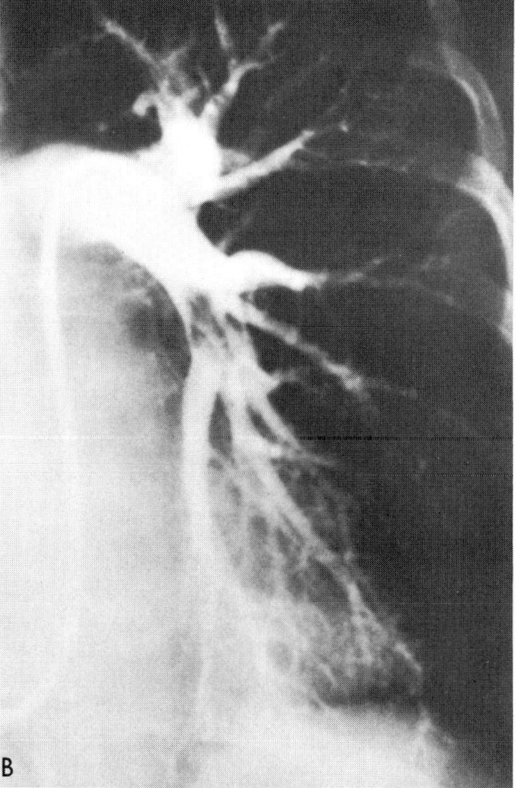

Figure 4–13. *A*. Pulmonary arteriogram following main pulmonary artery injection demonstrates relatively less filling and smaller vessels in the left lower lobe. All but the segmental branches of the left lower lobe artery are obscured by a combination of slight reflux of contrast media into the right ventricular outflow tract and overlapping by the main pulmonary artery. *B*. Selective left pulmonary arteriogram demonstrates a large embolus in the lower lobe artery.

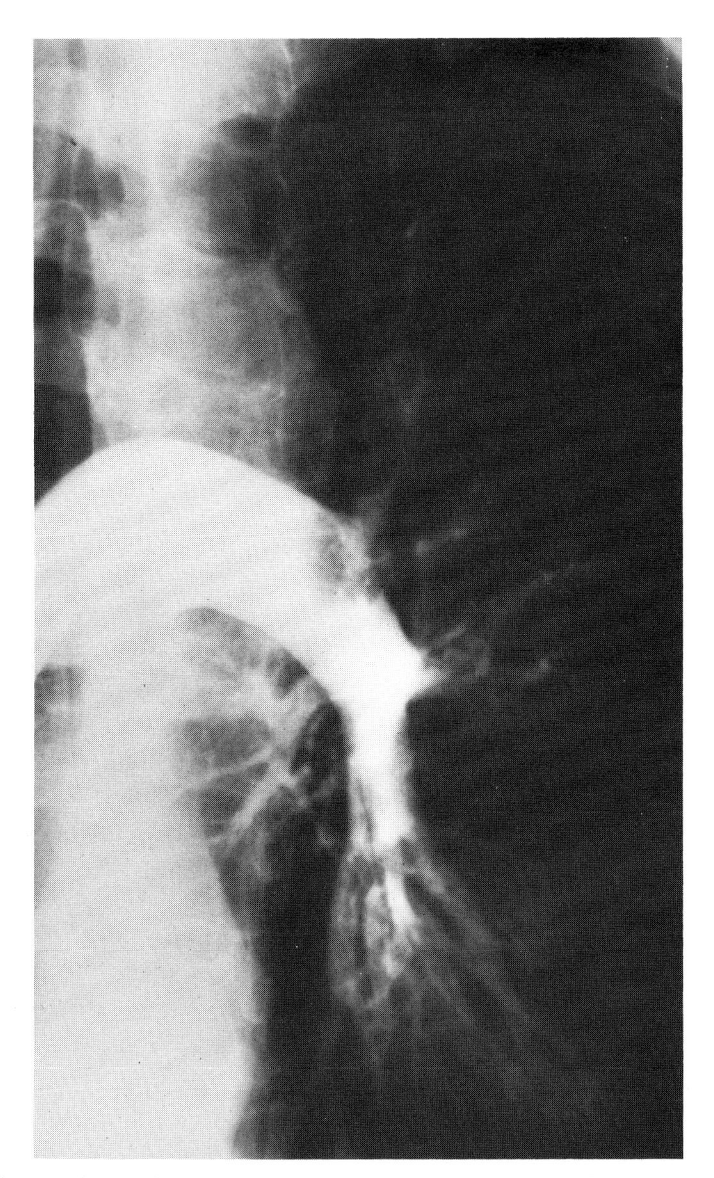

Figure 4–14. Selective left pulmonary arteriogram in right posterior oblique projection demonstrates an embolus occluding the orifice of the upper lobe artery. Only absence of perfusion to the left upper lobe was demonstrable on the anteroposterior angiogram after main pulmonary artery injection.

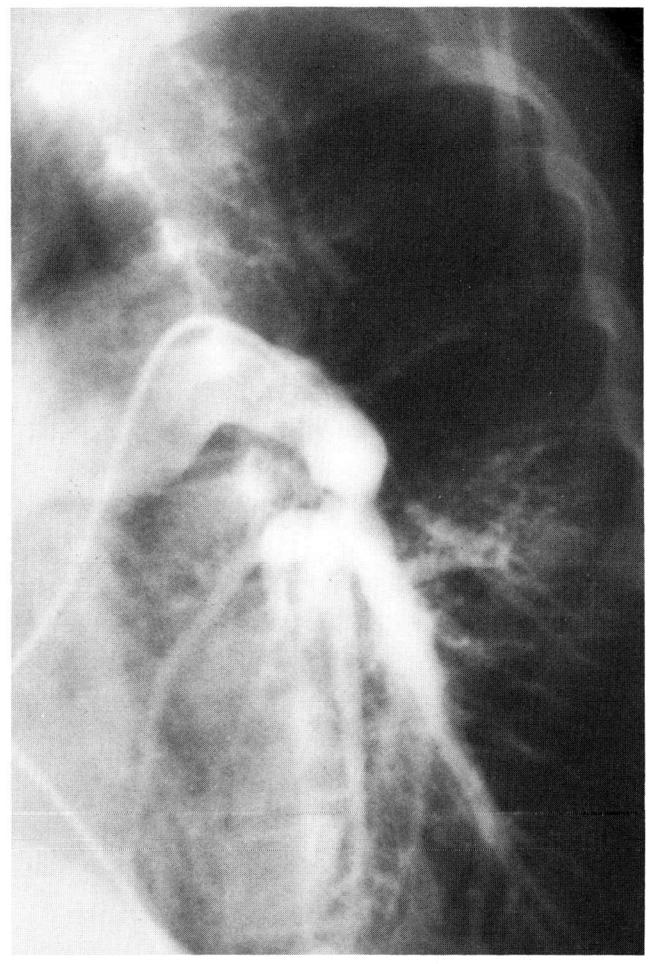

Figure 4–15. An 8 year old boy with the post-rubella syndrome. Selective left pulmonary arteriogram in right posterior oblique projection demonstrates stenosis at the origin of the lower lobe artery.

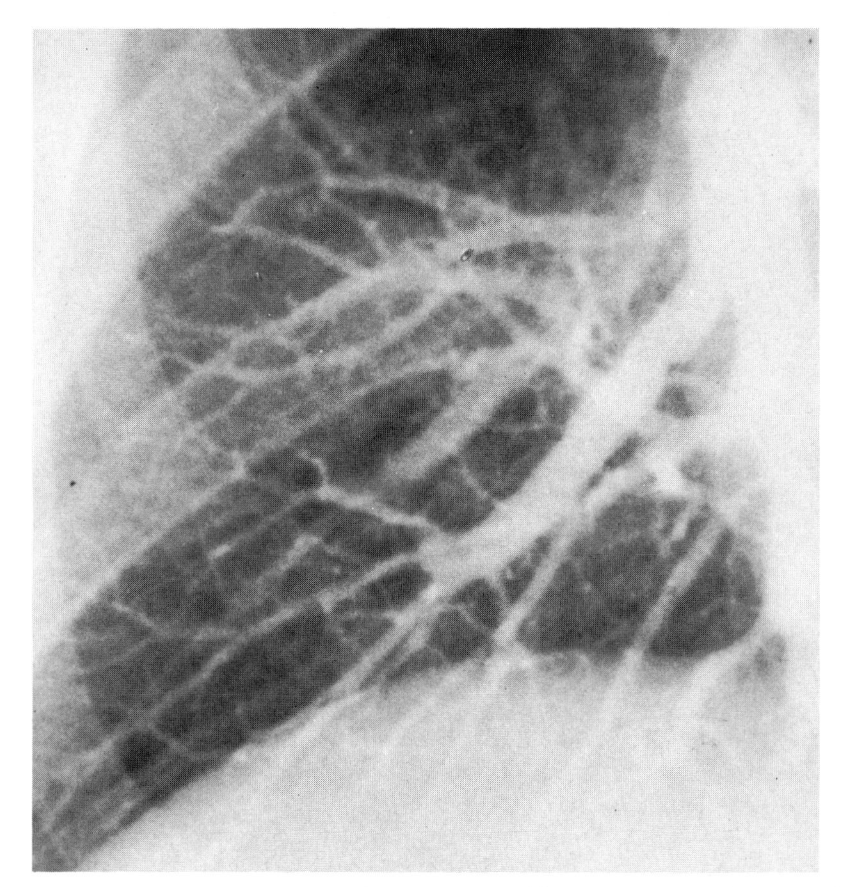

Figure 4–16. A 49 year old woman with pulmonary arterial hypertension. Selective right lower lobe pulmonary arteriogram demonstrates irregularity of the segmental arteries with eccentric areas of constriction along their course, consistent with pulmonary atheromata. The angle between some bifurcating vessels is rounded and widened by plaques, rather than forming a normal pointed acute angle.

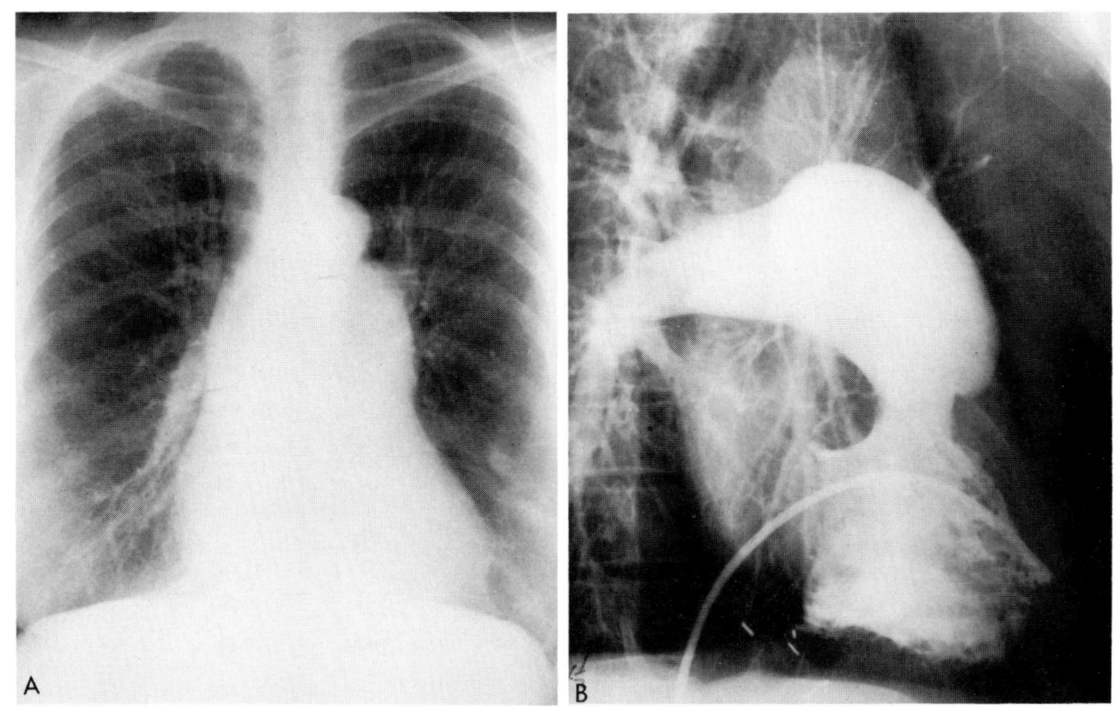

Figure 4–17. A 58 year old woman with peptic ulcer disease and no cardiopulmonary symptoms. *A*. Posteroanterior chest radiograph demonstrates apparent enlargement of the main pulmonary artery. No murmur was detected. In order to exclude occult pulmonary valvular stenosis or a tumor mass about the pulmonary artery, angiography was performed. *B*. Right ventricular injection demonstrates normal outflow tract and valve with a markedly dilated main pulmonary artery. Normal right-sided pressure and absence of a hemodynamic gradient across the valve led to the exclusion diagnosis of idiopathic dilatation.

Regional redistribution of flow can occur from any number of causes. A common condition encountered in pulmonary angiography is redistribution of flow secondary to pulmonary venous hypertension, since these patients frequently are studied for the diagnosis of pulmonary embolism. This form of pulmonary vascular alteration is characterized by slowed and diminished flow to the lower lobes[4, 20] (Fig. 4–20). Detection of an elevated pulmonary artery pressure should lead to determination of the pulmonary wedge pressure to confirm the diagnosis. Because of the poor lower lobe flow in these patients, exclusion of a possible pulmonary embolism frequently requires lower lobe selective injections.

EXTRA VESSELS

Arteriovenous Malformation. Large malformations fill quite early in the arterial phase and present as well opacified round densities in the lung. Generally, there is a reflection of the increased flow to these structures: large arteries feeding the malformation as well as large and early draining veins. Angiography is of value in this disease for demonstration of smaller and less prominent malformations in patients with well known large lesions[13] (Fig. 4–21).

II. Abnormalities Which Present Predominantly in the Parenchymal Phase

Increased Parenchymal Density. Slow flow of the pulmonary circulation is the mechanism which accounts for this abnormality. Any form of pulmonary infiltrative process which prolongs the circulation time in the lungs can give rise to this appearance. Patchy increased density also can be seen in atelectasis[4] (Fig. 4–19). Unaffected portions of lung in patients with massive pulmonary embolism may have this increased flow and may show a dense parenchymal stain in the area supplied by the unoccluded vessels.

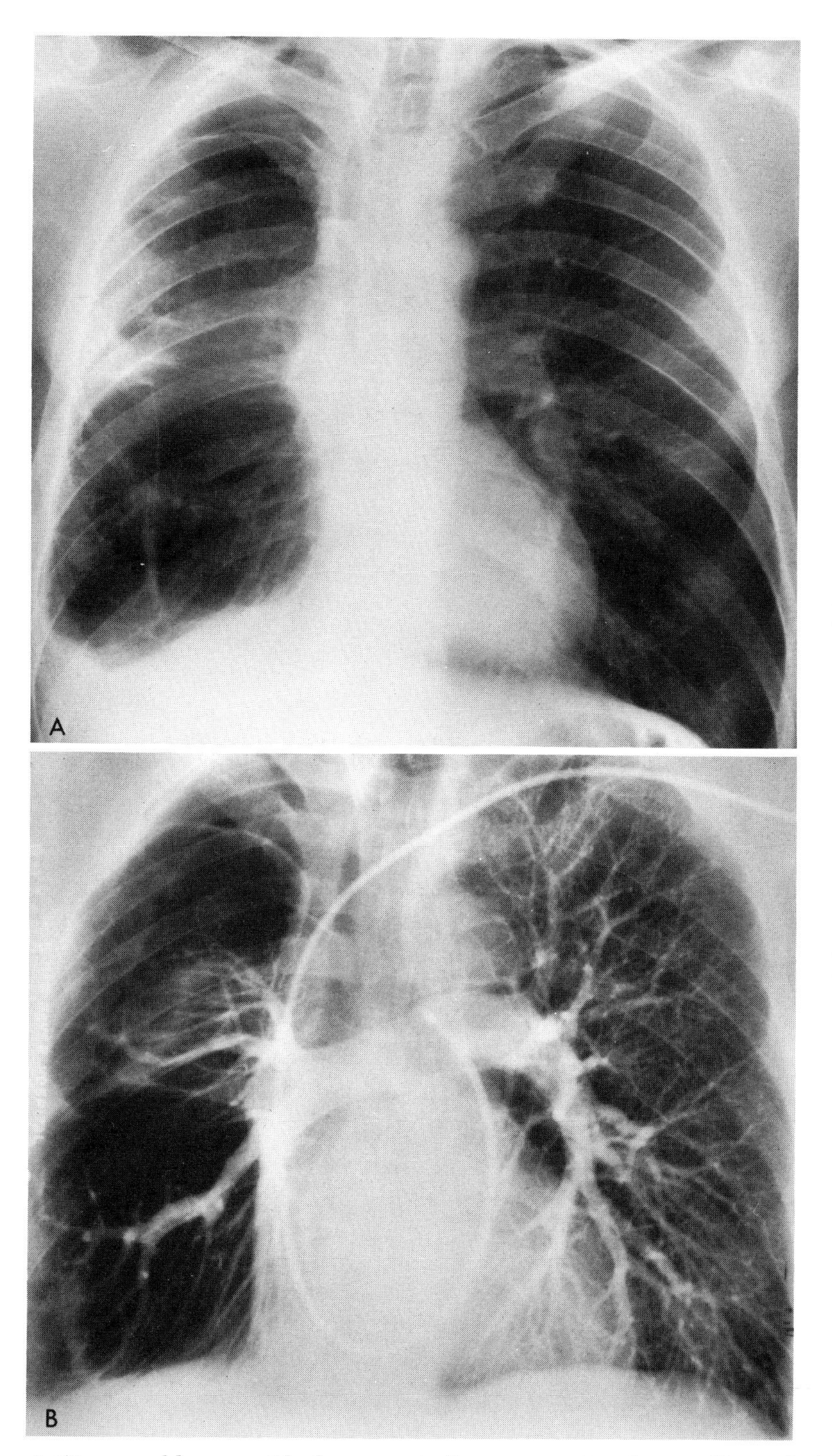

Figure 4–18. A 52 year old man with dyspnea. *A.* Posteroanterior chest radiograph demonstrates obstructive airways disease with extensive bullous changes in the right lung. *B.* Pulmonary arteriogram demonstrates the pulmonary arteries displaced and distorted around large avascular areas in the right lung. There is little or no fill of the smaller pulmonary vessels. Filling defects in the parenchymal phase with diminished venous fill would also be expected.

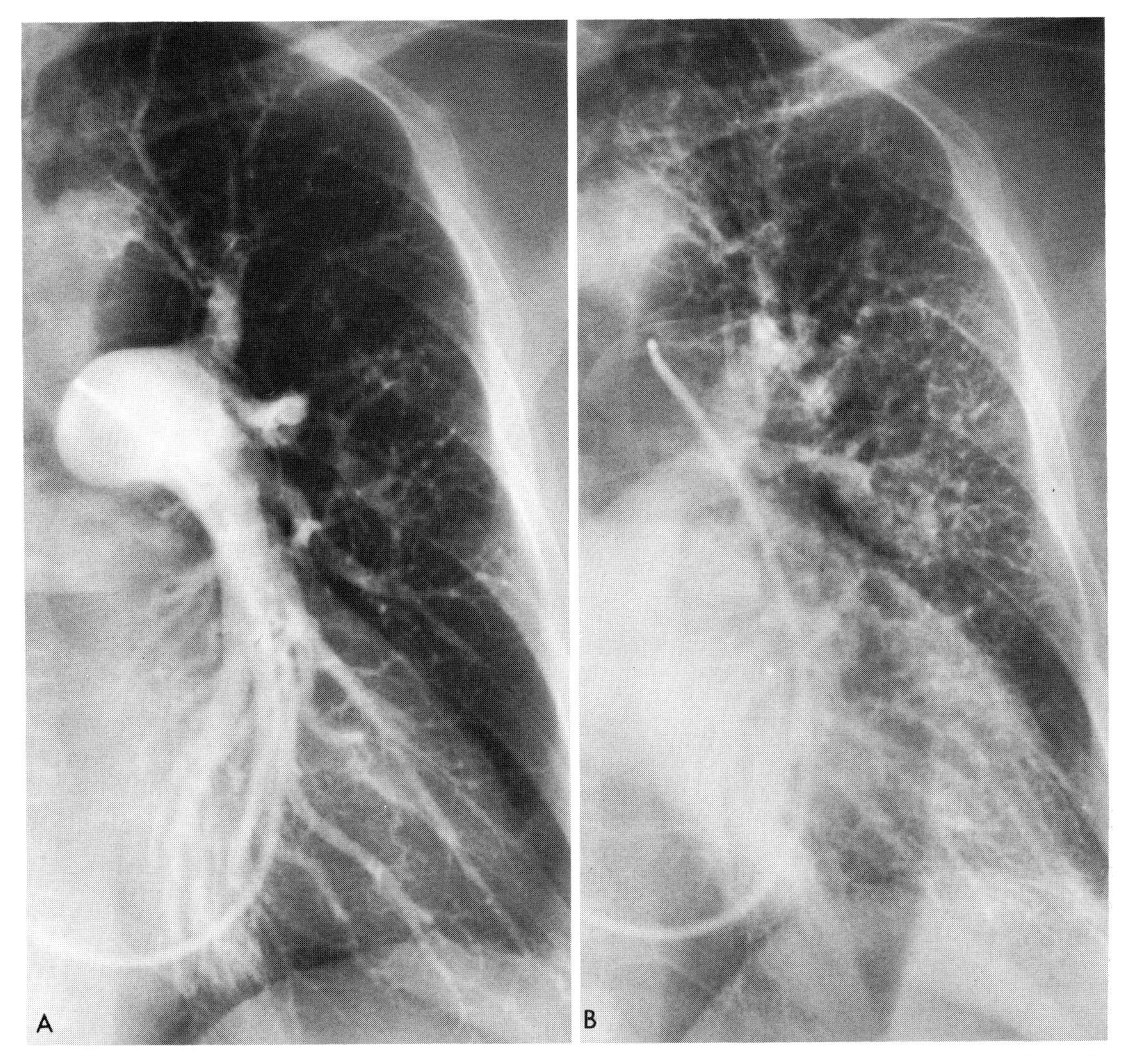

Figure 4–19. A. Left pulmonary arteriogram shows crowding together of pulmonary vessels in the medial portion of the lower lobe. *B*. The levogram phase demonstrates a persistent dense stain in the atelectatic segment. Delayed flow in that segment is indicated because the veins from the remainder of the left lung and the left atrium are opacified.

Decreased Parenchymal Density. Local patches of decreased density are seen in areas without blood supply, whether the vessels are obliterated by intrinsic vascular disease or parenchymal destruction or are simply displaced.

III. Abnormalities Which Present in the Venous Phase

Anomalous Pulmonary Venous Return. This is a condition in which one or more pulmonary veins drain to the right atrium, or to the superior or inferior vena cava. This can be diagnosed by the abnormal course which the anomalous vein takes.

Meandering Pulmonary Veins. Occasionally, pulmonary veins may have an unusual course through the lung, with an appearance similar to an anomalous vein, but with normal drainage into the left atrium.[9] This is frequently a plain film finding; pulmonary angiography is performed to opacify a bizarre, snake-like structure passing through the lung. The diagnosis is

Text continued on page 118

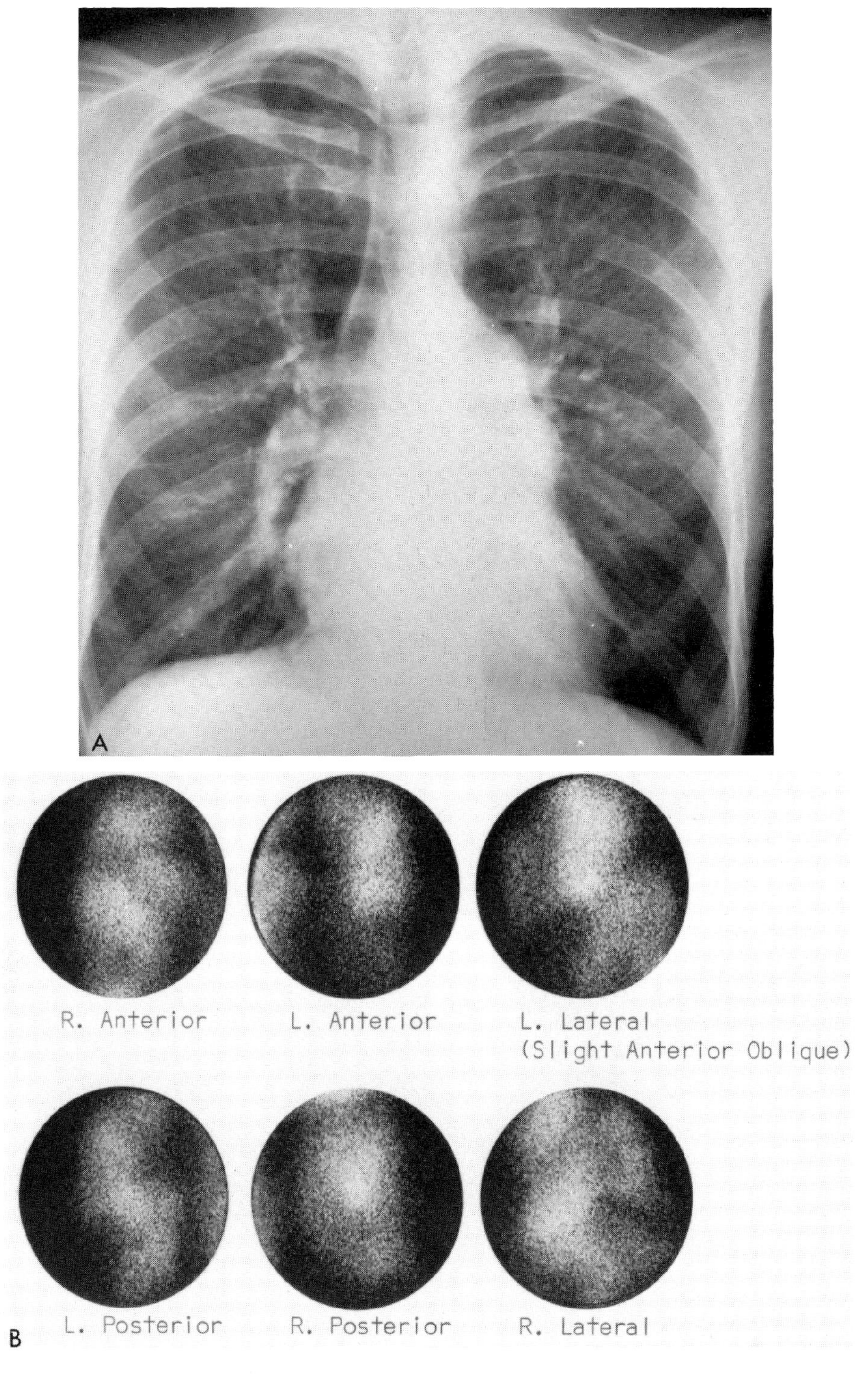

Figure 4–20. A 26 year old man, 2 months after mitral valve replacement, with wheezing and dyspnea. *A*. Posteroanterior chest roentgenogram shows diversion of blood flow to the upper lobes. *B*. Radioisotopic perfusion scintiphotogram demonstrates multiple perfusion defects, most prominent at the lung bases.

Illustration and legend continued on the following page

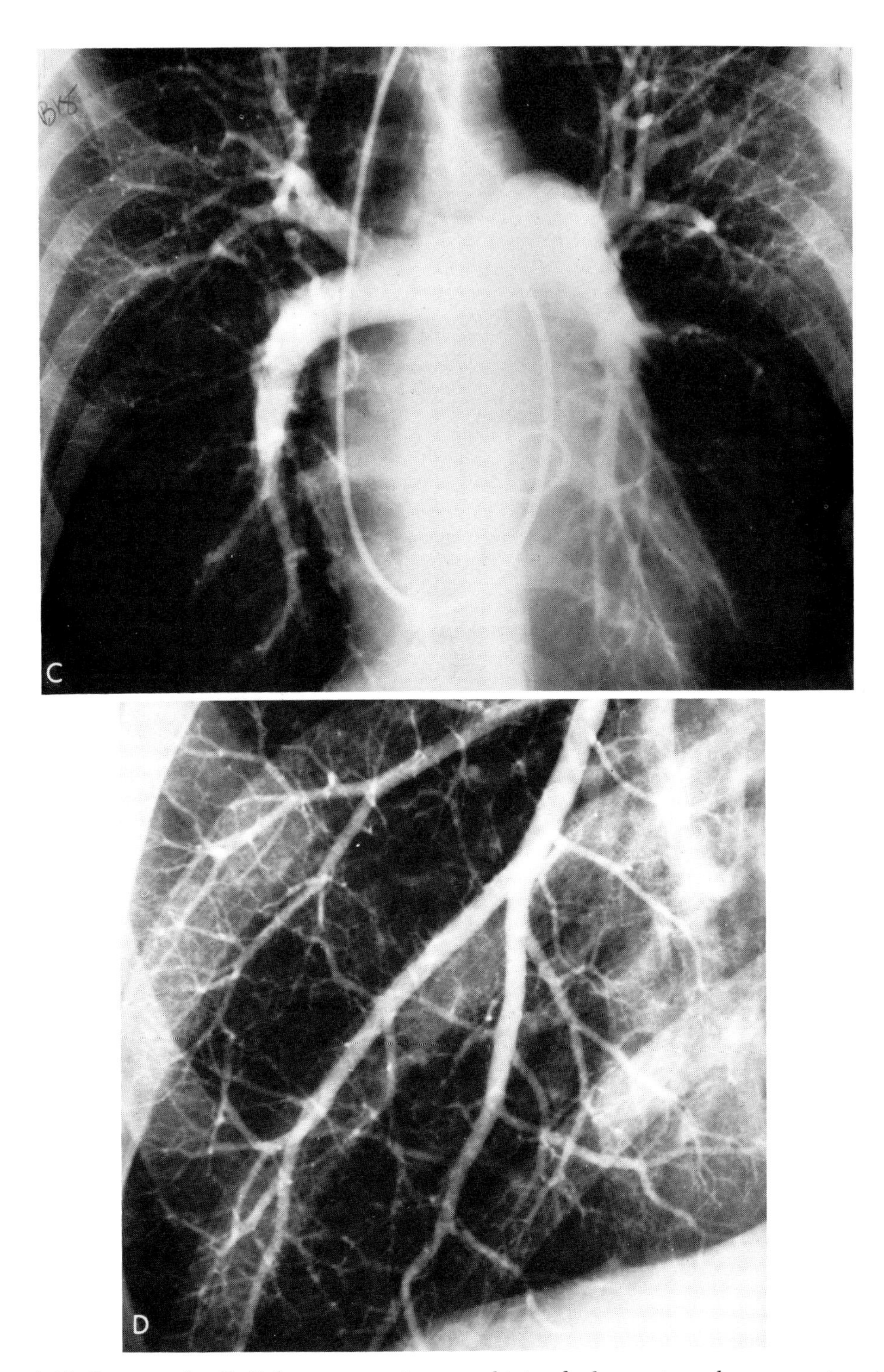

Figure 4–20 Continued. *C.* Pulmonary angiogram obtained after main pulmonary artery injection shows diversion of blood flow to the upper lobes, with underfill and poor visualization of small lower lobe vessels. *D.* Selective middle lobe and right lower lobe (not illustrated) arteriograms, obtained with magnification technique, demonstrate patency of all peripheral arteries, without evidence of pulmonary emboli.

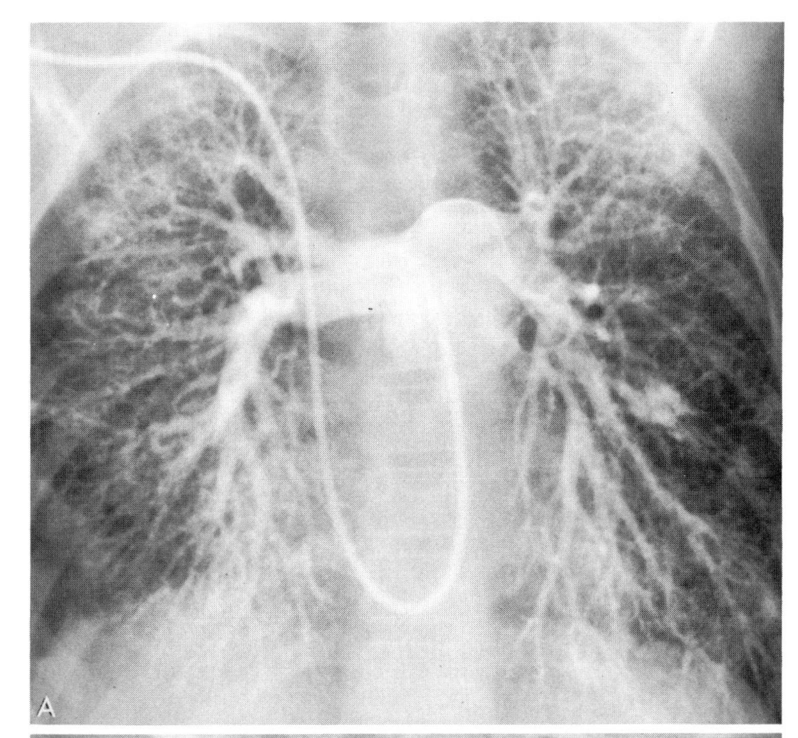

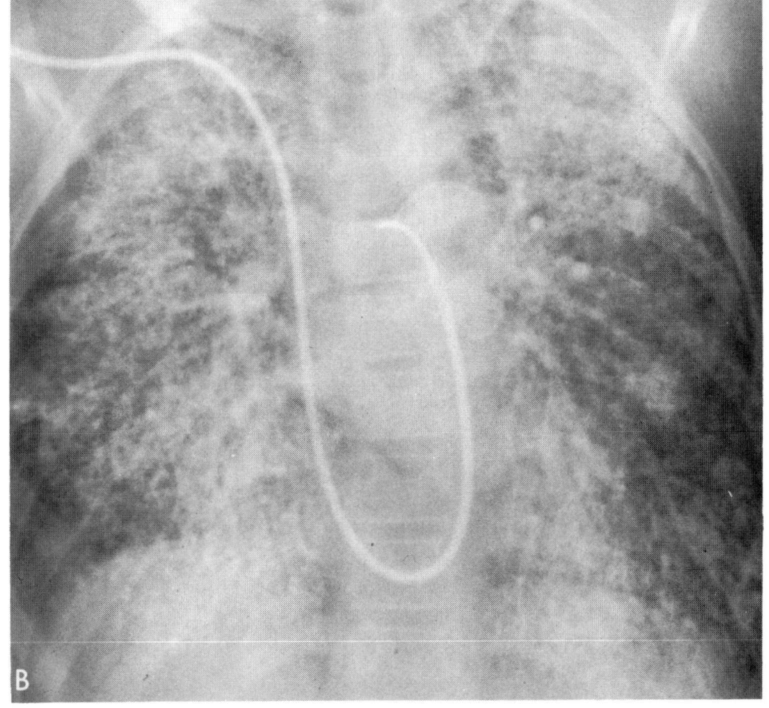

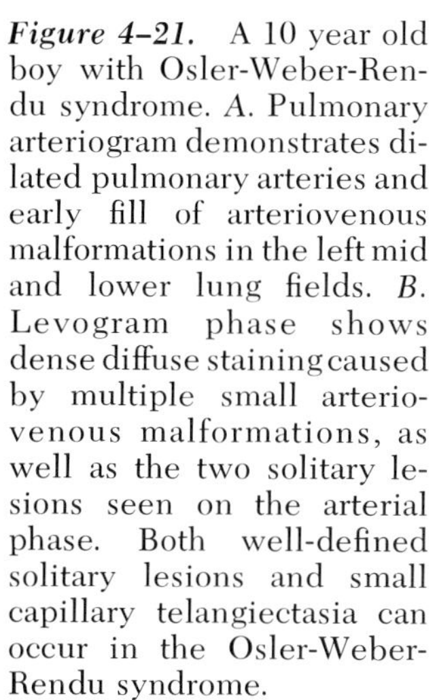

Figure 4–21. A 10 year old boy with Osler-Weber-Rendu syndrome. *A*. Pulmonary arteriogram demonstrates dilated pulmonary arteries and early fill of arteriovenous malformations in the left mid and lower lung fields. *B*. Levogram phase shows dense diffuse staining caused by multiple small arteriovenous malformations, as well as the two solitary lesions seen on the arterial phase. Both well-defined solitary lesions and small capillary telangiectasia can occur in the Osler-Weber-Rendu syndrome.

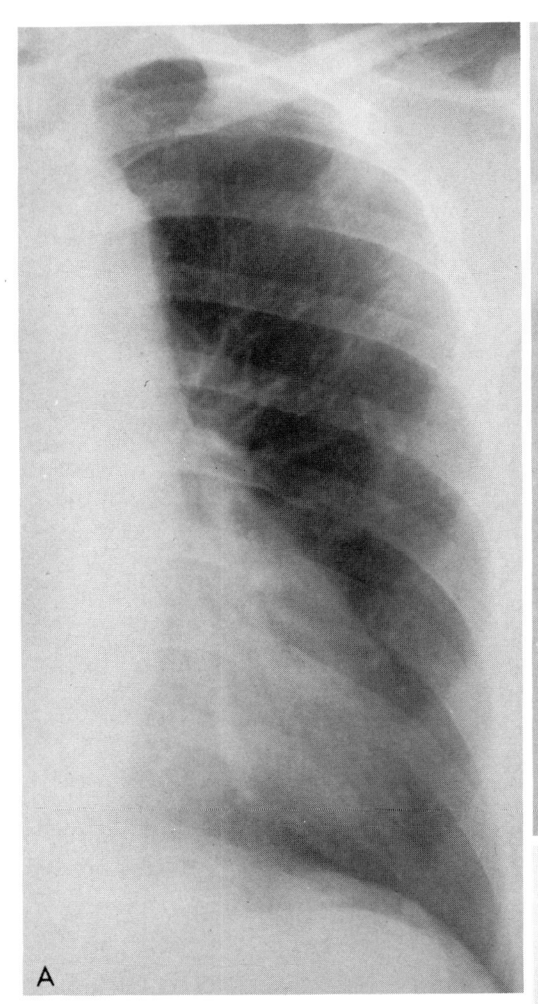

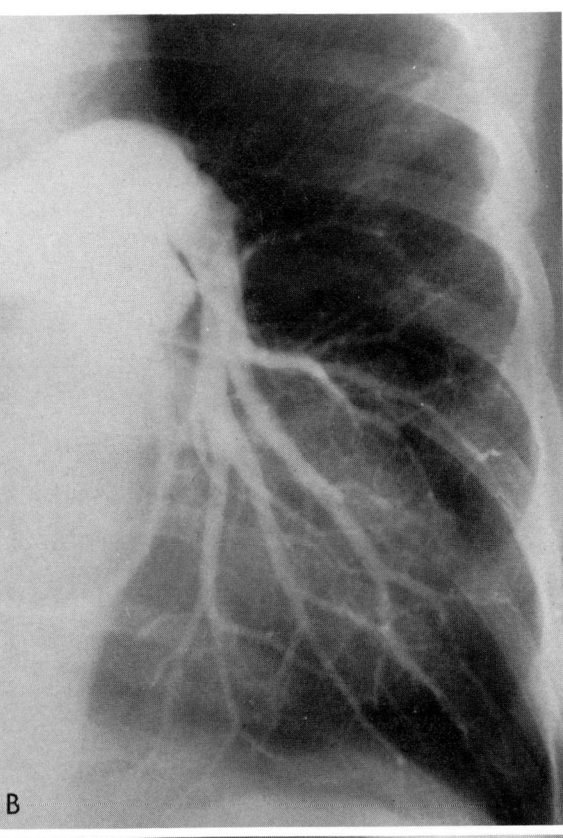

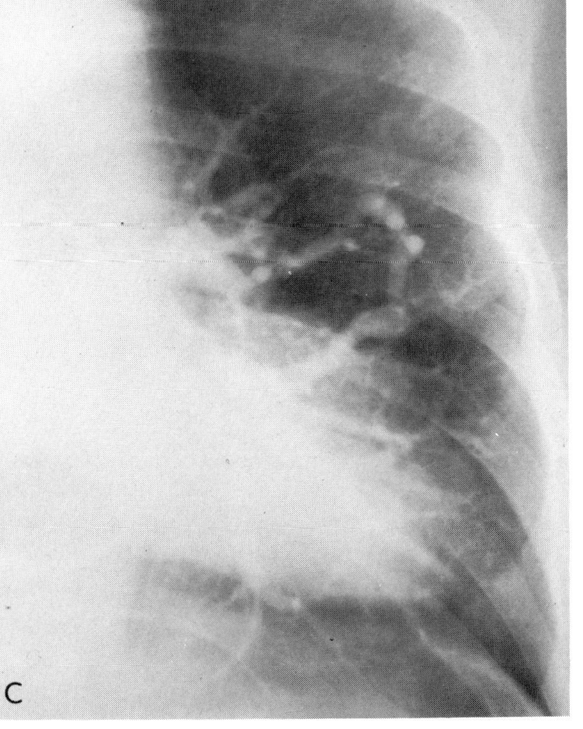

Figure 4–22. A 65 year old woman with suspected pulmonary embolism. *A.* Detail of left lung, posteroanterior roentgenogram, demonstrates an irregular serpiginous density in the mid lung field. *B.* Detail of left lung, pulmonary arteriogram, demonstrates occlusion of the left upper lobe artery by embolus. *C.* Levogram phase demonstrates opacification of a dilated meandering vein from the left lower lobe with normal drainage into the left atrium.

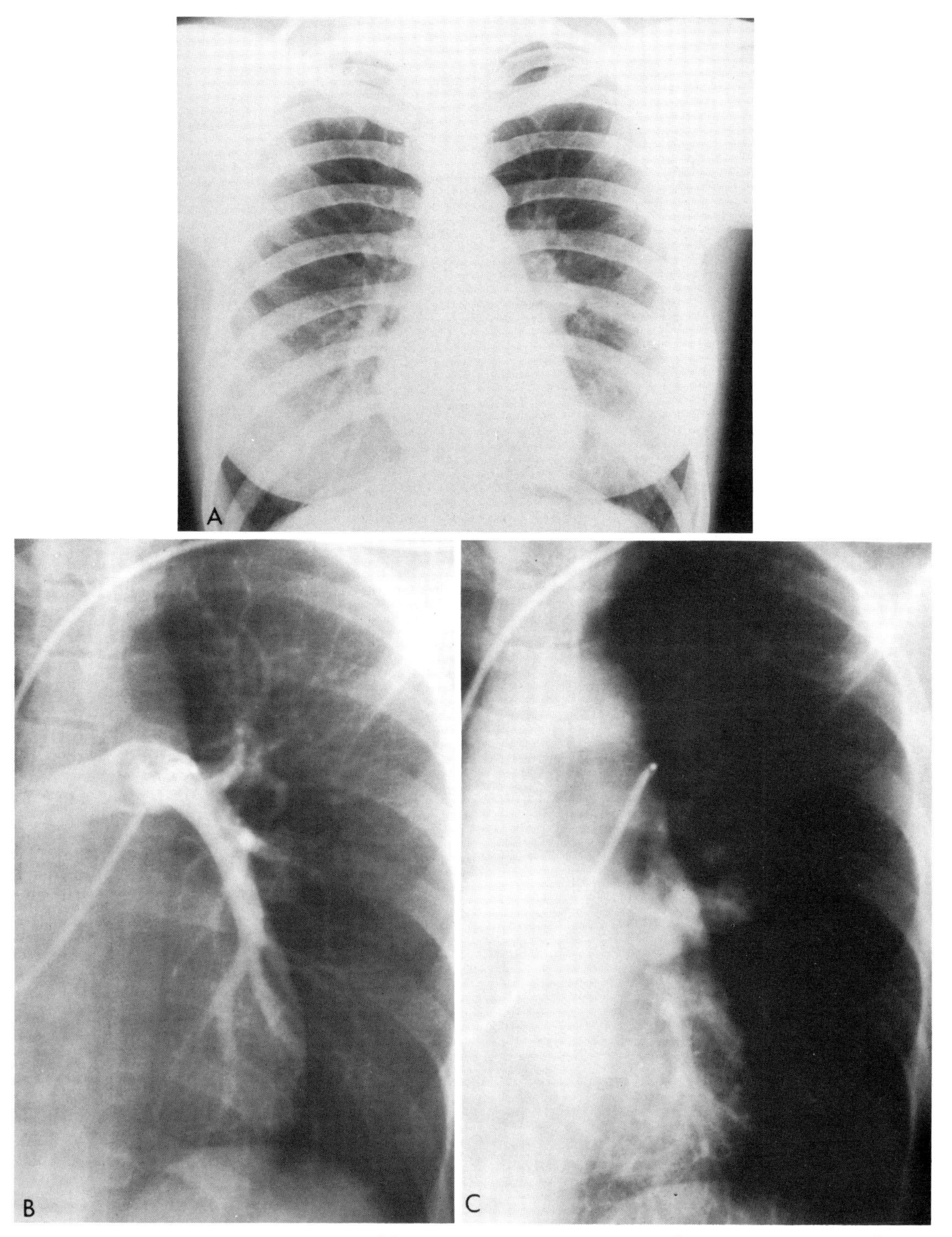

Figure 4–23. Asymptomatic 26 year old woman. *A.* Posteroanterior chest roentgenogram demonstrates a left perihilar mass. *B.* Selective left pulmonary arteriogram shows a normal arterial phase. *C.* Levogram phase demonstrates opacification of a large venous varicosity emptying into a normal left atrium.

quite obvious in the levogram phase (Fig. 4–22).

Pulmonary Venous Varices. Patients with long-standing pulmonary venous hypertension may have localized dilatation in the pulmonary veins. Most frequently, the location is in the veins just before entry into the left atrium. The angiogram is usually performed for the diagnosis of a hilar or perihilar nodule (Fig. 4–23), although varices may occur slightly more peripherally in the lung fields.[1]

BIBLIOGRAPHY

1. Bartram, C. M., and Strickland, B.: Pulmonary varices. Brit. J. Radiol., 44:927–935, 1971.
2. Bookstein, J. J.: Segmental arteriography in pulmonary embolism. Radiology, 93:1007–1012, 1969.
3. Bookstein, J. J.: Pulmonary thromboembolism with emphasis on angiographic pathologic correlation. Seminars in Roentgen., 5:291–305, 1970.
4. Bookstein, J. J., and Silver, T. M.: The angiographic differential diagnosis of acute pulmonary embolism. Radiology, 110:25–33, 1974.
5. Brammell, H. L., Vogel, J. H. K., Pryor, R., and Blount, S. G., Jr.: The Eisenmenger syndrome. A clinical and physiologic reappraisal. Amer. J. Cardiol., 28:679–692, 1971.
6. Challis, T. W., and Fay, J. E.: Isolated dilatation of the main pulmonary artery. A report of three cases and a review of the literature. J. Canad. Assoc. Radiol., 20:180–184, 1969.
7. Dalen, J. E., Brooks, H. L., Johnson, L. W., Meister, S. G., Szucs, M. M., and Dexter, L.: Pulmonary angiography in acute pulmonary embolism: Indications, techniques and results in 367 patients. Amer. Heart J., 81:175–185, 1971.
8. Gay, B. B., Jr., Franch, R. H., Shuford, W. H., and Rogers, J. V., Jr.: The roentgenologic features of single and multiple coarctations of the pulmonary artery and branches. Amer. J. Roentgen., 90:599–613, 1963.
9. Goodman, L. R., Jamshidi, A., and Hipona, F.: Meandering right pulmonary vein simulating the scimitar syndrome. Chest, 62:510–512, 1972.
10. Greenough, W.: The role of pulmonary angiography in carcinoma of the lung. Chest, 62:206–210, 1972.
11. Greenspan, R. H., and Steiner, R. E.: The radiologic diagnosis of pulmonary thromboembolism. *In* Simon, M., Potchen, E. J., and LeMay, M., editors: Frontiers of Pulmonary Radiology. New York, Grune and Stratton, 1969, pp. 222–245.
12. Johnson, B. A., James, A. E., Jr., and White, R. S., Jr.: Oblique and selective pulmonary angiography in diagnosis of pulmonary embolism. Amer. J. Roentgen., 118:801–808, 1973.
13. Kinkhabwala, M. N., Becker, J. A., and Rabinowitz, J. G.: Osler-Weber-Rendu syndrome with multiple angiographic findings. Brit. J. Radiol., 45:534–536, 1972.
14. Miller, R. E.: Internal jugular pulmonary arteriography and removal of catheter emboli. Radiology, 102:200–202, 1972.
15. Moffat, R. E., Chang, C. H., and Slavin, J. E.: Roentgen considerations in primary pulmonary artery sarcoma. Radiology, 104:283–288, 1972.
16. Moses, D. C., Silver, T. M., and Bookstein, J. J.: The complementary roles of chest radiography, lung scanning and selective pulmonary angiography in the diagnosis of pulmonary embolism. Circulation, 49:179–188, 1974.
17. Raphael, M. J., and Steiner, R. E.: Selective cinefluoroscopic studies of pulmonary circulatory disorders. Brit. Heart J., 28:523–530, 1966.
18. Rutishauser, M., Egli, F., and Wiler, F.: Juvenile liver cirrohosis with multiple arteriovenous aneurysms of lung. Schweiz. Med. Wschr., 102:514–517, 1972.
19. Sagel, S. S., Sheft, D. J., Amberg, J. R., and Margulis, A. R.: Recent advances in clinical diagnostic roentgenology. *In* Welch, C. E., and Hardy, J. D., editors: Advances in Surgery. Chicago, Year Book Medical Publishers, Inc., 1971, pp. 63–69.
20. Sagel, S. S., and Greenspan, R. H.: Nonuniform pulmonary arterial perfusion. Radiology, 99:541–548, 1971.
21. Sherrick, D. W., Kincaid, O. W., and DuShane, J. W.: Agenesis of a main branch of the pulmonary artery. Amer. J. Roentgen., 87:917–928, 1962.
22. Snider, G. L., Ferris, E., Gaensler, E. A., Messer, J. V., Hayes, J. A., Gersten, M., and Coutu, R. E.: Primary pulmonary hypertension: A fatality during pulmonary angiography. Chest, 64:628–635, 1973.
23. Stein, M. A., Winter, J., and Grollman, J. H., Jr.: The value of the pulmonary-artery-seeking catheter in percutaneous selective pulmonary angiography. Radiology, 114:299–304, 1975.
24. Stein, P. D.: Wedge arteriography for the identification of pulmonary emboli in small vessels. Amer. Heart J., 82:618–623, 1971.
25. The Urokinase-Pulmonary Embolism Trial, a national cooperative study. Circulation, 47(suppl 2):1–108, 1973.

Chapter 5

THORACIC AORTOGRAPHY

by Robert C. McKnight, M.D., and Stuart S. Sagel, M.D.

INTRODUCTION

Thoracic aortography is utilized to delineate or exclude congenital or acquired lesions of the aorta and its major branches that cannot be clarified by conventional radiologic methods. Fluoroscopy is generally of limited usefulness in diseases of the aorta, either to make or to exclude a diagnosis. Similarly, while ultrasonic techniques and intravenous radionuclide angiography are occasionally helpful, at present problems with significant false-positive and false-negative diagnosis rates limit their routine use. Aortography is also an integral part of the investigation of certain acquired and congenital heart diseases, but this chapter will be restricted to primary aortic lesions. Conditions which will be discussed include:

A. Congenital anomalies
   1. Coarctation of the aorta
   2. Pseudocoarctation
   3. Aortic arch anomalies
   4. Pulmonary sequestration
B. Acquired aortic disease
   1. Aneurysm
   2. Dissection
   3. Traumatic injury
   4. Aortic arch syndrome
C. Clarification of thoracic mass

TECHNIQUE

Thoracic aortography is performed at our hospital under local anesthesia, following premedication with mild sedation and atropine. The percutaneous transfemoral artery approach is most often utilized. Large bore, thin-walled catheters of approximately No. 8 French size and 100 cm. length, with "pigtail" or "J-shaped" tips containing four to six side holes, are used. These catheters permit adequate flow rates without undue pressures.

In some elderly patients with extensive atherosclerotic disease, when coarctation of the aorta is suspected, or if the femoral pulses are absent or barely palpable, percutaneous axillary (usually right) artery entry is used. Smaller catheter diameters (No. 7 French) and shorter length (50 to 80 cm.) will allow adequate study with little risk, provided meticulous technique is used.

Initial thoracic aortograms are generally performed with the catheter tip in the mid-ascending aorta. When aortic dissection or insufficiency is suspected, the end is placed just above the aortic valve.

Contrast media. Either Renografin-76 or Hypaque-M 75% is generally employed as the contrast agent in adults. Utilizing these agents, a 20% contrast–blood mixture is optimal for visualization of the central aorta adjacent to the catheter. Contrast-blood levels of 30 to 40 per cent are frequently necessary for opacifying the distal branches which are remote from the catheter tip or for providing optimal identification of small amounts of extravasation from the aorta or its branches. With normal aortic flow of about 100 ml. per second in the average adult, injection flow rates of 20 to 40 ml. per second will achieve these concentrations of contrast. A common error in aortographic technique resulting in inadequate radiographic contrast is the selection of an inadequate flow rate for contrast injection. This problem cannot be remedied by increasing the contrast dose. Proportionately lower flow rates are used

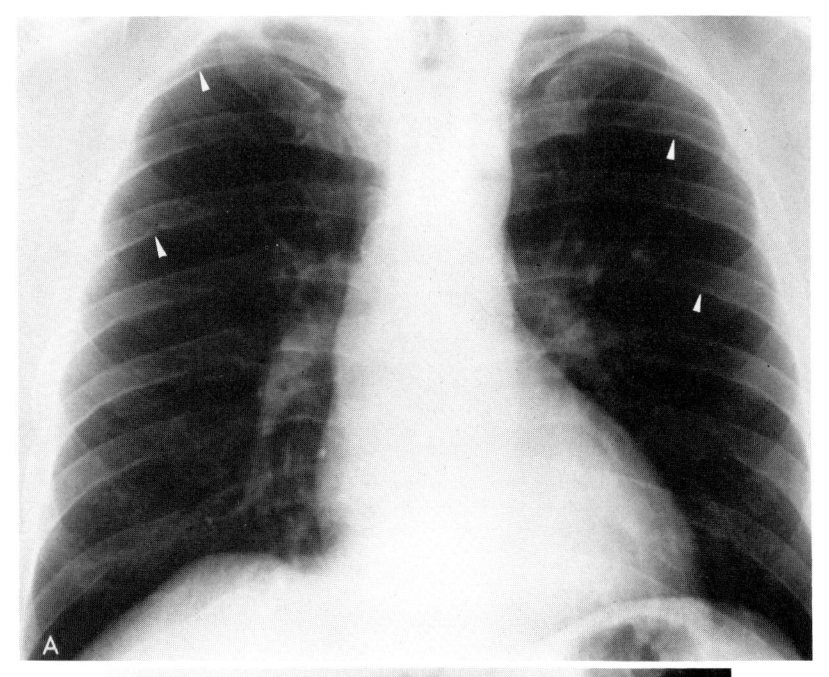

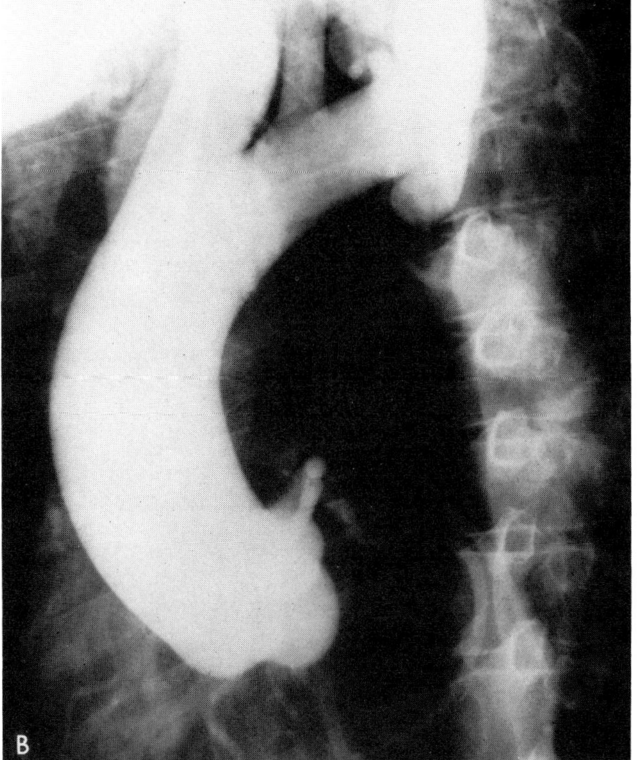

Figure 5–1. Coarctation of the aorta. *A*. Posteroanterior chest radiograph in a 39 year old man demonstrates a prominent ascending aorta, a small aortic knob with an enlarged left subclavian artery, a bulging descending aorta, and rib notching (arrows). *B*. Aortogram, right posterior oblique projection, early film, showing complete interruption of the aorta.

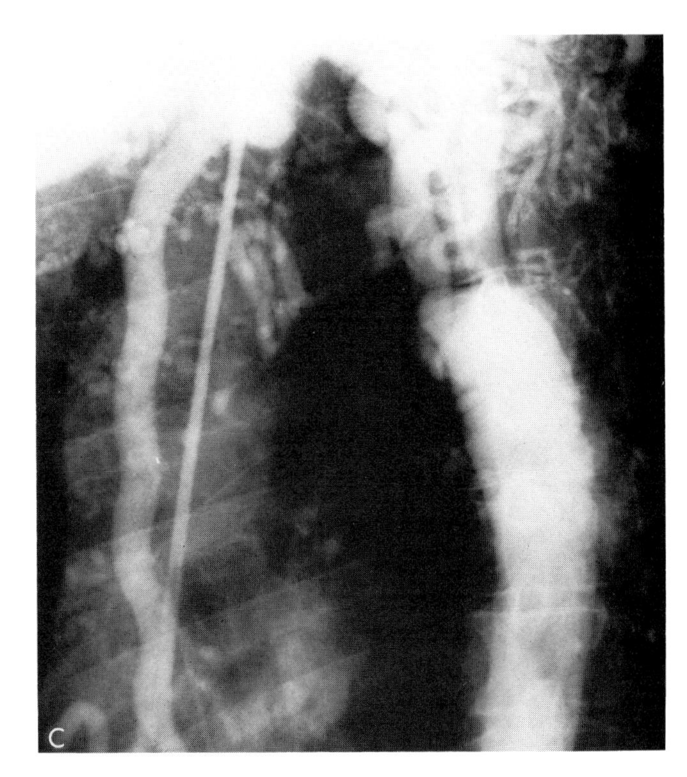

Figure 5–1 Continued. *C*. Later film from aortogram shows refilling of the descending aorta by collaterals.

for infants and young children. We have found a simple ratio of the body weight to that of an adult to be an entirely satisfactory method of estimating aortic flow and contrast injection rates in almost all circumstances.

A dose of 0.8 ml. per kg. body weight (with an upper limit of 80 ml.) will usually provide optimal opacification for a single injection. Total doses of 4 ml. per kg. body weight are usually well tolerated in the absence of severe renal disease or congestive heart failure, and generally serve as the upper limit in our hospital.

FILMING. Film changers covering an exposure area of 14 × 14 inches or 10 × 14 inches are generally satisfactory for aortography of adult patients. A repetition rate of 3 or 4 films per second is often necessary to adequately visualize the aorta. Normally we obtain 4 films per second for 2 seconds following injection of contrast medium, and then 2 films per second for 3 additional seconds. The later exposures may give important information about collateral and branch vessels.

Biplane filming provides the most satisfactory method of study, frequently obviating turning the patient into a different projection for additional examinations as well as shortening the duration of a procedure. In larger adults biplane examinations may be somewhat compromised owing to cross fogging of the films by scatter from the closely placed larger body. This problem may be partially alleviated by alternate firing of the biplane X-ray tubes (3 or 4 films per second are produced in each plane, while the changer moves at speeds of 6 or 8 films per second).

The 45° to 60° right posterior oblique projection is best for demonstrating the aortic arch and the major brachiocephalic branches, and is the primary view obtained in most studies. If biplane facilities are available, this view can be obtained in conjunction with a left posterior oblique projection. In studying possible anomalies of the aortic arch, we have found standard anteroposterior and lateral projections generally the most helpful.

Exposure times should be as short as practical for the generator and tube in use. An exposure of 0.025 second will usually produce diagnostic films in adult patients.

ANCILLARY EQUIPMENT. Continuous

oscilloscopic electrocardiographic monitoring of the patient is mandatory. Monitoring of catheter tip pressure provides an additional margin of safety. Insertion of a stable intravenous line before the procedure is strongly recommended, should prompt treatment of the patient become necessary. The angiographic room should be fully equipped to treat cardiorespiratory arrest.

COMPLICATIONS

One would expect thoracic aortography, like all catheter procedures involving the intravascular injection of contrast media, to cause some morbidity and mortality. The hazards of this study over a considerable period of time and by a variety of techniques have been extensively summarized, with a mortality ranging from 0.7 to 1.35 per cent.[1] In our institution, 321 patients (ages 14 to 89) were studied by percutaneous femoral or axillary aortography between 1971 and 1975. While there were three deaths within twenty-four hours of the procedure (0.9 per cent), two of these deaths were in patients with extensive aortic dissections with aortic insufficiency and renal failure, and the third patient expired when his ascending aortic aneurysm ruptured while the groin was being prepared for femoral artery puncture. There was one femoral artery thrombosis necessitating surgical embolectomy (0.3 per cent). No local complications occurred in 41 transaxillary catheterizations, despite that potential.[18]

COARCTATION OF AORTA

In most adults, the area of stenosis is situated at the aortic isthmus (site of the ligamentum arteriosum peripheral to the origin of the left subclavian artery). The type of surgical correction will often be influenced by the information obtained from aortography regarding the anatomy of the coarcted segment. Knowledge of the length and severity of the stenosis is extremely valuable (Figs. 5–1 and 5–2). The radiologist should realize that it is usually not possible to distinguish between severe constriction and complete interruption. Many apparently complete obstructions seen on aortography are actually anatomically moderate strictures. The ligamentum arteriosum binds the pre-stenotic segment forward, causing a kink and subsequent complete obstruction to blood flow as demonstrated on the aortogram. When the ligament is severed surgically, forward displacement of the aorta is relieved, and an absolute obstruction often becomes a moderate one. Other anatomic details important to ascertain are the width, length, and direction and degree of forward displacement of the aortic segments between the left carotid and left subclavian arteries and also between the left subclavian and the maximal area of stenosis.

While the ascending aorta may be normal, it is usually dilated, often quite markedly. The presence of aortic valve deformity and insufficiency should always be evaluated. When aortic regurgitation is present, it is usually mild and will commonly disappear after resection of the stenotic area.

The poststenotic segment of the descending aorta may be dilated, with incomplete stenosis producing the most severe expansion as the result of turbulence arising distal to the constriction. The most common and effective collateral pathway in adult coarctation is formed by the first pair of posterior intercostal arteries supplied by the subclavian arteries via the costocervical trunk. Longer collateral pathways include the internal mammary artery and lower intercostal arteries. If collaterals are lacking or very small, then the stenosis is of mild degree. The presence, size, and location of collaterals is important preoperative information.

PSEUDOCOARCTATION

In this condition, also called kinking of the aorta, the descending part of the aortic arch is angulated sharply forward, downward and to the right at the point of attachment of the ligamentum arteriosum. Proximal to this kink, the aortic arch rises high in the mediastinum.

This entity may simulate true coarctation of the aorta or a superior mediastinal mass on plain chest roentgenograms. The aortic knob may not be seen on the posteroanterior chest radiograph, and the trachea and

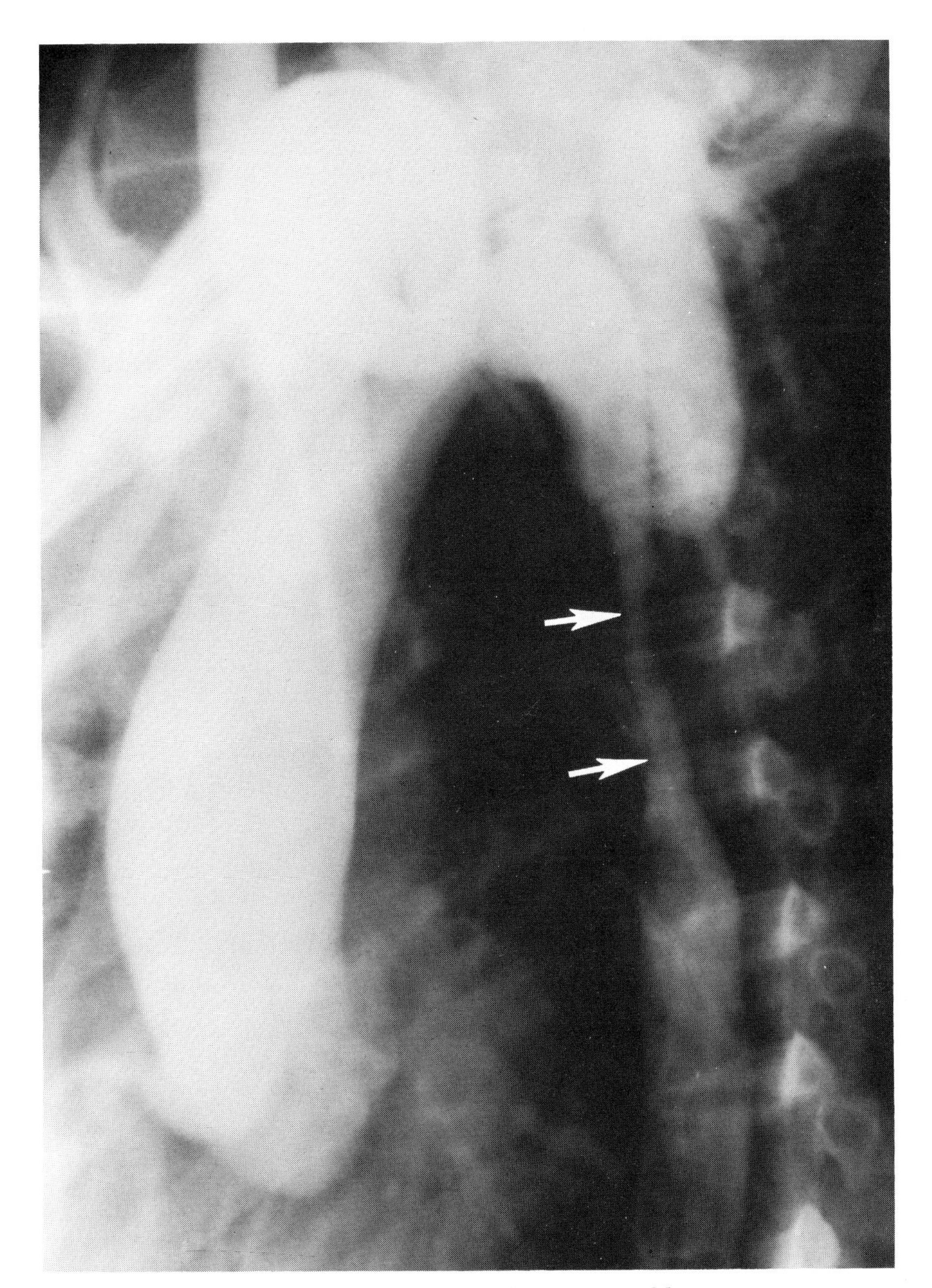

Figure 5–2. Coarctation of the aorta. Aortogram, right posterior oblique projection, in an asymptomatic 22 year old woman demonstrates a long coarcted segment beyond the left subclavian artery. A bicuspid aortic valve is present.

barium-filled esophagus may be displaced forward on lateral projection. No diminution in pressure or pulse in the lower extremities occurs, as the lesion has no hemodynamic significance, but a systolic ejection murmur may be present.[5]

While ultrasonography may be used as a non-invasive technique to make the diagnosis,[15] aortography with pressure measurements permits definitive diagnosis and excludes true luminal narrowing (Fig. 5–3).

This condition is felt to be due to an embryologic variation in development similar to true coarctation, and may have associated cardiovascular lesions, especially in children.[25]

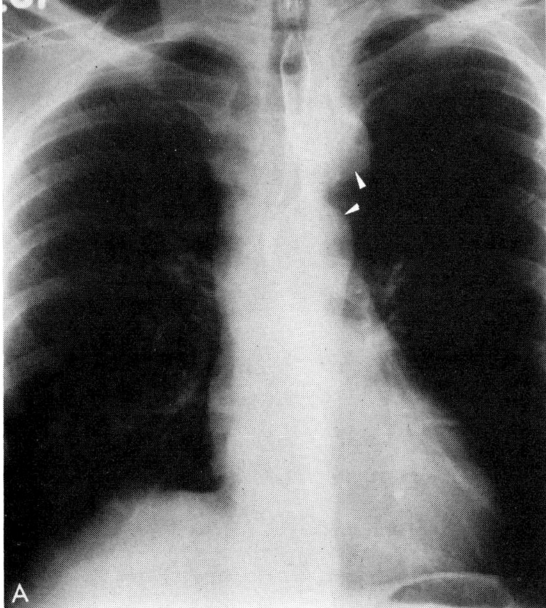

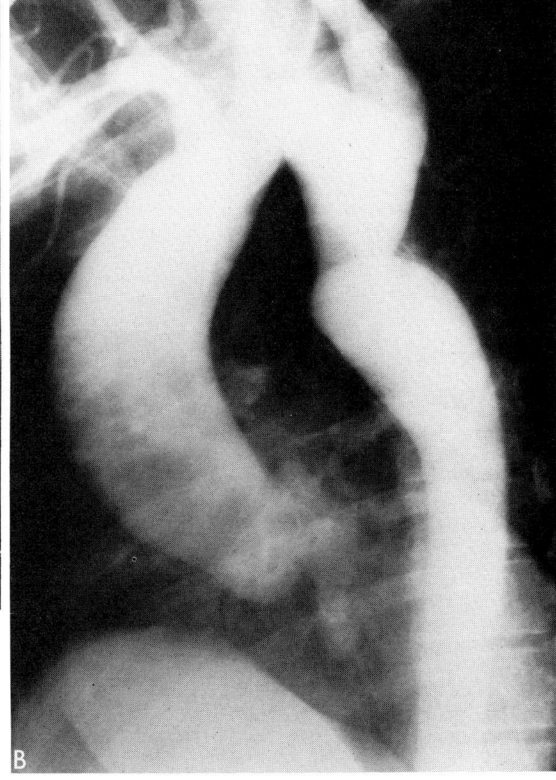

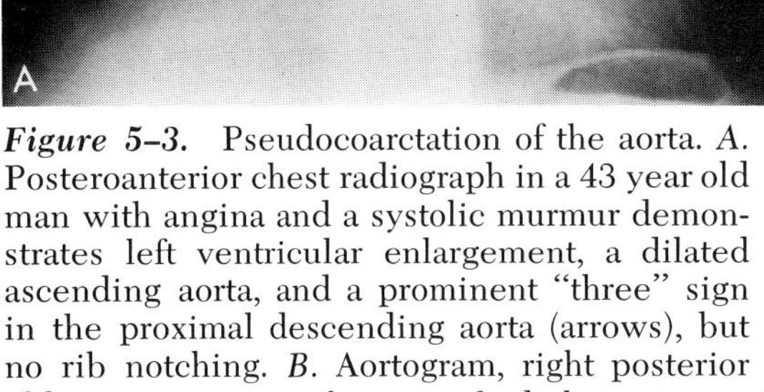

Figure 5–3. Pseudocoarctation of the aorta. *A.* Posteroanterior chest radiograph in a 43 year old man with angina and a systolic murmur demonstrates left ventricular enlargement, a dilated ascending aorta, and a prominent "three" sign in the proximal descending aorta (arrows), but no rib notching. *B.* Aortogram, right posterior oblique projection, shows marked elongation and bending of the aorta but no significant narrowing. No pressure gradient was present.

AORTIC ARCH ANOMALIES

Most vascular anomalies of the aortic arch do not disturb circulatory dynamics significantly and are asymptomatic. When symptoms are produced, they usually result from esophageal or tracheal obstruction. Complete plain film radiographic and fluoroscopic study of the aortic arch and its major branches in relation to the trachea and barium-filled esophagus usually suffices to identify the nature of the anomaly.[26] If the diagnosis is still uncertain or surgical treatment is considered, aortography permits specific anatomic definition of the anomaly. In the presence of double aortic arch, the patency and relative size of both arches may be established, permitting differentiation of vascular from ligamentous rings.[24] Although frequently not symptomatic (Fig. 5–4), the right aortic arch with retroesophageal aberrant left subclavian artery and left ductus ligament may produce dysphagia. Right aortic arches without an aberrant subclavian artery are rarely involved in ring syndromes, but have an extremely high incidence of associated congenital heart disease.

PULMONARY SEQUESTRATION

One or more anomalous branches of the aorta, usually the descending thoracic portion, supply the abnormal pulmonary tissue (usually lower lobe) that has been partially or completely separated from the normal bronchial tree. Suspicion of this entity is raised by the presence of an apparent paravertebral mass, pulmonary consolidation, or cystic changes in the lower lobes on plain chest roentgenograms, especially if the patient has a history of recurrent pulmonary infections. Aortography may be of value for definitive diagnosis or if surgical resection is contemplated (Fig. 7–2). Aberrant aortic branches may prove troublesome at surgery if there is no prior knowledge of their site or number, particularly if the anomalous arteries arise from the sub-

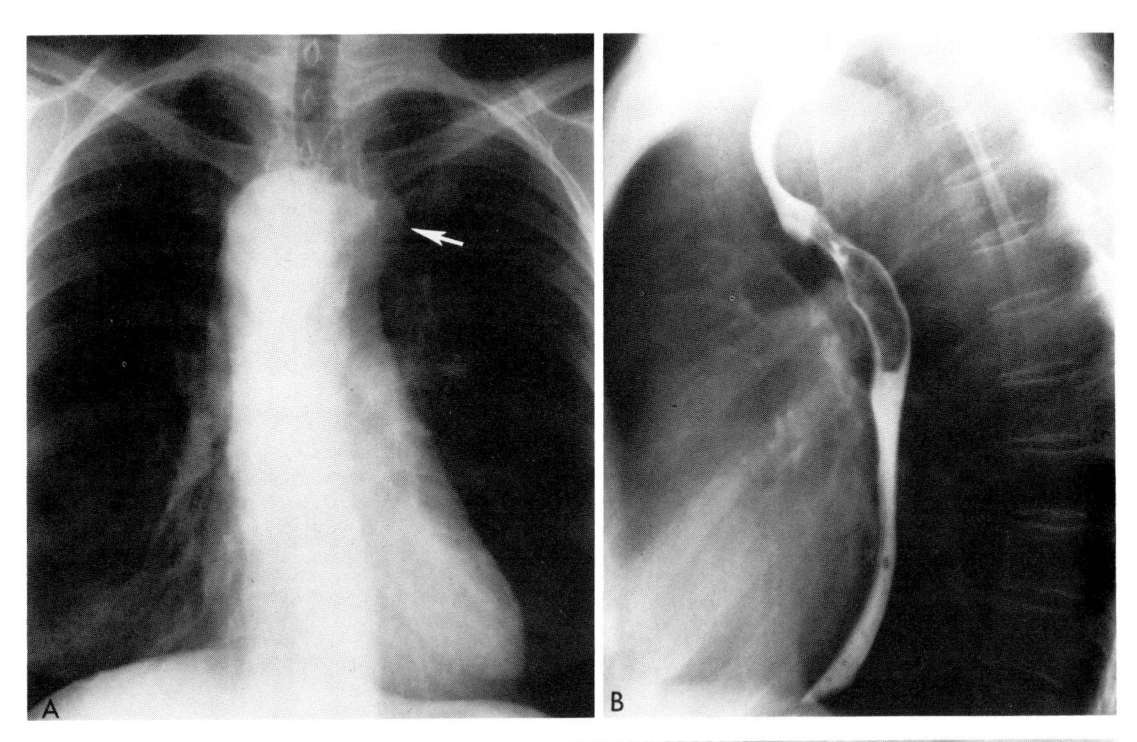

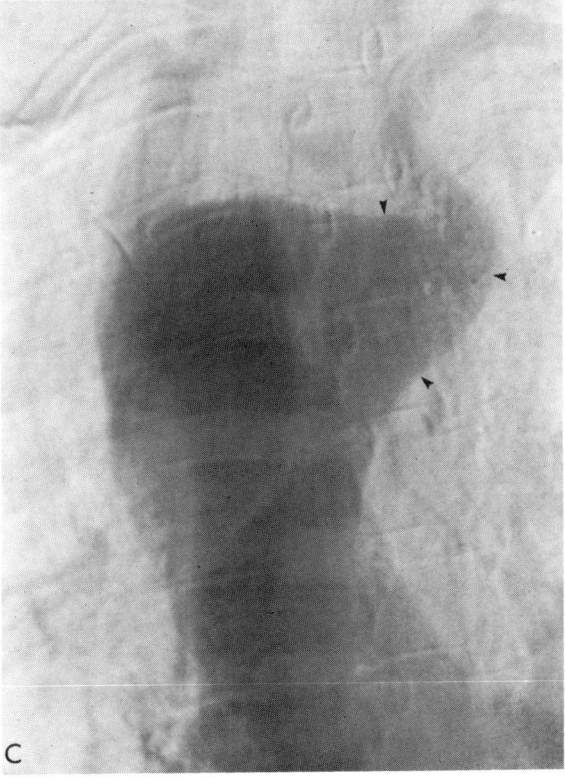

Figure 5–4. Right aortic arch with retroesophageal left subclavian artery and left ductus ligament. *A.* Posteroanterior chest radiograph in a 65 year old woman without symptoms of tracheal or esophageal obstruction shows enlargement of the large anomalous left subclavian root (arrow). *B.* Lateral chest radiograph demonstrates indentation of posterior aspect of barium-filled esophagus by aberrant left subclavian artery. *C.* Anteroposterior subtraction film from levophase of a pulmonary angiogram (performed to exclude pulmonary embolism) shows the dilated infundibulum of the retroesophageal left subclavian artery.

diaphragmatic aorta. The association with the scimitar syndrome and other congenital cardiac anomalies should be remembered.[21]

ANEURYSMS OF THE THORACIC AORTA

Diagnosis and appropriate treatment of thoracic aortic aneurysms is extremely important because of an eventual mortality of 30 to 50 per cent with these lesions. An aortic aneurysm often can be suspected from the plain chest radiograph. The value of fluoroscopic pulsations to distinguish aneurysms from solid mediastinal masses has been greatly overrated in our opinion. Calcification in the margin of a mediastinal mass strongly suggests an aneurysm, but is

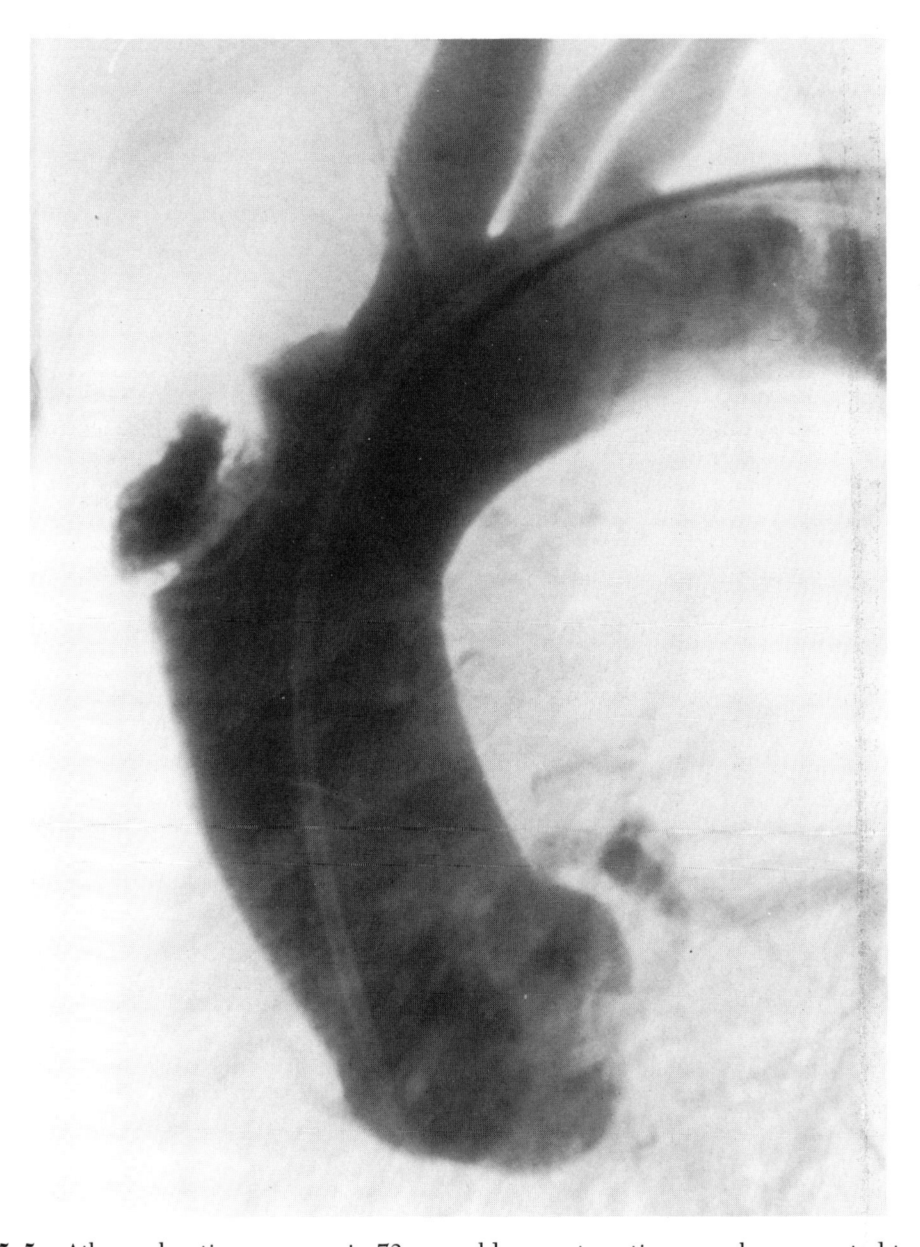

Figure 5–5. Atherosclerotic aneurysm in 72 year old asymptomatic man who was noted to have an anterior bulge in the ascending aorta on a lateral chest roentgenogram. Subtraction film, aortogram, right posterior oblique view, demonstrates an aneurysm of the ascending aorta with mural clot formation. While the patient's serology was positive, pathologic examination of the resected specimen was most consistent with an atherosclerotic aneurysm.

not pathognomonic, as mediastinal tumors or cysts may demonstrate peripheral calcification.

Aortography not only can definitively distinguish between aneurysm and other mediastinal masses, but is of value in determining the exact morphology of an obvious aneurysm when surgical management is contemplated. The relationship of the brachiocephalic vessels and surrounding structures to the aneurysm can be ascertained, as well as the detection of early aneurysm formation elsewhere in the aorta.

ATHEROSCLEROTIC ANEURYSMS. Atherosclerosis is the commonest cause of thoracic aortic aneurysm (Fig. 5–5). Generally, these aneurysms are easily detectable on plain chest roentgenograms. Although occasionally they may remain unchanged for long periods of time, their stability cannot be predicted and they represent a potential threat to the patient's life.[16]

LUETIC ANEURYSMS. The incidence of aneurysms due to syphilis has decreased markedly in recent years. These lesions carry a grave prognosis, the average time from appearance of symptoms to death being 6 months. Luetic aneurysms can involve any portion of the thoracic aorta (Figs. 5–6 and 5–7), sometimes in multiple sites.

Differentiation of luetic from atherosclerotic aneurysm on radiographic grounds alone is often impossible (Fig. 5–5). Certainly the presence or location of calcification is no help.[13]

MYCOTIC ANEURYSMS. These aneurysms are rarely seen in the aorta since the advent of widespread antibiotic use. They most commonly occur engrafted upon atherosclerotic aneurysms in elderly patients, with *Salmonella* being the most frequent causative organism. Radiologic findings are indistinguishable from aneurysms of other etiologies. The diagnosis may be suggested when fever and chills accompany a rapidly enlarging aneurysm. Prognosis is dismal.

CYSTIC MEDIAL NECROSIS. Most cases occur in Marfan's syndrome or a forme fruste of this disease. Aortography classically reveals aneurysmal dilatation of the aorta starting at the annulus and extending upward, usually to a point just proximal to the innominate artery, but sometimes into the arch.[4] Aortic regurgitation is frequently present (Fig. 5–8). The cardiovascular changes in this condition may be seen relatively early in life (Fig. 5–9). Incompetence of the atrioventricular valves may also be present in this connective tissue disorder.

AORTIC DISSECTION

Various disease processes causing degeneration of the arterial media may ultimately result in aortic dissection. Etiologies include arteriosclerosis, genetic predisposition (cystic medial necrosis associated with Marfan's syndrome or a forme fruste of the disease), giant cell aortitis, syphilis, and coarctation of the aorta.

Dissection is initiated by rupture of the vasa vasorum into the aortic media, with the resultant medial hematoma progressing to longitudinal cleavage of the media. The hematoma usually dissects distally, but may also go proximally. In most cases the medial hematoma communicates with the aortic lumen through intimal perforation, often in two sites (so-called "entry" and "re-entry").[12] The ascending aorta 1 to 2 cm. superior to the aortic valve cusps is the initial site of the dissection in two thirds of cases: the aorta just distal to the left subclavian artery is the site in one third[7] (Table 5–1). The dissection usually involves a localized area of the aorta but sometimes may extend around the entire aortic circumference.[12] Most often, dissections are located on the anterolateral aspect on the right side in the ascending aorta, superiorly in the aortic arch, and on the posterolateral aspect on the left side in the descending thoracic aorta.[3]

The terms "aortic dissection" and "dissecting hematoma" are preferable to "dissecting aneurysm." In some cases the medial hematoma (false lumen) is so thin that no aneurysm is present. Only when the medial hematoma becomes quite large is the resultant false aneurysm recognizable on plain chest roentgenograms. Also, the term "dissecting aneurysm" is misleading because it suggests that dissection starts from a pre-existing aneurysm, which is usually true only of cases secondary to cystic medial necrosis. In the majority of cases the true lumen is not dilated but actually compressed by the false lumen; the true lumen may remain wider than normal in

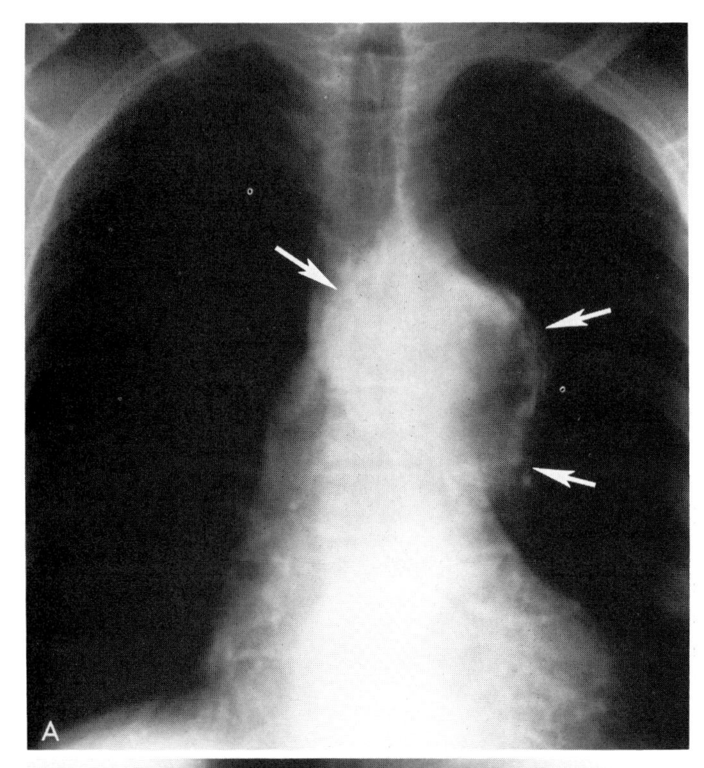

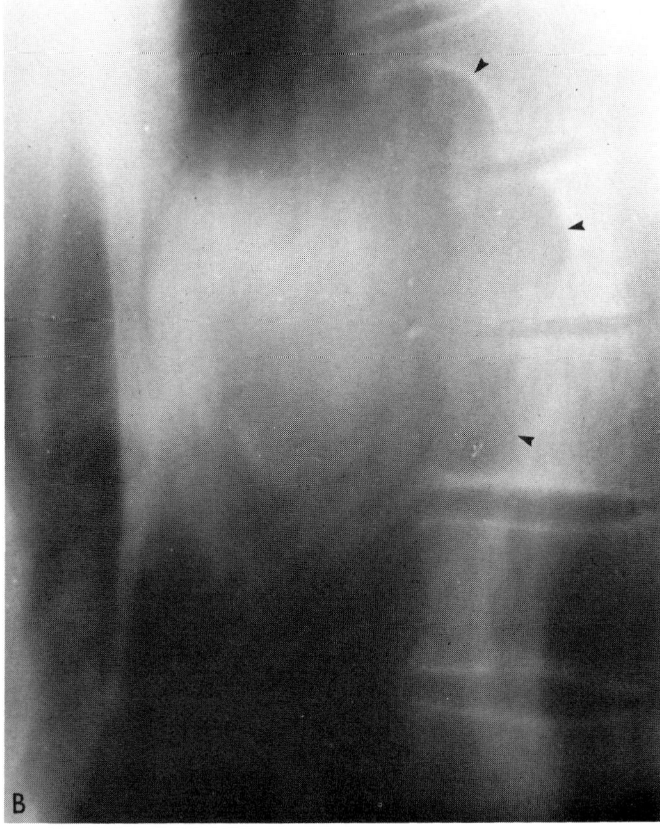

Figure 5–6. Luetic aortitis. *A*. Posteroanterior chest radiograph in a 59 year old man with back pain and a history of syphilis demonstrates a calcified aneurysmal aorta (arrows). *B*. Lateral thoracic spine laminogram shows extensive bone erosion (arrows).

Legend continued on the opposite page

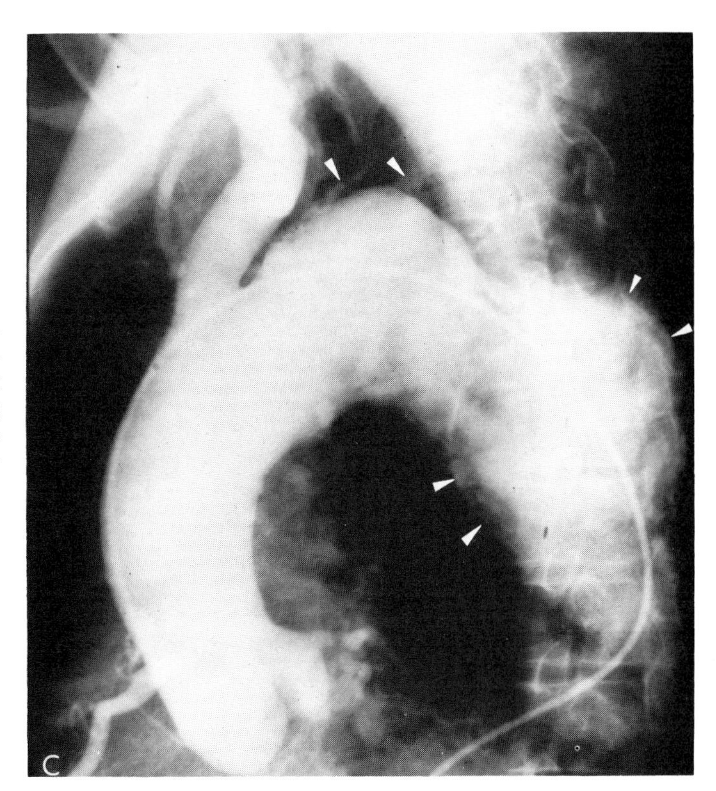

Figure 5–6 Continued. *C.* Aortogram, right posterior oblique projection, shows aneurysmal involvement of the arch and proximal descending aorta (4 arrows), with occlusion of the left carotid and left subclavian arteries (2 arrows).

cases due to pre-existing cystic medial necrosis.

The diagnosis of aortic dissection can be a serious problem, as classic symptoms may not occur. Plain chest roentgenography may be suggestive. Local dilatation of a portion of the aorta or widening of the superior mediastinum may be seen. These findings assume especial importance if there has been a change in configuration in comparison to previous radiographs. If the aortic intima is calcified, measurement of the thickness of the aortic wall can be done. Roentgenographic measurements over 6 mm. suggest thickening of the wall and support the diagnosis (Fig. 5–10), but many pitfalls exist in the application of this sign since the calcification may not be in the lateral intimal wall and causes other than dissection may apparently "thicken" the aortic wall.[19]

As advances in hypotensive and surgical therapy have greatly improved the dismal prognosis of untreated cases, angiographic study of the aorta and its branches has assumed a major role in confirming the diagnosis and clarifying the anatomy of the particular dissection.

TECHNIQUE. Aortography in suspected dissection is generally performed by using a retrograde femoral artery approach, assuming a good femoral pulse is present. A precaution taken is that only guide wires or catheters with J-shaped tips are advanced proximally. If femoral pulses are absent, an axillary artery approach is utilized. Intravenous aortography is rarely if ever used at our hospital.

The initial contrast injection is into the ascending aorta, usually with biplane filming (simultaneous anteroposterior and lateral projections or right and left posterior oblique views). Complete study usually requires visualization of the aorta from its root down to the bifurcation of the iliac arteries (Figs. 5–10 and 5–11). Important information necessary for possible surgical management of patients with dissection includes the location of the initial dissection, the site of any subsequent re-entry from the false lumen, evaluation of aortic valve competence, coronary, arch and vis-

Text continued on page 134

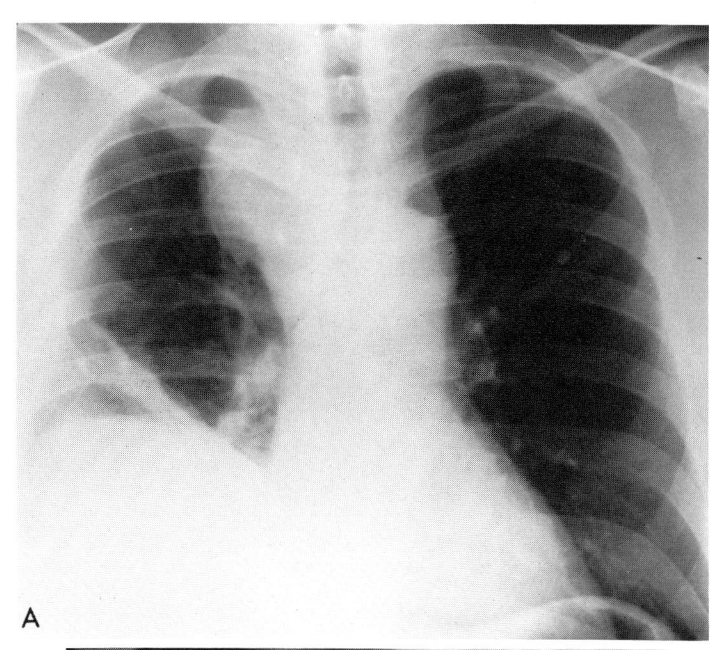

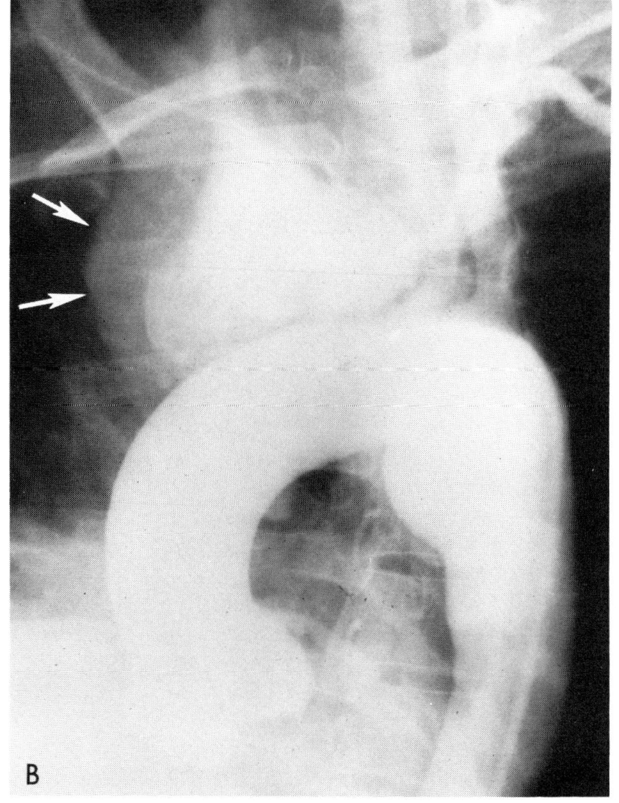

Figure 5–7. Luetic aortitis in a 42 year old man who had a recent thoracotomy at another hospital because of a suspected malignant tumor on a chest radiograph. *A.* Posteroanterior chest roentgenogram demonstrates postoperative changes in the right hemithorax, a paralyzed right hemidiaphragm due to phrenic nerve injury, and a large right paratracheal mass. *B.* Aortogram, right posterior oblique view, shows a large aneurysm of the root of the innominate artery surrounded by a soft tissue mass (arrows). The soft tissue mass in this case was due to 2 cm. thick laminar thrombus, although a similar density may simply represent the laterally displaced innominate vein and superior vena cava. Pathologic examination was consistent with luetic etiology.

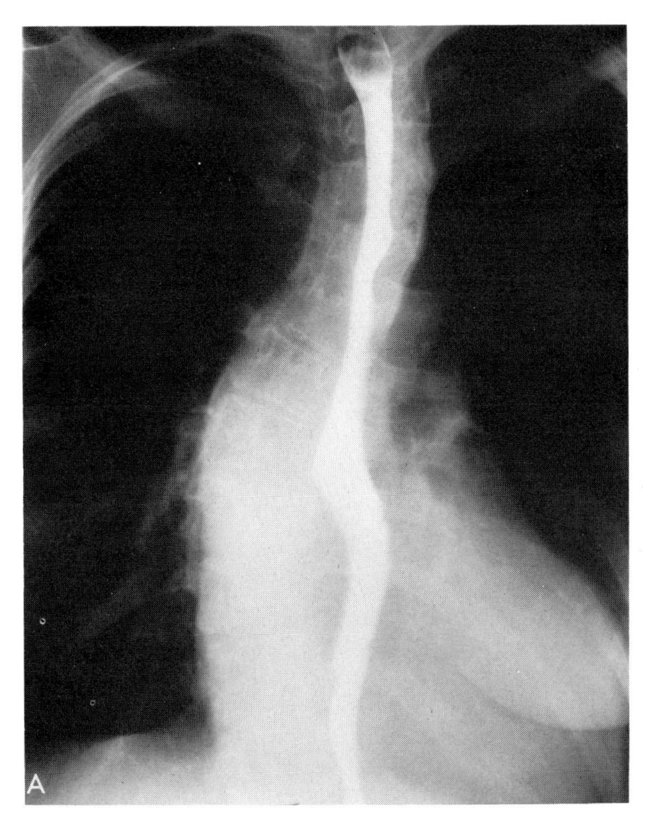

Figure 5–8. Cystic medial necrosis. *A*. Posteroanterior chest radiograph in a 39 year old woman with Marfan's syndrome and murmur of aortic regurgitation shows scoliosis and left ventricular enlargement.

Illustration and legend continued on the following page

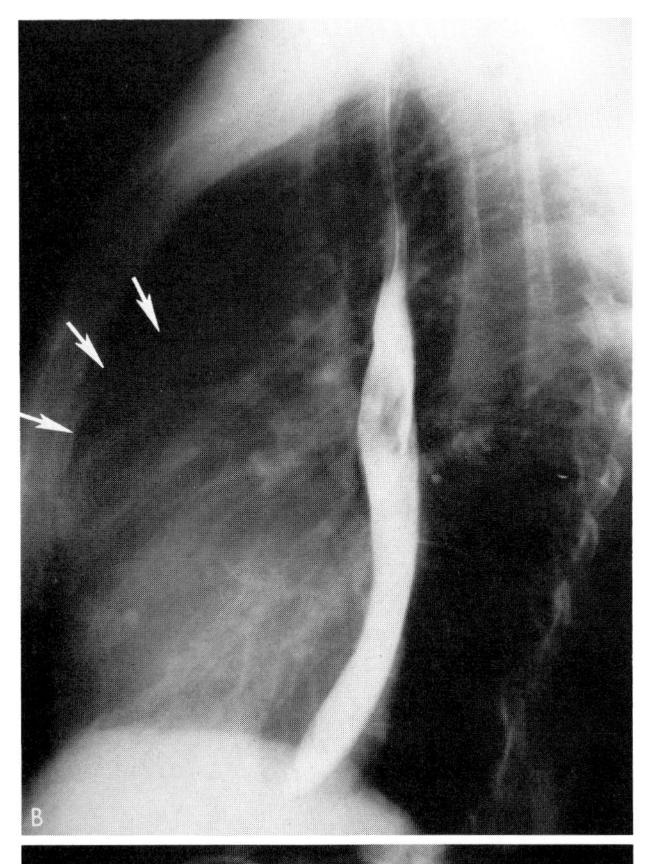

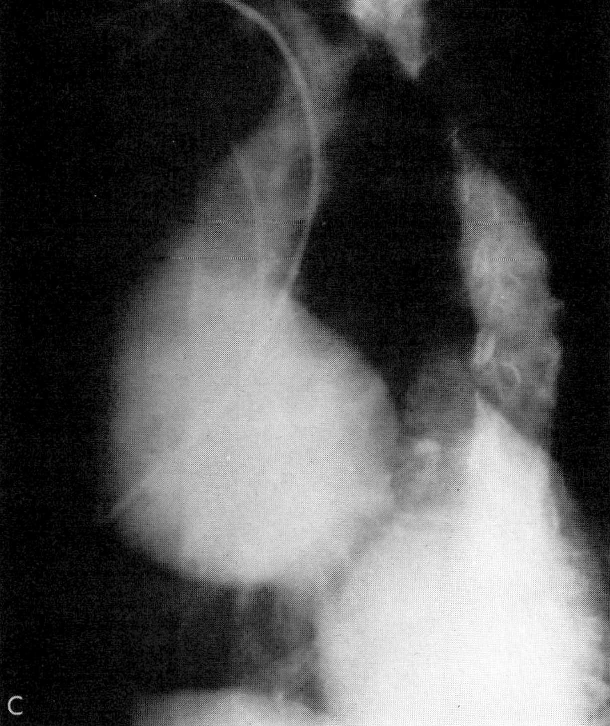

Figure 5–8 Continued. *B.* Lateral chest radiograph demonstrates dilated ascending aorta filling the retrosternal space (arrows). *C.* Aortogram, right posterior oblique view, shows massive enlargement of the aortic root with severe aortic regurgitation.

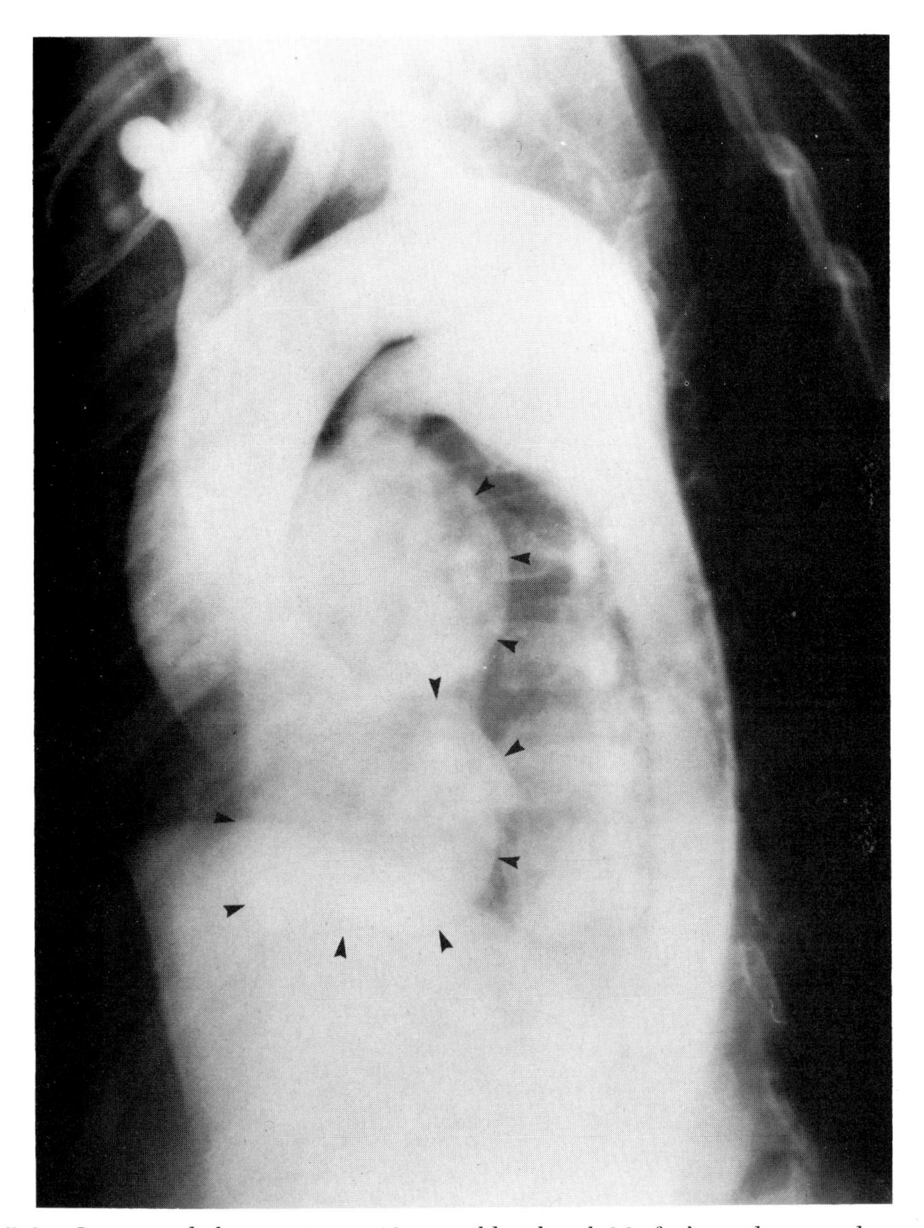

Figure 5–9. Cystic medial necrosis in a 10 year old girl with Marfan's syndrome and murmur consistent with patent ductus. Aortogram, right posterior oblique projection, demonstrates early dilatation of both the aortic and pulmonary roots (arrows). No valvular insufficiency is present. Aneurysmal dilatation of the aorta at the site of the patent ductus is shown.

TABLE 5–1. Classification of Aortic Dissection*

Type I	Dissection begins in ascending aorta and extends across the aortic arch to the descending aorta, often down to the iliac arteries (most common).
Type II	Dissection limited to ascending aorta (usually seen in cystic medial necrosis).
Type III	Dissection begins distal to left subclavian artery and extends a variable distance.

*Modified from DeBakey, M. E., Henly, W. S., Cooley, D. A., Morris, G. C., Jr., Crawford, E. S., and Beall, A. C., Jr.: Surgical management of dissecting aneurysms of the aorta. J. Thorac. Cardiovasc. Surg., 49:130–149, 1965.

ceral artery origins, and the lower extent of the dissection. Surgical treatment has been advocated with massive aortic valve insufficiency, continued severe pain (suggesting impending rupture), uncontrollable hemorrhage, and occlusion of major vessels.[7]

It is not particularly rare for the catheter to enter the false lumen. If backflow through the catheter is satisfactory and rapid dispersal of hand-injected contrast medium occurs, angiography can be safely performed in this location. When false luminal opacification is recognized on the initial set of films, the catheter should be withdrawn and then re-advanced in an attempt to enter the true lumen. If this is impossible, a second puncture into the opposite femoral artery or axillary artery should be performed. Aortic insufficiency may be present and not recognized if injection is into the false lumen.

FINDINGS. The aortographic findings in aortic dissection are listed in Table 5–2.

The demonstration of both false and true channels within the opacified aorta is the hallmark of aortic dissection (Fig. 5–12). Without this finding, a diagnosis of aortic dissection is subject to error unless there is clear-cut compression of the opacified aortic lumen. Double channels can be recognized when a thin radiolucency (torn or separated intima and inner media) is seen separating the two channels; the two channels are opacified in different density or timing; or catheterization of each lumen is accomplished and contrast medium is injected separately.[12]

Simultaneous and equal opacification of both true and false lumina could be a cause of false negative diagnosis. Under these circumstances, the two lumina will appear as one, and only a diagnosis of aortic dilatation will be made.[3, 12] The linear radiolucency representing the torn intima and media will be seen only when it is tangential to the X-ray beam. This factor constitutes a strong argument for biplane filming in cases of questionable dissection. Also, during pressure injection the catheter will recoil and abut against the outer wall of the ascending aorta and aortic arch. When dissection is present, the separated intima and media do not allow the catheter to recoil to the outer wall of the aorta. Thus, an abnormal catheter position in which the catheter during injection is more than 4 mm. from the outer opacified lumen in the distal ascending aortic arch (especially as noted on the lateral projection) is strong suggestive evidence of dissection should simultaneous opacification of the true and false lumina occur.[6]

The so-called site of entry (most proximal intimal tear) is sometimes clearly identified by contrast media passing from one lumen to another (usually true to false) (Fig. 5–12B) and rarely by the catheter passing through the intimal tear. Generally, it is reasonable to consider that the tear is located in the most proximal portion of the demonstrated dissection when it cannot clearly be seen.[3]

The false lumen may not be opacified when it is filled with blood clot, the intimal tear is located more distal than the area filmed, and the dissection has proceeded proximally and distally, or when there is no intimal tear.[12] In these circumstances, narrowing of the opacified lumen and thickening of the aortic wall may be the major aortographic findings of dissection. It should be emphasized that aortic wall thickening alone is a reliable criterion of dissection only when a relatively long segment of the aorta (particularly the descending thoracic portion) is involved. Excessive application of this sign will result in some false-positive diagnoses, since apparent thickening of the wall may be due to causes other than dissection, including severe atherosclerosis or clot within an atherosclerotic aneurysm, mediastinal hematoma from any etiology, neoplasm or fat along the aortic wall, or aortitis.[19] Aortic wall thickness should not

Text continued on page 139

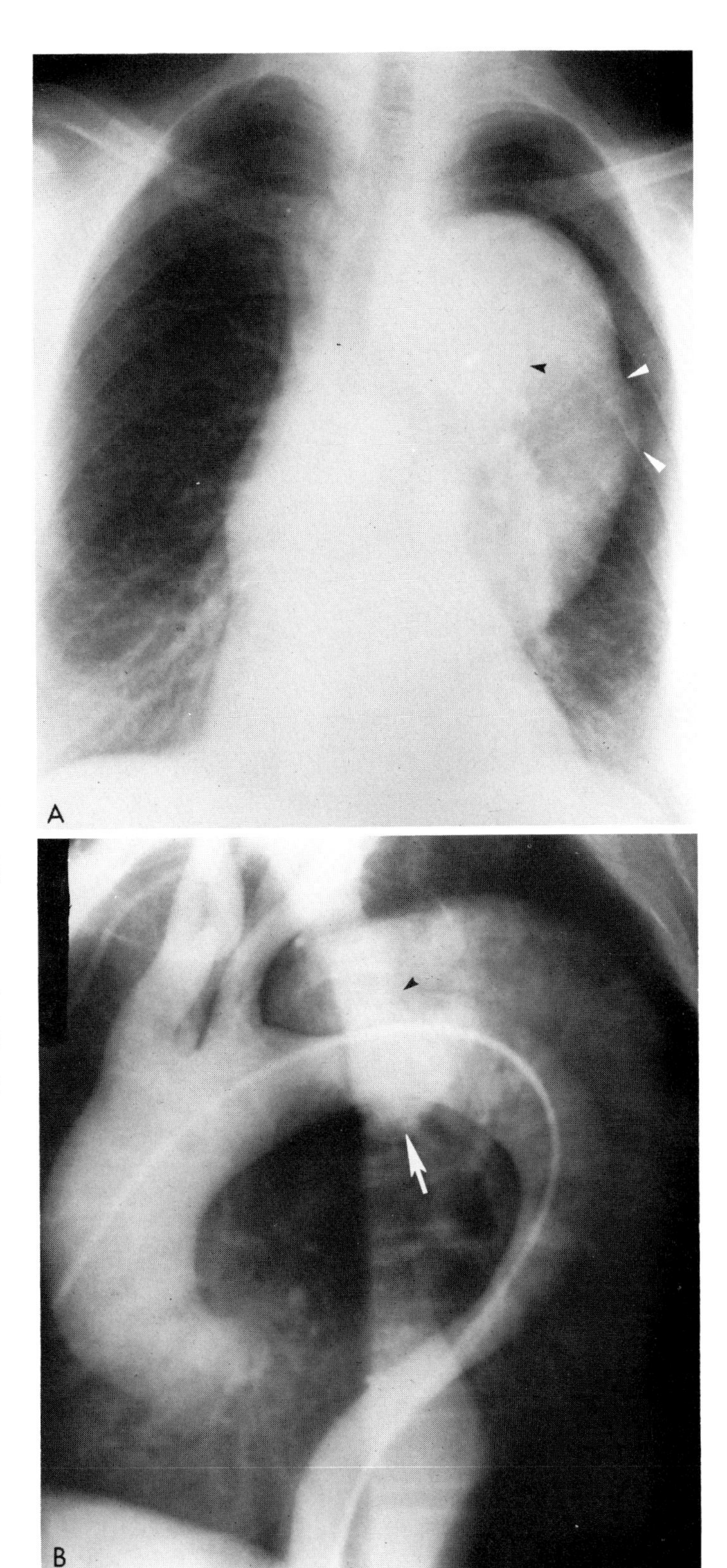

Figure 5–10. Aortic dissection. *A.* Posteroanterior chest radiograph in a 67 year old woman with recent onset of sudden severe chest pain shows a large aortic mass with an irregular left border (white arrows). The mass extends well beyond calcification in the aortic intima (black arrow). *B.* Aortogram, steep right posterior oblique view, shows a dissection starting just beyond the left subclavian artery, with a portion of the false lumen projecting circumferentially inferior to the true lumen (white arrow) as well as superiorly. The thin radiolucent intima and media separating the two channels more distally is seen beginning at the black arrow.

Illustration and legend continued on the following page

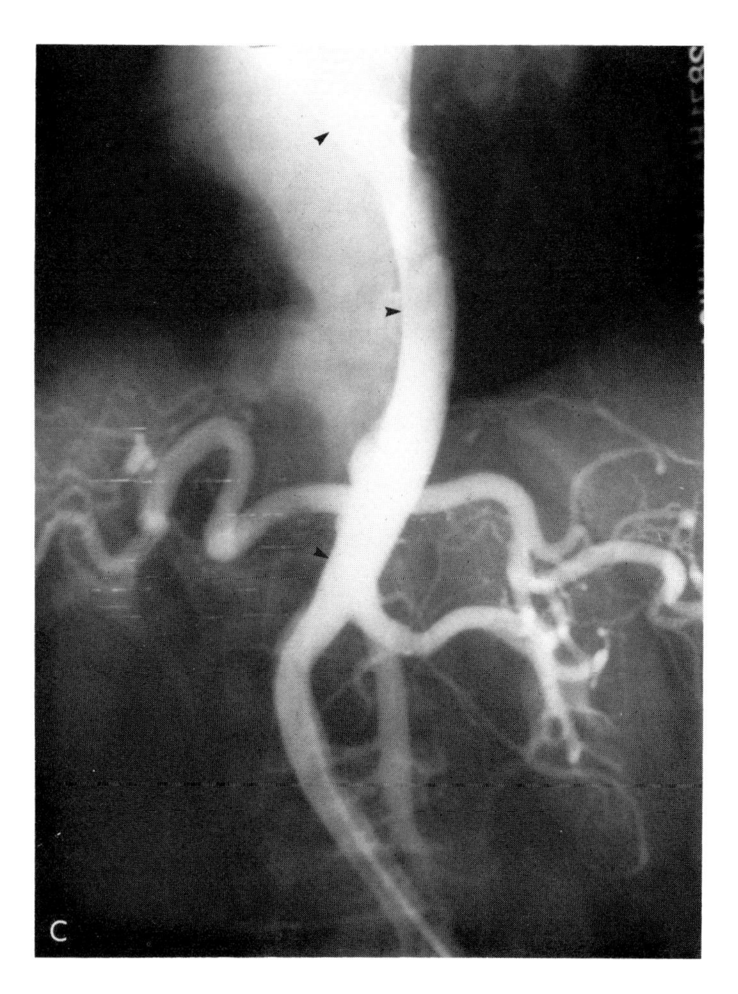

Figure 5–10 Continued. *C.* Abdominal aortogram, anteroposterior view, shows extension of the dissection into the abdominal aorta with narrowing of the true lumen (arrows) and no filling of the right renal or iliac arteries.

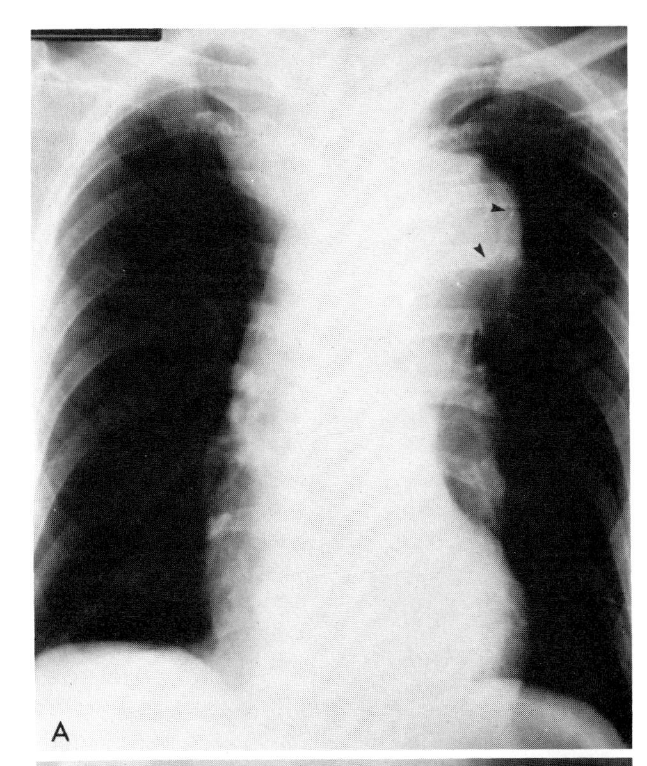

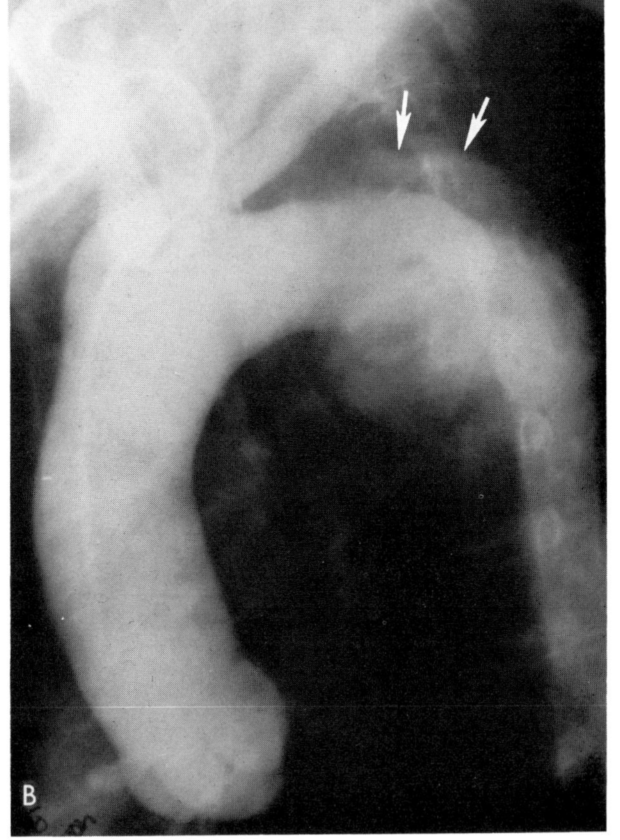

Figure 5–11. Aortic dissection. *A.* Posteroanterior chest radiograph in a 68 year old man with sudden onset of severe chest pain and neck swelling shows widening of the superior mediastinum. Enlargement of the aorta is present, with the lateral margin of the descending portion extending well beyond the intimal calcification (arrows). *B.* Aortogram, right posterior oblique view, demonstrates a large dissection starting distal to the left subclavian artery (arrows). Some extravasation of contrast media into the mediastinum was noted.

Illustration and legend continued on the following page

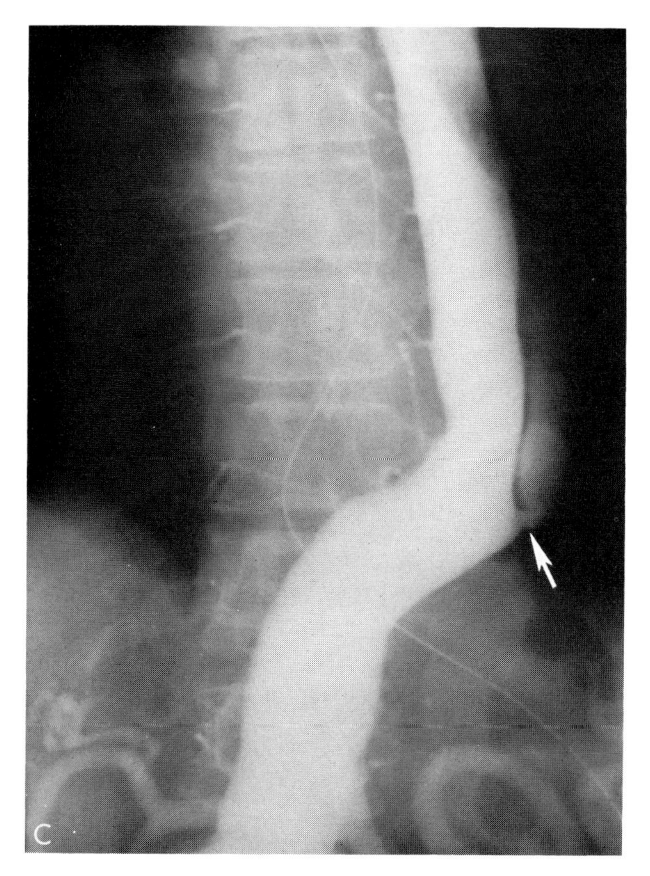

Figure 5–11 *Continued. C.* Thoracolumbar aortogram, anteroposterior projection, shows re-entry of false lumen into true lumen (arrow) at level of diaphragm.

TABLE 5–2. Aortographic Findings in Aortic Dissection

1. Opacification of false lumen.
2. Identification of faint radiolucent septum between the two channels.
3. Narrowing of the opacified true lumen by the false lumen.
4. Catheter does not hug the wall of aorta during injection.
5. Thickening of extraluminal soft tissue (aortic wall) about the opacified true lumen by greater than 6 mm.
6. Occlusion or narrowing of side branches.

be measured in the ascending aorta, as normal mediastinal structures or fat can produce factitious widening.[3, 19]

Opacification of the false lumen may have prognostic value. In one series, opacification of the false lumen was associated with a 43 per cent survival, whereas a 90 per cent survival occurred when no opacification of the false channel was seen.[8]

Branch arteries from the aorta may be narrowed or occluded, often appearing as "ulcer-like" projections from the true lumen.[12] If a renal artery is not opacified, a delayed abdominal film may be of value to determine whether the kidney is functioning (implying arterial supply from the false lumen).

TRAUMATIC INJURY

Non-penetrating injuries of the thoracic aorta usually result from rapid deceleration in vehicular accidents. While the minimal lesion that can occur is a transverse intimal tear, most surviving patients sustain circumferential tears of both the intima and media. Massive fatal hemorrhage may be prevented because the adventitia and mediastinal connective tissue contain the bleeding, forming a false aneurysm.[10] It has been estimated that about 10 per cent of patients survive acute rupture of the aorta temporarily owing to pseudoaneurysm formation, but the majority of these patients will die within three weeks from a secondary hemorrhage if untreated.[14] Approximately 3 per cent of these patients may live long enough to develop a chronic aneurysm.[22] Sites of traumatic tears are the relatively mobile portions of the aorta near points of fixation. Ninty-five per cent of patients surviving the immediate injury sustain damage to the aorta in the region of the aortic isthmus (site of the ligamentum arteriosum), with the remaining 5 per cent occurring just above the aortic valve.[22]

Prompt recognition of this injury is important, because the local nature of the damage is generally amenable to surgical repair.[20] Clinical findings which should lead to suspicion of the diagnosis of aortic tear include chest pain, shock, different or elevated blood pressure in an upper extremity, or a harsh systolic murmur over the precordium or interscapular area. Dysphagia or respiratory distress may result from compression of the esophagus or tracheobronchial tree by the mediastinal hematoma. The most common plain chest roentgenographic finding is mediastinal widening (Fig. 5–13A). But because the radiograph is often performed in the supine position with a short focal-film distance, the mediastinum may be difficult to evaluate. Other more suggestive plain film findings include a localized mass or distortion of the normal contour about the aortic arch, depression and deviation of the left main stem bronchus to the right, widening of the paraspinal line, and left pleural effusion (hemothorax).[22] Rib fractures, especially of the upper three ribs, may occur in 50 per cent of patients.[14]

However, not all patients with clinical or plain chest radiographic evidence consistent with a mediastinal hematoma have aortic rupture. Such findings may follow tear of smaller arteries or veins, and aortography is mandatory for definitive diagnosis. We prefer the retrograde femoral artery approach, but only advance a guide wire or catheter with a J-shaped end through the injured area. If difficulty is encountered advancing a guide wire or catheter past the aortic isthmus the femoral approach is abandoned, and retrograde right axillary artery entry is used. The aortographic appearance of aortic tear ranges from slight irregularity in contour of the aortic isthmus, to slight fusiform widening just distal to the arch, to a large saccular false aneurysm (Fig. 5–13B). A sharply defined linear defect, produced by protrusion of the transected intima and media into the opacified lumen, may sometimes be seen at the proximal or distal margin of the aneurysm.[22] Because most traumatic aneurysms occur in the area of the aortic

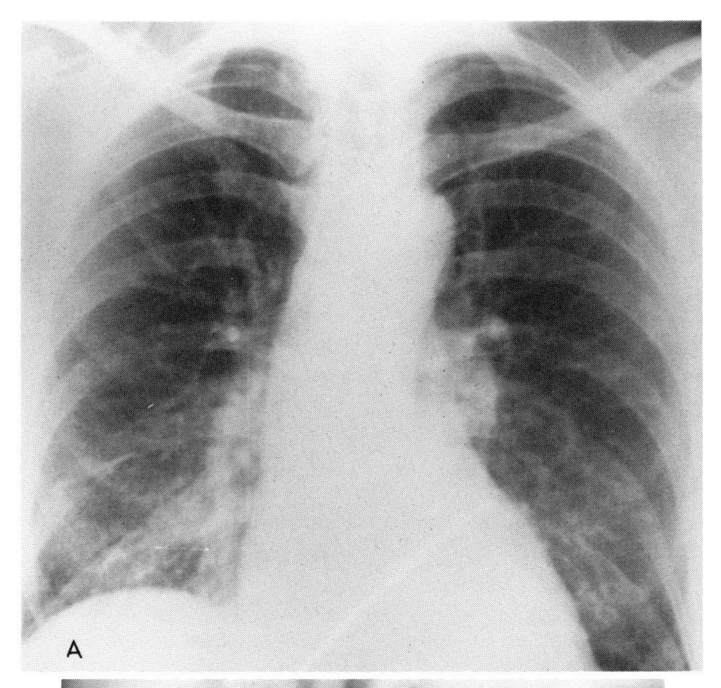

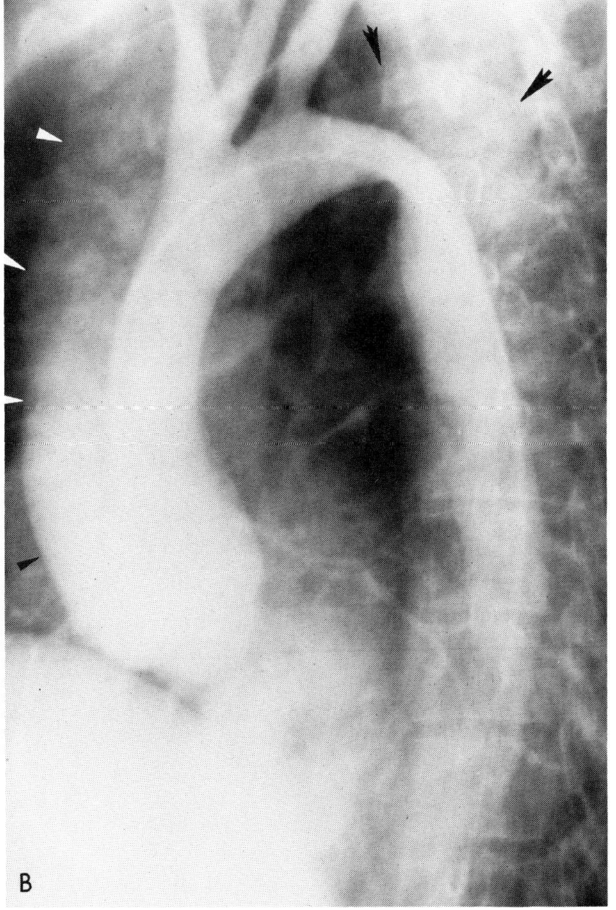

Figure 5–12. Aortic dissection. *A.* Posteroanterior chest radiograph in a 48 year old hypertensive man with sudden severe chest pain shows some mild left ventricular enlargement. The aortic shadow is unremarkable. No change had occurred from a roentgenogram performed eight years before. *B.* Aortogram, right posterior oblique projection, during ventricular systole demonstrates a dissection starting just above the aortic cusps with some opacification of the false lumen (arrows) and mild aortic regurgitation.

Legend continued on the opposite page

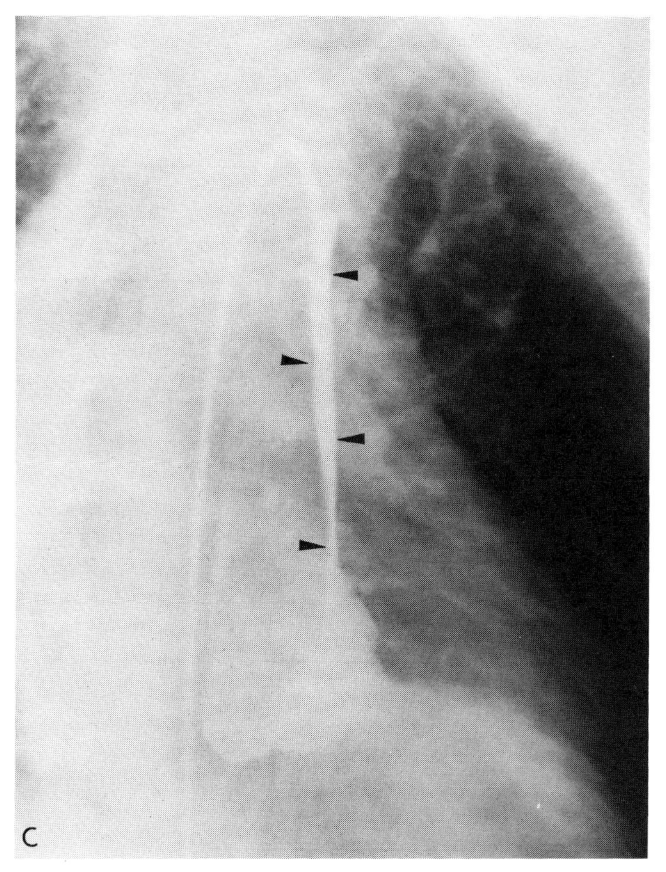

Figure 5-12 Continued. *C.* Aortogram, biplane left posterior oblique view, during ventricular diastole demonstrates narrowing of the true lumen by the blood-filled false lumen.

isthmus, aortic insufficiency is rarely found.

Nonpenetrating trauma may result in tears in the innominate or subclavian arteries as well as in the aorta.[2,9] The plain chest radiographic findings are similar, and aortography is necessary to show the site(s) and extent of such vascular injuries. Bulbous dilatation of the great vessel is seen just distal to its origin, often associated with a thin lucent line across its base.

Traumatic aneurysms secondary to penetrating wounds of the thorax (Fig. 5-14) are much less common because laceration through the adventitia and adjacent tissues usually results in immediate fatal hemorrhage.

AORTIC ARCH SYNDROME

A nonspecific inflammatory disease of unknown etiology (Takayasu's disease, giant cell arteritis) may involve the great vessels arising from the arch. While the brachiocephalic arteries are predominantly involved, any artery with an elastic media may be affected. This disease has a predilection for young women, especially Orientals.

The early pathologic changes consist of inflammatory cell infiltration (lymphocytes, plasma cells, giant cells) of the arterial wall. Nonspecific systemic symptoms may occur in this phase, including fever, night sweats, pleuritis, abdominal pain, and skin rash.[17] Later, intimal proliferation and superimposed thrombosis may result in arterial stenosis or obstruction. Where the muscle and elastic lamina in the media are destroyed, dilatation and aneurysm formation take place.[11] Late symptoms are a reflection of the arterial area involved, consisting of various ischemic manifestations. Brachiocephalic arteritides may result in cerebral, ocular, or upper extremity symptoms.

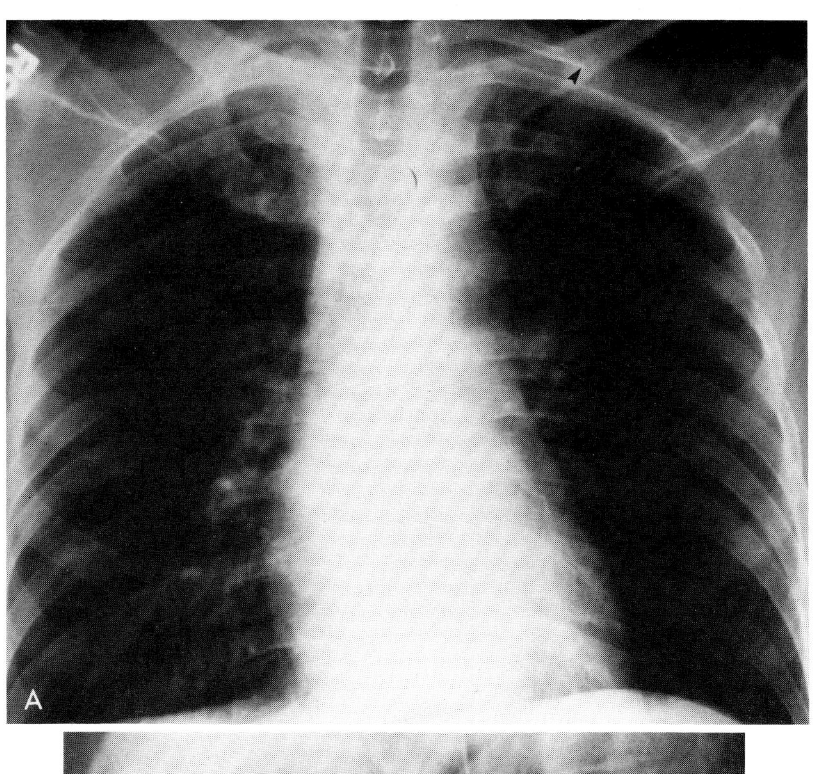

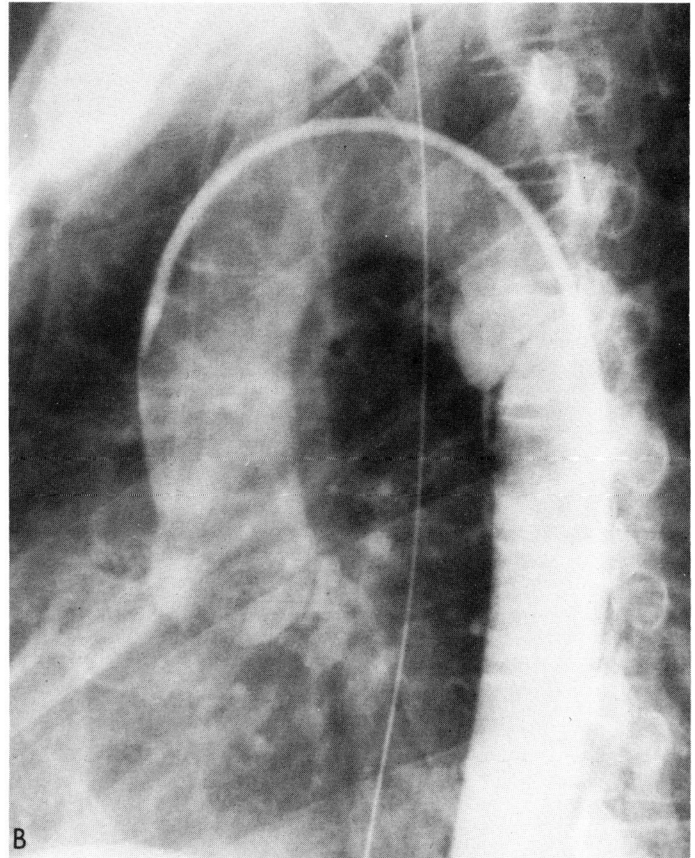

Figure 5–13. Traumatic aortic laceration. *A.* Anteroposterior chest radiograph, in a 35 year old patient who collided with the rear of a parked truck at "low speed" while on a motorcycle and suffered no apparent injury other than a wrist fracture, shows mediastinal widening and a fracture of the left first rib (arrow). *B.* Aortogram, right posterior oblique projection, demonstrates a false aneurysm near the ductus ligament with an intimal flap seen at its distal end. At surgery, almost complete circumferential transection of the intima and media was present.

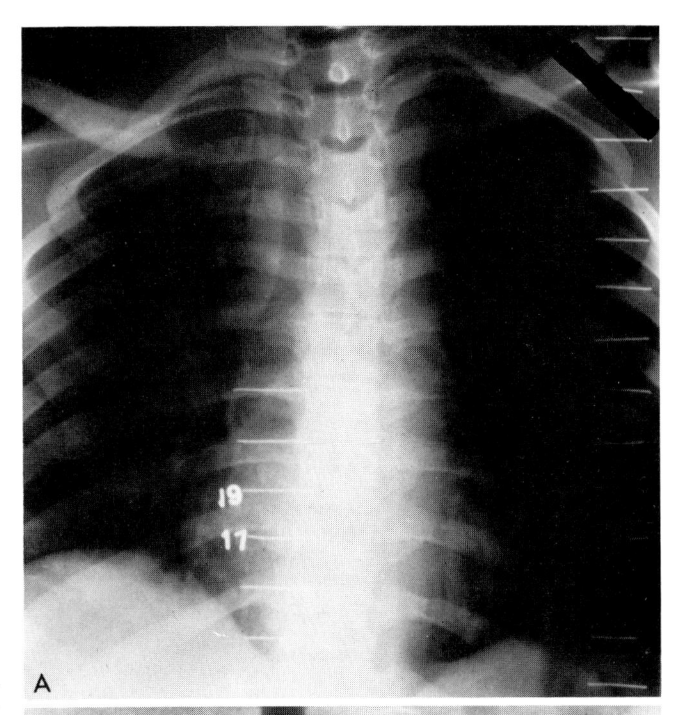

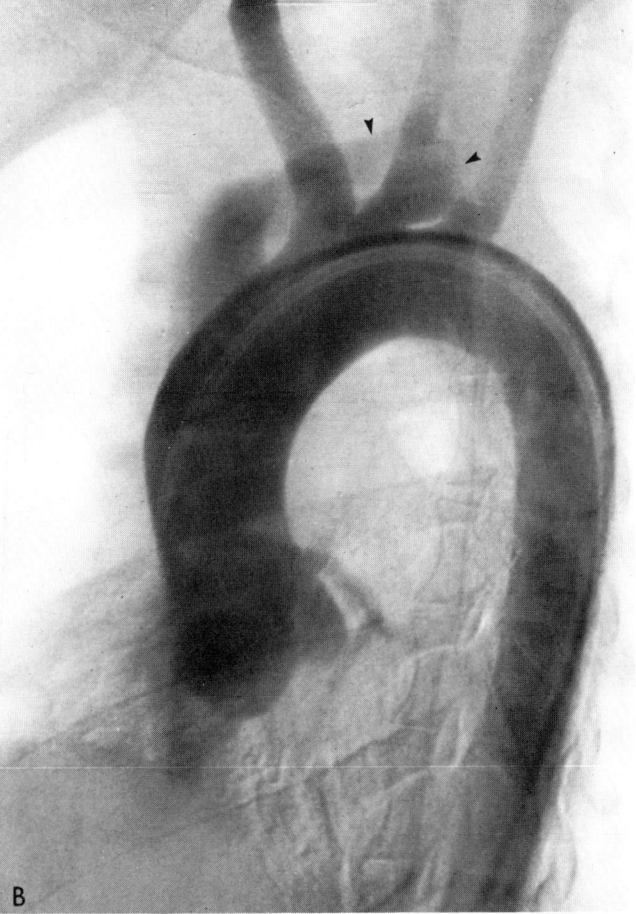

Figure 5–14. Traumatic false aneurysm and arteriovenous fistula. *A.* Supine anteroposterior chest radiograph in a 32 year old man who was stabbed with a knife in the left side of the neck shows some mediastinal widening. *B.* Subtraction film, aortogram, right posterior oblique view shows extravasation from a false aneurysm of the left carotid artery with a fistula to the innominate vein (arrows), with subsequent flow into the superior vena cava.

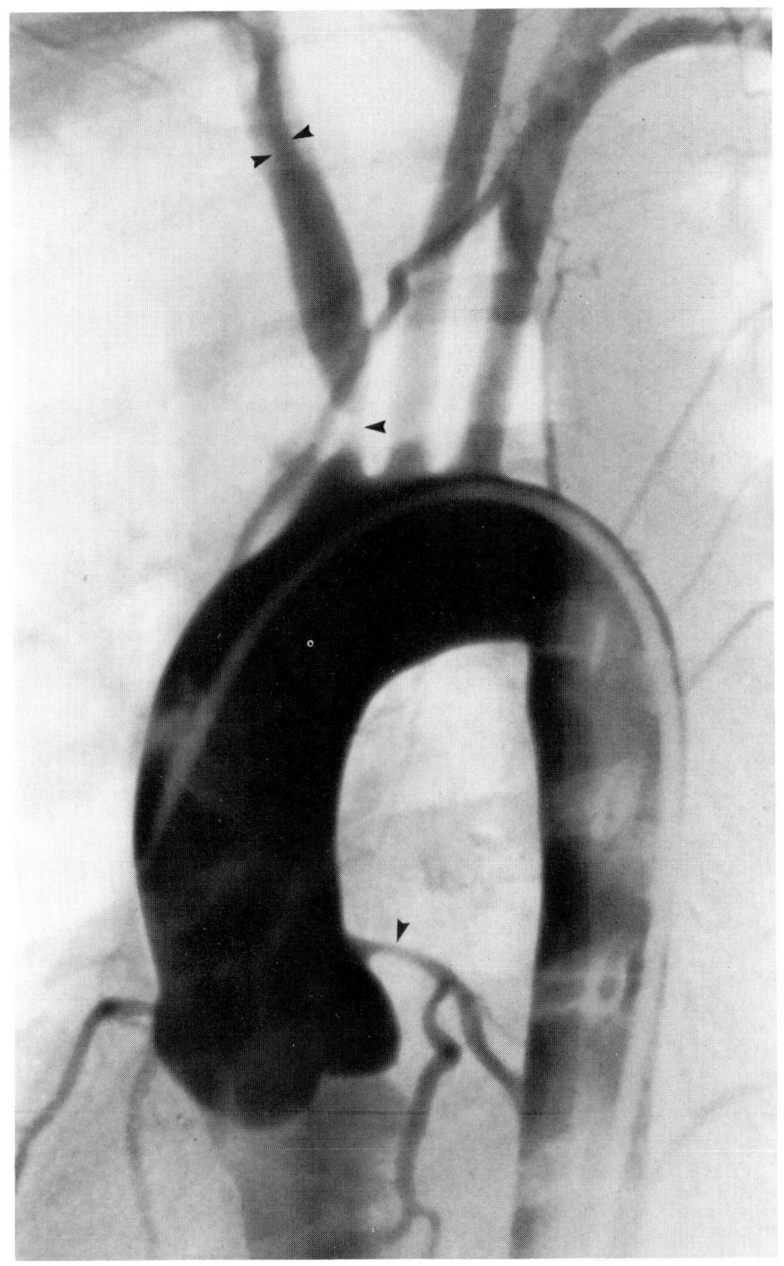

Figure 5–15. Aortic arch syndrome, arteritis, in a 26 year old woman with symptoms of cerebral ischemia, who had previous surgery for ischemic disease involving her superior mesenteric and left renal artery. Aortogram, subtraction film, right posterior oblique projection shows stenotic areas in the left coronary (lower arrow), innominate (middle arrow), and right vertebral (upper arrows) arteries.

Aortography reflects the pathologic lesions – demonstrating narrowing (Fig. 5–15) (or occlusion) or dilatation (or aneurysm). Abdominal as well as thoracic aortography is recommended for complete assessment.[17, 23] Renal artery involvement can lead to hypertension, which results in superimposed atherosclerosis, sometimes making histologic diagnosis difficult.[17] However, advanced atherosclerosis by itself may cause occlusive disease of the brachiocephalic arteries (Fig. 5–16).

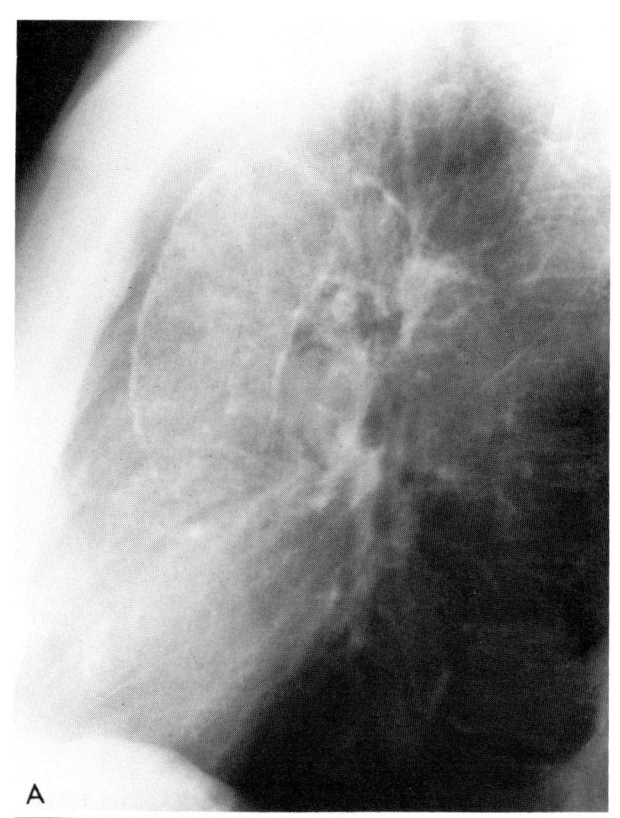

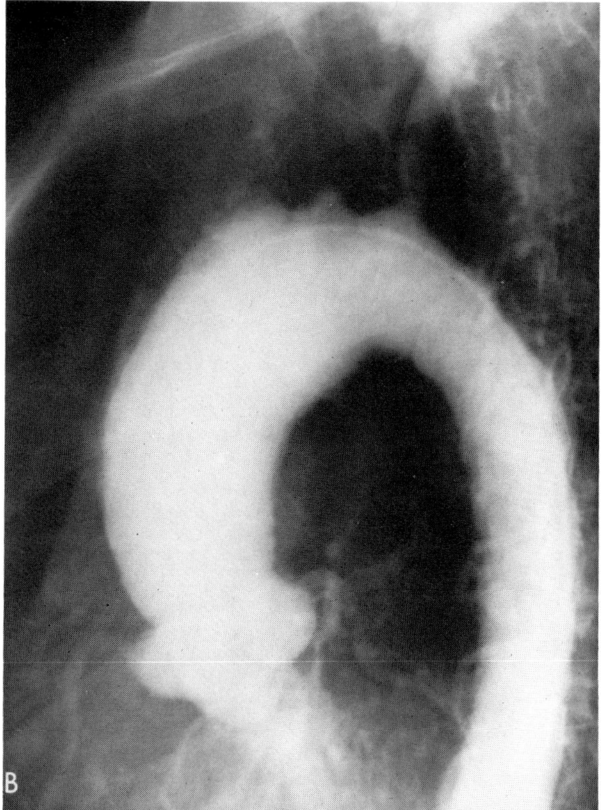

Figure 5–16. Aortic arch syndrome, atherosclerosis. *A*. Lateral chest radiograph in a 59 year old woman with cerebral ischemic symptoms demonstrates dense aortic calcification. *B*. Aortogram, right posterior oblique view, shows occlusion of the innominate and left carotid arteries. Histology of these vessels and temporal artery biopsy demonstrated atherosclerosis.

CLARIFICATION OF THORACIC MASS

An aneurysm of the aorta or one of the arch vessels may be mistaken for an intrathoracic neoplasm, and vice versa. Aortography usually can clearly distinguish between these two possibilities (Fig. 5–7).

In the elderly patient, tortuous innominate or carotid arteries may mimic an aneurysm or superior mediastinal mass. Pulsations detected clinically in the neck are usually of no help in distinguishing buckling of the brachiocephalic vessels from an aneurysm. Careful study of the plain chest radiographs, often in conjunction with oblique views, will usually enable recognition of simple tortuous vessels, but rarely aortography may be required to exclude an aneurysm or neoplastic mass.

BIBLIOGRAPHY

1. Abrams, H. L.: The hazards of thoracic aortography. *In* Abrams, H. L., editor: *Angiography,* Second Ed. Boston, Little, Brown and Company, 1971, p. 295.
2. Bar-Ziv, J., Eger, M., Fauchtwanger, M., and Hirsch, M.: Angiography in diagnosis of subclavian vessel injury. Clin. Radiol., 23:471–473, 1972.
3. Beachley, M. C., Ranniger, K., and Roth, F. J.: Roentgenographic evaluation of dissecting aneurysms of aorta. Amer. J. Roentgen., 121:617–625, 1974.
4. Chapman, D. W., Beazley, H. L., Peterson, P. K., Webb, J. A., and Cooley, D. A.: Annulo-aortic ectasia with cystic medial necrosis. Amer. J. Cardiol., 16:679–687, 1965.
5. Cheng, T. O.: Pseudocoarctation of the aorta—An important consideration in the differential diagnosis of superior mediastinal mass. Amer. J. Med., 49:551–555, 1970.
6. Cramer, G. G., and Amplatz, K.: Catheter position: An aid in diagnosis of dissecting aneurysm of the thoracic aorta. Amer. J. Roentgen., 98:836–839, 1966.
7. DeBakey, M. E., Henly, W. S., Cooley, D. A., Morris, G. C., Jr., Crawford, E. S., and Beall, A. C., Jr.: Surgical management of dissecting aneurysm of the aorta. J. Thorac. Cardiovasc. Surg., 49:130–149, 1965.
8. Dinsmore, R. E., Willerson, J. T., and Buckley, M. T.: Dissecting aneurysm of the aorta: Aortographic features affecting prognosis. Radiology, 105:567–572, 1972.
9. Eller, S. L., and Ziter, F. M. H., Jr.: Avulsion of the innominate artery from the aortic arch. Radiology, 94:75–78, 1970.
10. Freed, T. A., Neal, M. P., Jr., and Vinik, M.: Roentgenographic findings in extracardiac injury secondary to blunt chest automobile trauma. Amer. J. Roentgen., 104:424–432, 1968.
11. Gotsman, M. S., Beck, W., and Schrire, V.: Selective angiography in arteritis of the aorta and its major branches. Radiology, 88:232–248, 1967.
12. Hayashi, K., Meaney, T. F., Zelch, J. V., and Tarar, R.: Aortographic analysis of aortic dissection. Amer. J. Roentgen., 122:769–782, 1974.
13. Higgins, C. B., and Reinke, R. T.: Nonsyphilitic etiology of linear calcification of the ascending aorta. Radiology, 113:609–613, 1974.
14. Kirsh, M. M., Crane, J. D., Kahn, D. R., Gago, O., Moores, W. Y., Redman, H., Bookstein, J. J., and Sloan, H.: Roentgenologic evaluation of traumatic rupture of the aorta. Surgery, Gynecology and Obstetrics, 131:900–904, 1970.
15. Kronzon, I., Mehta, S. S., and Zelefsky, M.: Cervical aorta presenting as superior mediastinal mass: diagnosis by echography. Brit. J. Radiol., 47:900–902, 1974.
16. Litwak, R. S., Lev, R., Baron, M., and Gadbays, H. L.: The surgical treatment of aortic aneurysms. Geriatrics, 22:105–121, 1969.
17. Lande, A., and Rossi, P.: The value of total aortography in the diagnosis of Takayasu's arteritis. Radiology, 114:287–297, 1975.
18. Molnar, W., and Paul, D. J.: Complications of axillary arteriotomies. Radiology, 104:269–276, 1972.
19. Price, J. E., Jr., Grey, R. K., and Grollman, J. H., Jr.: Aortic wall thickness as an unreliable sign in the diagnosis of dissecting aneurysm of the thoracic aorta. Amer. J. Roentgen., 113:710–712, 1971.
20. Reul, G. J., Rubio, P. A., and Beall, A. C.: The management of acute injury to the thoracic aorta. J. Thorac. Cardiovasc. Surg., 67:272–281, 1974.
21. Saegesser, F., and Besson, A.: Extralobar and intralobar pulmonary sequestrations of the upper and lower lobes. Chest, 63:69–73, 1973.
22. Sanborn, J. C., Heitzman, E. R., and Markarian, B.: Traumatic rupture of the thoracic aorta. Radiology, 95:293–298, 1970.
23. Sano, K., Aiba, T., and Saito, I.: Angiography in pulseless disease. Radiology, 94:69–74, 1970.
24. Shuford, W. H., Sybers, R. G., and Ween, H. S.: The angiographic features of double aortic arch. Amer. J. Roentgen., 116:125–140, 1972.
25. Steinberg, I., Engle, M. A., Holswade, G. R., and Hagstrom, J. W. C.: Pseudocoarctation of the aorta associated with congenital heart disease, Report of ten cases. Amer. J. Roentgen., 106:1–20, 1969.
26. Stewart, J. R., Kincaid, O. W., and Titus, J. L.: Right aortic arch: Plain film diagnosis and significance. Amer. J. Roentgen., 97:377–389, 1966.

Chapter 6

NUCLEAR MEDICINE IN LUNG DISEASE

by Roger H. Secker-Walker, M.B., M.R.C.P.

INTRODUCTION

Radionuclides provide unique opportunities to study the disturbances in blood flow and ventilation that accompany most disease processes affecting the lungs. Perfusion imaging is widely used, but the altered relationships between blood flow and ventilation, which are found in pulmonary disease, make the combined examination of both aspects of lung function a virtual necessity, if any logical interpretation is to be made of a perfusion scan.

Recognition of the disturbance in physiology rarely leads to a precise pathological diagnosis, but when it is combined with the relevant clinical and roentgenographic findings appropriate further action can usually be taken on the course of the patient's management.

PHYSIOLOGY AND PATHOPHYSIOLOGY

A number of factors influence the distribution of blood flow and ventilation in healthy people. Blood flow is largely determined by the direction of gravitational forces, so that whatever posture is adopted, the more dependent regions have the greater blood flow. In any region the distribution depends on the balance between alveolar pressure, pulmonary arterial pressure, pulmonary venous pressure, and interstitial pressure. Normally in the upright position there is a gradient of one to three or more between the upper and lower zones, and this gradient changes at different lung volumes[40] (Fig. 6–1). Exercise increases pulmonary arterial blood flow so that proportionately more blood goes to the upper parts of the lung, so that the regional distribution is more uniform. Local hypoxia is associated with a shift of blood flow away from the hypoxic region owing to local pulmonary arteriolar constriction.

Because of the effect that the weight of the lungs has on the distribution of pleural pressure, gravity also influences the distribution of ventilation, but the gradient is less than that for blood flow.[7] Basal alveoli are smaller than apical ones, and for a given change in pressure they expand relatively more, causing more air to be exchanged in the lower zones than in the upper zones. At residual volume, however, the basal airways are functionally closed so that little ventilation takes place there until functional residual capacity is approached. The volume at which these airways seem to close—"closing volume"—is least toward the end of the second decade. It is relatively larger in childhood and begins increasing again in the third decade. The increase is related to the loss of elastic recoil that occurs as lungs age.[26] By the age of 60, closing volume has reached functional residual capacity, so that even during normal respiration ventilation is uneven in the lower zones. A similar effect is seen in obese individuals and also in subjects in the supine position. The rate and depth of respiration also influence the distribution of ventilation. As the rate of air flow in-

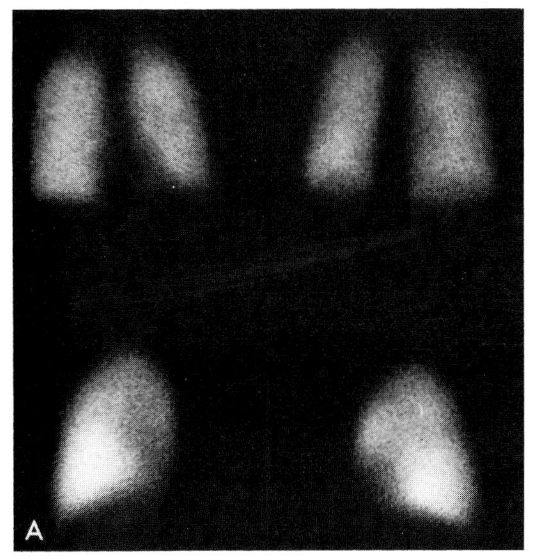

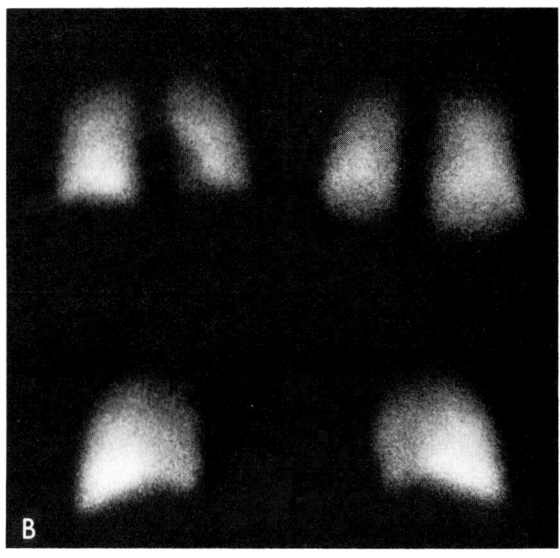

Figure 6–1. The effect of posture on the regional distribution of blood flow. *A*. The left-hand group of perfusion images were obtained after the intravenous injection of 99m Tc labeled particles, with the subject lying *supine*. There is an even distribution of activity from apex to base in the anterior and posterior views. *B*. The right-hand group of perfusion images were obtained the following day, after the injection of labeled particles, with the patient in the *upright position*. Perfusion is clearly diminished in the upper one third of the lungs and increased toward the base, compared to the "supine" images. NOTE: In these perfusion images, and in subsequent perfusion images, the format is as follows: Top left, anterior view; top right, posterior view. Bottom left, right lateral view; bottom right, left lateral view.

creases, airway resistance increases, and this happens more in the lower zones than the upper zones, causing the latter to contribute to a larger fraction of ventilation.

Abnormal patterns of pulmonary arterial blood flow are seen in conditions affecting the pulmonary vessels themselves, such as pulmonary embolism (from thrombus, tumor, or fat), vasculitis, arteriovenous malformations, or compression or invasion of the vessels in the hilum by inflammatory or malignant conditions such as granulomata, lymphoma, or carcinoma.

Regional hypoxia is another important mechanism and is associated with reflex vasoconstriction which causes a shift of blood flow away from the hypoxic region.[5] Changes in pulmonary blood flow due to this mechanism are seen in chronic bronchitis, emphysema, bronchial asthma, and bronchiectasis as well as in localized bronchial obstruction. In addition, structural changes may take place in the blood vessels in the more chronic conditions. In bronchiectasis, the bronchial arteries enlarge and provide collateral flow to the affected segments, and back flow into the pulmonary arterial branches may occur.

As would be expected, compression or displacement of lung parenchyma is associated with diminished blood flow; and this may be seen in patients with cardiomegaly, pleural effusion, emphysematous bullae, or a pneumothorax.

In pneumonic consolidation, blood flow is usually reduced, the blood flowing through the consolidated region acting as a right-to-left shunt, but the reduction is not usually as extensive as that seen with pulmonary infarction.

Increasing left atrial pressure, as can be seen in patients with mitral stenosis or left ventricular failure, is accompanied by a redistribution of pulmonary arterial blood flow, with a greater proportion flowing to the upper zones and a smaller proportion to the lower zones compared to normal. The change in distribution is proportional to the elevation of left atrial pressure, and is related to the increase in vascular resistance in the lower zones which accompanies the perivascular edema of the extraalveolar vessels.[16]

Abnormal regional ventilation is seen most commonly in those diseases that affect the airways, such as acute or chronic bronchitis, bronchial asthma, emphysema, and bronchiectasis.[25] Defects may be seen in single breath studies, after a washin period and more commonly during the washout of the tracer gas.

Airway obstruction by tumor, foreign body, or mucus plugs is accompanied by abnormalities of ventilation which are localized to the affected lobe or segment. The degree of impairment depends on the completeness of the obstruction. Regions with alveolar consolidation, such as are seen in pneumonia, pulmonary infarction, or pulmonary edema, have no ventilation.

In conditions in which lung compliance is decreased, clearance of xenon may be more rapid than usual, for in these conditions minute volume is increased. Patients who hyperventilate will also show more rapid clearance than normal.

REGIONAL PERFUSION

Images of the distribution of pulmonary arterial blood flow can be obtained following the intravenous injection of either radioactive particles or xenon-133 in saline. Both the particulate and gaseous tracers are well mixed with blood as they pass through the right atrium and right ventricle. Approximately 85 per cent of labeled particles, which usually measure 20 to 40 μ in diameter, are trapped in the terminal arterioles and capillaries during their first passage through the lungs, while 95 per cent of the xenon-133 comes out of solution as it passes air-containing alveoli. Strictly speaking, the labeled particles give an indication of relative pulmonary arteriolar blood flow, while the xenon-133 shows the relative distribution of capillary blood flow to air-containing alveoli. In regions of lung that are collapsed or consolidated, the use of xenon-133 in saline will underestimate the relative blood flow to these areas.

The particles gradually break up, pass through the lungs, and are removed from the circulation in the liver and spleen. The xenon-133 is cleared by ventilation.

AGENTS USED FOR PERFUSION IMAGING. Table 6–1 shows some of the preparations available for lung scanning together with their physical characteristics.

Macroaggregates of human serum albumin labeled with iodine-131 are still widely used. The lungs receive a relatively large dose of radiation, which limits the quantity of radioactivity that can be given to 250 to 300 μCi, and the quality of these

TABLE 6–1. Radiopharmaceuticals Used for Perfusion Lung Scanning*

AGENT	DOSAGE	PHYSICAL HALF-LIFE	BIOLOGICAL HALF-LIFE	PRINCIPAL GAMMA ENERGY	PARTICLE SIZE	RADIATION ABSORBED DOSE/mCi
Iodine-131 Macroaggregated Albumin	250–300 μCi	8 days	2–9 hours	364 Kev	5–100 μ	1–6.3 rads
Technetium-99m Macroaggregated Albumin	1–3 mCi	6 hours	2–9 hours	140 Kev	5–100 μ	150 mrad
Technetium-99m Albumin Microspheres	1–3 mCi	6 hours	7 hours	140 Kev	20–40 μ	400–600 mrad
Technetium-99m Ferric Hydroxide	1–3 mCi	6 hours	27 hours	140 Kev	5–60 μ	150–620 mrad
Indium-113m Ferric Hydroxide	1–3 mCi	1.7 hours	27 hours	393 Kev	5–60 μ	550–750 mrad
Xenon-133	5–10 mCi	5.3 days	30 seconds	80 Kev	Gaseous	100 mrad

*Adapted from Taplin, G. V., and MacDonald, N. S.: Sem. Nuc. Med., 1:132–152, 1971.

scans tends to be inferior to those obtained with technetium-99m or indium-113m labeled particles. In addition, the thyroid should be blocked with Lugol's iodine (10 drops three times daily for 10 days) to reduce the uptake of the iodine-131 released by metabolism of the particles.

At the present time, the agent of choice is technetium-99m labeled macroaggregates of albumin or albumin microspheres. Kits are commercially available for labeling human albumin macroaggregates, microspheres, or ferric hydroxide particles with technetium-99m. There is evidence that the ferric hydroxide particles have a longer biological half-life in the lungs than do the albumin preparations. Microspheres are more uniform than macroaggregates, but are harder, so that they have a longer residence time in the lung than do the soft albumin macroaggregates. The presence of chronic obstructive lung disease also delays the removal of these preparations from the lung capillaries, thereby increasing the radiation absorbed dose.

INSTRUMENTATION. Instrumentation for obtaining pulmonary perfusion studies using labeled particles varies from the relatively inexpensive rectilinear scanner to multiple-detector systems to highly sophisticated computer-assisted radionuclide cameras. If xenon-133 in saline is used, then only multiple-detector systems or the gamma camera can be used.

Rectilinear scanners offer no advantage other than price, and are limited to examination of the patient in the recumbent position, an undesirable situation when the patient is orthopneic or obese. The lateral views are often technically less satisfactory than those obtained with a gamma camera. With double-headed rectilinear scanners, the images obtained differ, depending on which part of the patient is closest to the lower probe; this image is smaller and its margins better defined than are those seen from the upper detector.

The gamma camera is most advantageous because of its maneuverability and the speed with which multiple images can be obtained. Radionuclide camera devices are capable of imaging the patient in any position, and can obtain four separate views even when the patient is restricted to one posture.

TECHNIQUE. As pulmonary blood flow is more evenly distributed from apex to base when the patient is in the supine position, the injections for lung scans are usually given in this position. If a comparison is to be made with ventilation, then the injection for the perfusion scan should be given with the patient in the same position that is used for the ventilation study. Ideally, the patient should be in the appropriate position for several minutes before the start of the procedure. The preparation of the particles should be shaken well before the injection and then given slowly over 20 to 60 seconds, taking care not to allow any clots to form from the withdrawal of blood into the syringe.

Images can be made at once. Anterior, posterior, and both lateral views should be obtained whenever possible. Some institutions prefer anterior and posterior oblique views from each side, instead of the laterals. These views have the advantage of avoiding the activity within the opposite lung contributing to the image of the lung being studied.

If xenon-133 in saline is being used, all air bubbles must be excluded from the syringe, for otherwise the xenon-133 would come out of solution into the bubble. In addition, glass syringes are better than plastic ones because xenon-133 is absorbed by the plastic. The patient should hold his breath at total lung capacity, shortly after the injection is given, while an image of the posterior chest is made. Other views are not possible with a single injection, because as soon as breathing is resumed the distribution of xenon is no longer proportional to blood flow. However, if xenon-133 in saline is injected during normal breathing, an approximation to the distribution of blood flow can be obtained when the countrate over the lungs reaches a maximum.

PRECAUTIONS AND RISKS. Satisfactory perfusion scans, using labeled particles, can be made with 60,000 to 150,000 particles. Children present no special problems, but the number of particles should be reduced appropriately, especially for infants with their diminutive pulmonary vasculature. The safety of perfusion scans lies in the vastly greater number of terminal arterioles—about 250 to 300 million, so that less than 1 in 1000 vessels is blocked during a lung scan. A few deaths have occurred immediately after the injecton of particles for lung scanning in patients with severe pulmonary hypertension, so that this condition is a relative contraindication to a particulate-perfusion scan.[15] Xenon-133 in saline should not pose this hazard.

Right-to-left shunts are another relative contraindication, for the particles will pass through the shunt and become impacted in the cerebral, renal, and coronary circulations. No permanent sequelae have followed perfusion scans in such subjects; there is some evidence that human albumin microspheres are safer than albumin macroaggregates in these circumstances.

No measurable disturbances of either cardiac function or pulmonary function have been found following the administration of the regular quantity of macroaggregates.

ARTIFACTS. If the preparation of particles contains too many small aggregates, i.e., less than 10 μ in diameter, the liver and spleen are visualized, and this can make interpretation of the lung bases difficult. Similarly, if a few large particles form, or if clots form in the syringe at the time of administration, several large hot spots will be seen on the subsequent scan.

Metallic objects overlying the chest, such as pacemakers, some breast prostheses, and the nails inserted to support adolescent kyphoscoliosis, are usually readily recognized.

REGIONAL VENTILATION

Regional ventilation can be assessed only with radioactive gases (Table 6–2). Xenon-133 is most widely used, although its low gamma ray energy and solubility in blood and fat are disadvantages. Xenon-127 has a more favorable gamma ray emission, but the long half-life would mean trapping and perhaps recycling this gas, and at present production methods are expensive.

INSTRUMENTATION. Regional ventilation may be studied with multiple probe systems or with the gamma camera. The multiple detector systems may consist of any array of fixed probes viewing the posterior or anterior chest, or they may be arranged to scan the chest from base to apex during breath holding maneuvers. The fixed arrays may consist of 2, 4, 6, 8 or more probes viewing each lung. Such systems have excellent counting statistics, although their spatial resolution is inferior to that of a gamma camera. The output from the probes is best recorded on magnetic tape for subsequent analysis or computer processing.

The advantages of the gamma camera over the probe systems are the better spatial resolution, the images that can be obtained throughout the study, and the ease with which the camera can be positioned for seriously ill patients. The gamma camera can view the whole of each lung from one aspect when fitted with a diverging

TABLE 6–2. Radioactive Gases Used for Ventilation Studies

AGENT	DOSAGE	PHYSICAL HALF-LIFE	PRINCIPAL GAMMA ENERGY	RADIATION ABSORBED DOSE/mCi
Xenon-133	1 mCi/liter for rebreathing technique (up to 30 mCi for a single breath study)	5.3 days	80 Kev	300 mrad*
Xenon-135	0.2 mCi/liter	9.1 hours	250 Kev	250 mrad*
Xenon-127	0.5–1 mCi/liter (up to 10 mCi for a single breath study)	36.4 days	172 Kev 203 Kev 375 Kev	100 mrad*
Nitrogen-13	5 mCi	10 minutes	511 Kev	11 mrad
Oxygen-15	5 mCi	2 minutes	511 Kev	14 mrad

*The radiation absorbed dose has been estimated by assuming a rebreathing time of 5 minutes. For single breath studies it would be much smaller.

collimator, and its ability to do this more than makes up for poor counting statistics, particularly those during washout studies, that this collimator causes. If any numerical analysis is required, then the data should be stored on magnetic tape. Digital format is preferred, as this can be processed much more rapidly than videotape.

TECHNIQUE. There is as yet no established method of doing a ventilation study. Table 6–3 shows some of the methods that have been employed. In clinical practice, a washin period of 3 to 5 minutes using a rebreathing system, followed by a washout period of up to 10 minutes or more, provides enough information for the vast majority of studies.

A number of devices are commercially available for administering xenon-133 and for performing rebreathing and washout studies. Some of these are disposable, while others are extremely elaborate. It is essential that the exhaust from any system be properly vented, or the xenon-133 trapped and allowed to decay.

Ventilation studies can usually be obtained in children from about 5 or 6 years of age onward. Below this age they are unable to cooperate well enough to do inhalation studies. Similarly, feeble, demented, or stuporous subjects may be unable to cooperate sufficiently to enable an inhalation study to be performed. In these circumstances there are two ways of obtaining information about regional ventilation. The first is to give xenon-133 in saline intravenously and obtain washout images as the xenon-133 is cleared from the alveoli. A second method is to use nasal prongs and deliver the xenon-133 in air through them under slight positive pressure over the course of 2 to 3 minutes. Close-fitting anesthetic masks have been used successfully, but sometimes are unsatisfactory, for the child may struggle to get away from the mask.[39] Good exhaust systems are required for both types of study, as the xenon-133 will be freely exhaled.

Regional ventilation can be measured in two ways, either as a "static" index of the distribution of ventilation per unit volume or else as a "dynamic" index related to the rate at which the tracer gas enters or leaves the lung.[7] The static indices are obtained by comparing the regional distribution of a single breath of xenon-133 at total lung capacity to the regional distribution of xenon-133 after rebreathing the gas to equilibrium and again taking a breath to total lung capacity to give ventilation per unit volume.[11] The dynamic indices can be obtained from activity time curves of the washin or washout of xenon-133. The time to 50 or 90 per cent of the equilibrium count rate during washin has been used in the past, but it is more usual to measure some aspect of the regional clearance of xenon-133 either from a single breath, or following a rebreathing period or after an intravenous injection.[30]

A gamma camera fitted with a diverging

TABLE 6–3. Methods of Studying Ventilation Using Xenon-133

Method	Procedure
1. SINGLE BREATH 10–30 mCi	Followed by serial images of the washout
2. SINGLE BREATH* 10–30 mCi	Followed by rebreathing to equilibrium with a spirometer Followed by serial images of the washout
3. WASHIN FOR 3–5 MINUTES: 30–50 mCi with a Bag-Box System 10–20 mCi with a Rebreathing System	Image at equilibrium followed by serial images of the washout
4. BREATH-HOLD FOLLOWING I.V. XENON-133 IN SALINE 3–30 mCi	Followed by serial images of the washout *or* Followed by rebreathing to equilibrium and then serial images of the washout
5. BOLUS TECHNIQUES	In which a small volume of xenon is introduced during inspiration at different lung volumes or at different flow rates and its distribution studied at total lung capacity

*In this technique an image at total lung capacity is obtained at the end of the rebreathing period.

collimator permits both lungs to be viewed simultaneously and single breath images, images of the washin, equilibrium images representing lung volume, and serial images of the washout to be obtained. Of these, the serial washout images provide excellent qualitative evidence of both normal and impaired ventilation. In particular, regions of delayed clearance are readily visualized by comparison with the areas that have already cleared.[35] Although the quasi-static methods of measuring ventilation are well established, the figures obtained indicate what proportion of air enters a region in relation to the volume of that region (i.e., ventilation per unit lung volume), but do not show how efficiently the air is actually exchanged. Some measurement of the clearance of xenon-133 is more suitable, for such figures can be related to the fractional exchange of air and hence the efficiency with which air exchange is taking place. In healthy lungs, ventilation per unit volume and the fractional exchange of air are closely related, but in patients with chronic obstructive lung disease this is not so, with greatest disparity between the two methods being found in the most poorly ventilated regions.

NORMAL PERFUSION AND VENTILATION STUDIES

A normal perfusion scan shows an even distribution of activity throughout the lungs when the injection is given with the subject supine. Less activity is seen in the upper zones where the lung volume is smaller. The contours of the lung are smooth and correspond to the borders seen on the chest radiograph. The outline of the heart is clearly seen on the anterior view, less obviously on the left lateral view and even less well on the posterior view, unless it is enlarged. The aortic knob is sometimes seen as a defect on both anterior and posterior views, and a tortuous thoracic aorta may also be seen in the posterior view. In general, the chest radiograph gives an excellent idea of what to expect as far as the lung outlines are concerned. The lower border of each lung usually lies at the same level posteriorly, with only slightly blunted costophrenic angles on both posterior and lateral images. Obese subjects characteristically have rounded lateral margins to their bases. The hilar regions may be visualized as a central area of diminished activity in lateral views, especially with gamma camera images (Fig. 6–2).

If the injection for a perfusion scan is given with the subject sitting upright, the effect of gravity is usually clearly seen, especially in younger subjects, with diminished or absent activity in the upper zones and greater relative flow to the bases. The upper level of activity is horizontal, and this can be seen in all four views (Fig. 6–1).

Change in position may also influence detection of defects in blood flow. The redistribution of blood flow that takes place on assuming the upright position may be sufficient to overcome the vascular resistance offered by small pulmonary emboli, so that defects in perfusion seen following injections in the supine position may disappear when the injection is given in the upright position (Fig. 6–3).

It is important to recognize that apparently healthy people have been found to have small defects in the distribution of blood flow, especially in the upper zones. Such defects have been seen in about 20 per cent of young subjects. In an elderly population a larger number are found to have defects in blood flow—70 per cent in one series. The defects in older patients are probably related to airway obstruction or minor episodes of pulmonary embolism, but in almost half such subjects no cause was demonstrated.[22]

A normal ventilation study shows an even distribution of activity with a single breath inhalation and at the end of a washin. A little more activity can be seen in the upper zones at the end of a washin than in a single breath image, for the end of the washin represents lung volume. During the washout, clearance is even from each zone, with the bases clearing slightly faster than the mid and upper zones, if the study is done upright. Supine studies show no appreciable difference between zones. Normal subjects usually have clear lung fields 2 or 3 minutes after the washout has begun (Fig. 6–2). The rapidity of clearing depends on alveolar ventilation; the greater the tidal volume and frequency of respiration, the faster the clearing.

PULMONARY EMBOLISM

Because the pulmonary arteries and arterioles accompany the bronchi and bronchioles, the defects in blood flow seen in pulmonary embolism are usually segmental or subsegmental. Occasionally, lobar defects or even loss of blood flow to an entire lung may be seen. One advantage of lateral or oblique views is that the anatomical localization of the defects can then be appreciated. Another advantage is that additional defects may be seen in these views alone. The fissure sign is occasionally seen in patients with multiple small pulmonary emboli. However, this sign is seen more frequently with pleural fluid or pleural thickening and in patients with chronic obstructive lung disease, especially children with cystic fibrosis (Fig. 6–4).

Because most thrombi break up on their passage through the heart, several defects in blood flow may be seen following the passage of a single clot. The distribution of fragments is influenced by pulmonary arterial blood flow, so that usually more of them impact in the bases of the lung. However, defects in the upper lobes may be seen in one third to one half of patients with emboli, although rarely as the only abnormality. The multiplicity of fragments means that even if an individual embolus is missed, the others will betray the presence of the disease (Fig. 6–5).

Radiographic abnormalities, such as areas of consolidation, pleural effusions, pulmonary edema, or linear atelectasis, make the interpretation of a lung scan less reliable, for each is likely to be accompanied by a defect in blood flow. When the perfusion defect is larger than the radiographic abnormality, the presence of pulmonary embolism with infarction is more certain. If other defects in blood flow are seen in radiographically normal regions, then the diagnosis is again strengthened (Figs. 6–6 and 6–7).

Perfusion scans are nonspecific, and the chest radiograph can be normal in the presence of chronic obstructive lung disease.[2] In addition to the physiologic factors that influence the distribution of pulmonary arterial blood flow, virtually all pathological processes within the lungs can upset the pattern of perfusion. Of particular clinical importance are acute and chronic bronchitis, emphysema, and bronchial asthma and bronchiectasis. Each of these conditions may be accompanied by a normal chest radiograph, and although the clinical history and physical signs may help distinguish such illnesses from acute pulmonary

(Text continued on page 158.)

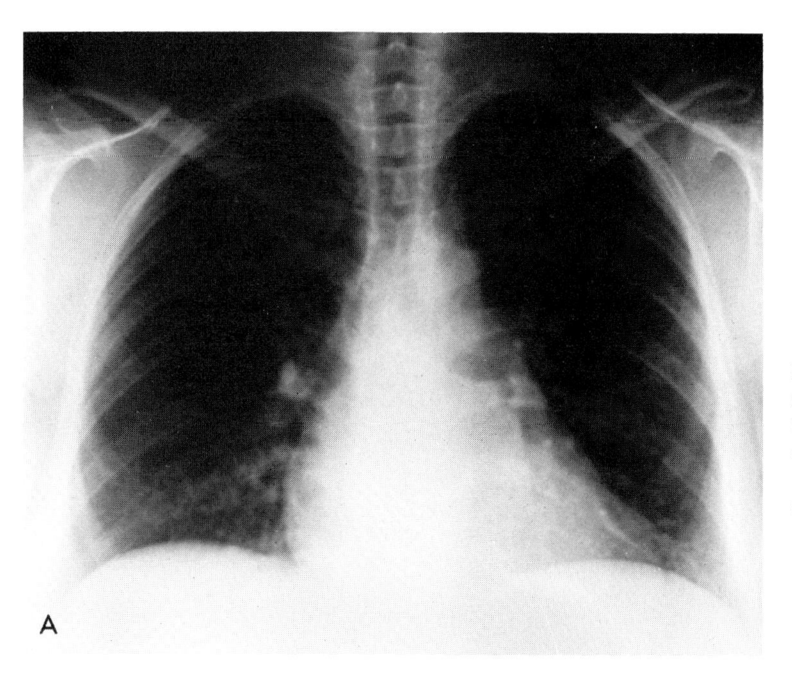

Figure 6–2. Normal perfusion and ventilation. A. Posteroanterior chest radiograph of a healthy woman, age 40.

Legend continued on the opposite page

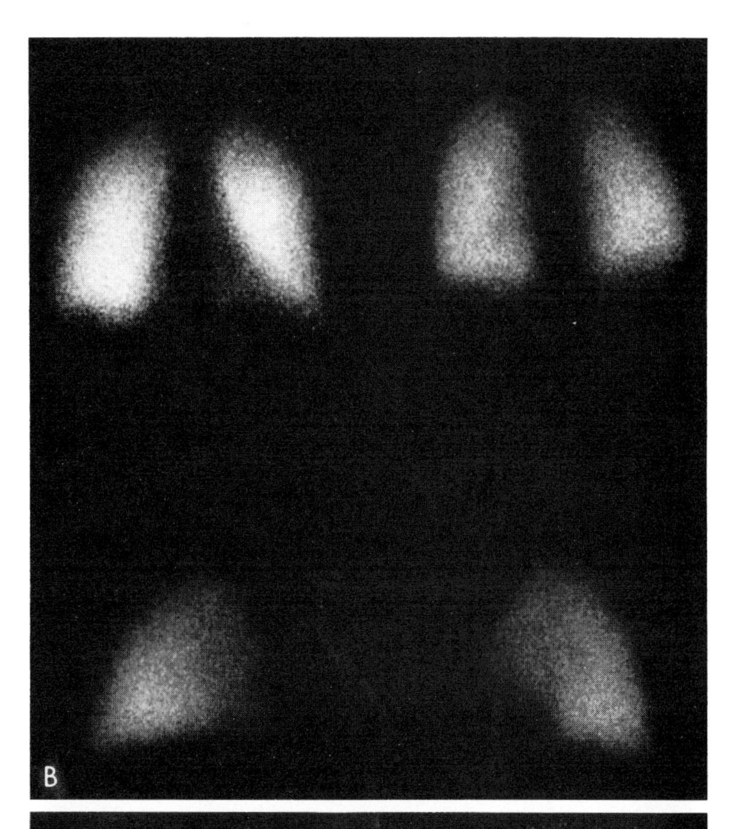

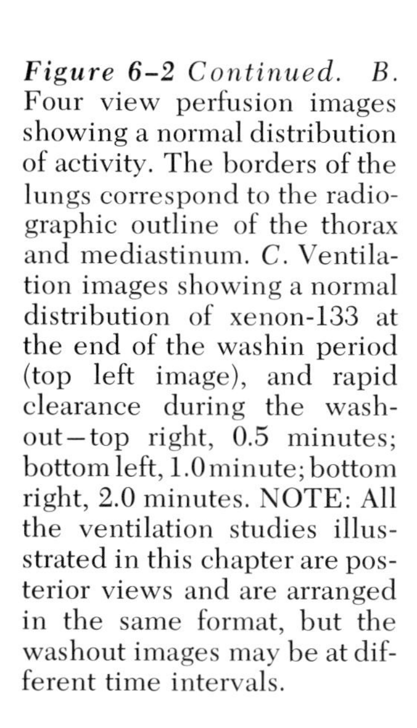
Figure 6–2 *Continued.* *B.* Four view perfusion images showing a normal distribution of activity. The borders of the lungs correspond to the radiographic outline of the thorax and mediastinum. *C.* Ventilation images showing a normal distribution of xenon-133 at the end of the washin period (top left image), and rapid clearance during the washout—top right, 0.5 minutes; bottom left, 1.0 minute; bottom right, 2.0 minutes. NOTE: All the ventilation studies illustrated in this chapter are posterior views and are arranged in the same format, but the washout images may be at different time intervals.

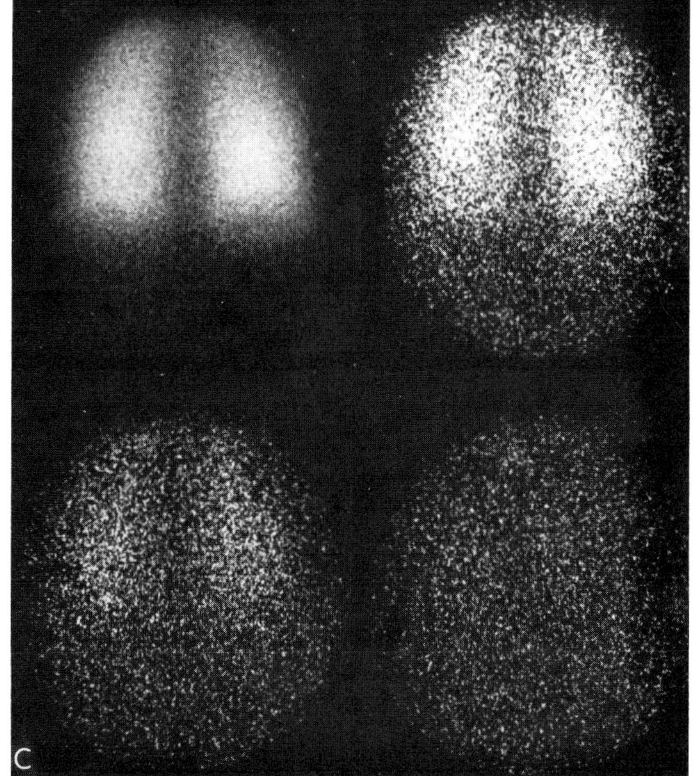

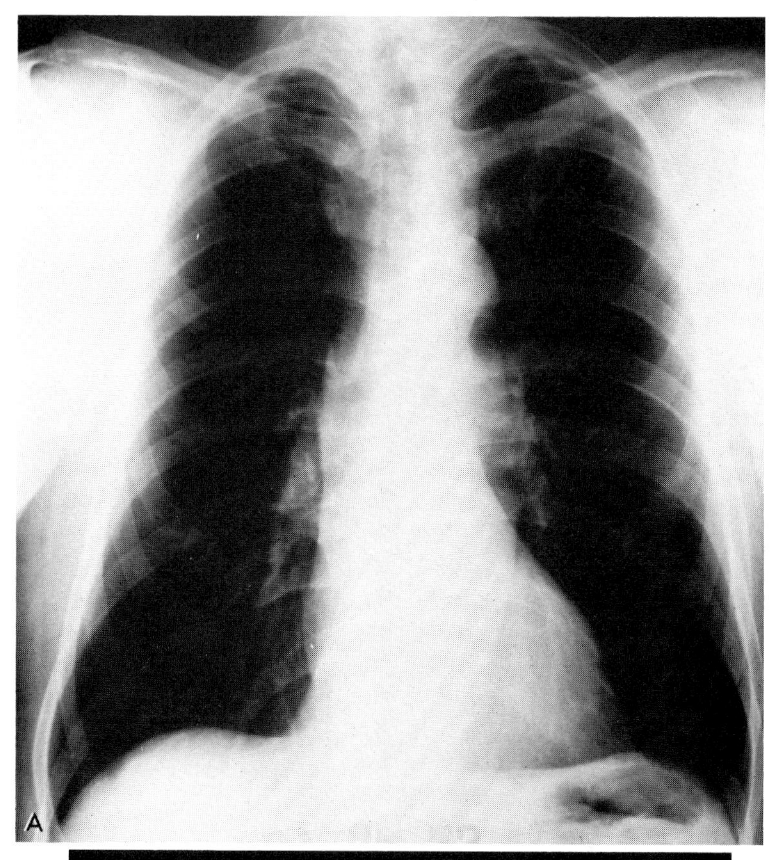

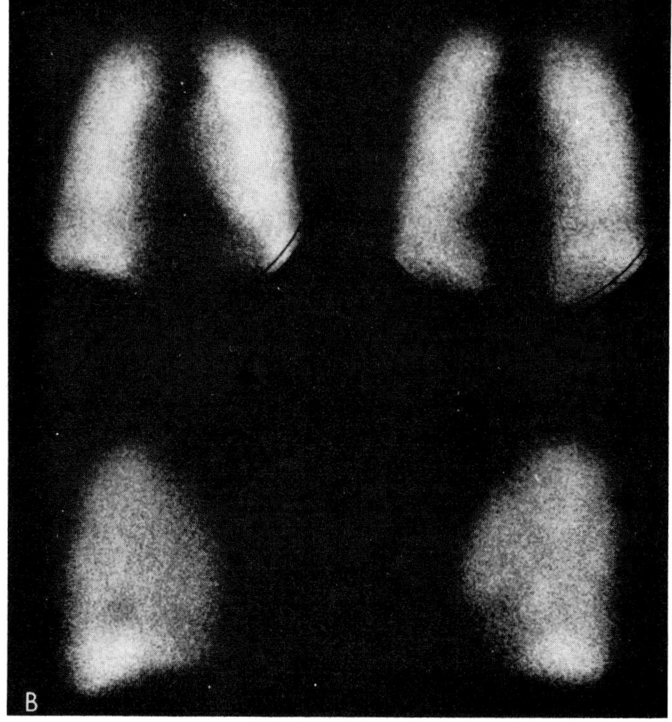

Figure 6–3. Effect of position at time of injection on detection of defects in blood flow. *A.* Posteroanterior chest radiograph of a 72 year old man who presented with right-sided pleuritic chest pain. The lung fields are clear. *B.* Initial perfusion images obtained following the intravenous injection of 99m Tc labeled particles with patient in the supine position. Defects in blood flow are visible at both bases.

Legend continued on the opposite page

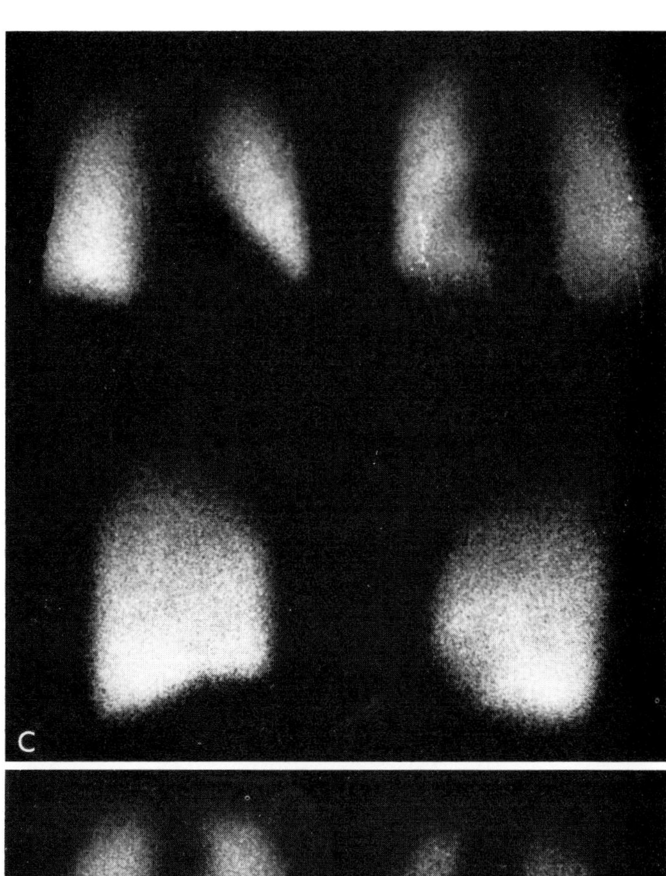

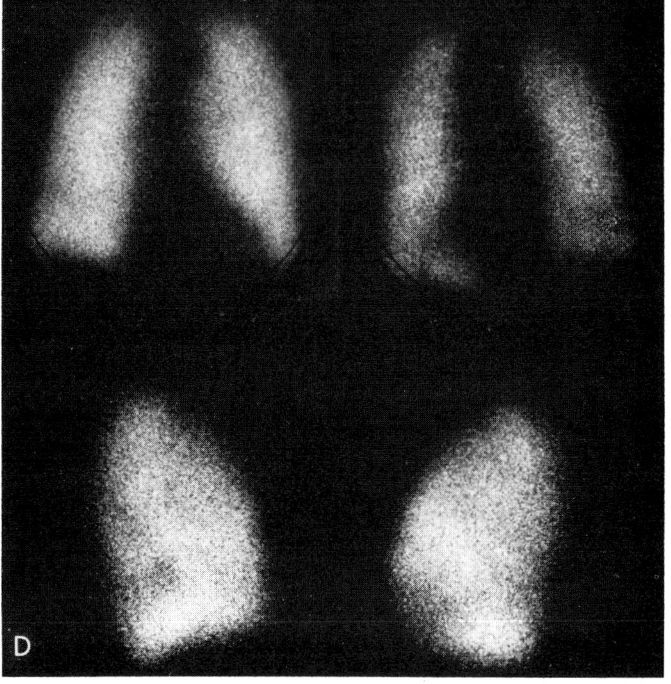

Figure 6–3 *Continued.* *C.* Second perfusion scan, obtained two days later; injection was given with patient seated in the upright position. The defects at the right base have disappeared, while those at the left base are much less obvious. Ventilation scan—not shown here—was normal. *D.* Third perfusion scan obtained five days later; injection was given with patient in the supine position. The original defects in blood flow are once more apparent.

embolism, difficulties in diagnosis are common.

Other acute and chronic inflammatory conditions such as pneumonia or tuberculosis disturb the pattern of blood flow, as do most bronchogenic cancers. Hilar lymphadenopathy from any cause, either benign or malignant, may be associated with perfusion defects. Although the presence of these latter conditions can be recognized from the chest radiograph, it is of considerable help to have a ventilation study accompanying each perfusion scan, especially when the patients may have airway obstruction.

Immediately after an embolus becomes impacted, ventilation is transiently shifted away from the affected region and there is evidence of bronchoconstriction associated with the local hypocarbia. However, this effect lasts only from 4 to 8 hours and often much less, so that by the time most patients have a lung scan, ventilation has returned to its previous pattern.[10,17] In some patients this effect could be sufficient to cause some difficulty in comparison with the perfusion images.[20] In almost all previously healthy lungs, a pulmonary embolus will show as a defect in blood flow accompanied by a normal pattern of ventilation—both in the distribution of a single breath and in the distribution of lung volume. Clearance may be normal or accelerated, because patients with pulmonary embolism tend to have increased alveolar ventilation (Fig. 6–5).

When obstructive airways disease and pulmonary embolism coexist, combined ventilation-perfusion studies may show evidence of both conditions. In this situation parts of the lung may have both impaired ventilation and impaired blood flow in the regions of airway obstruction, while in other embolized regions the ventilation may be normal or else less impaired than

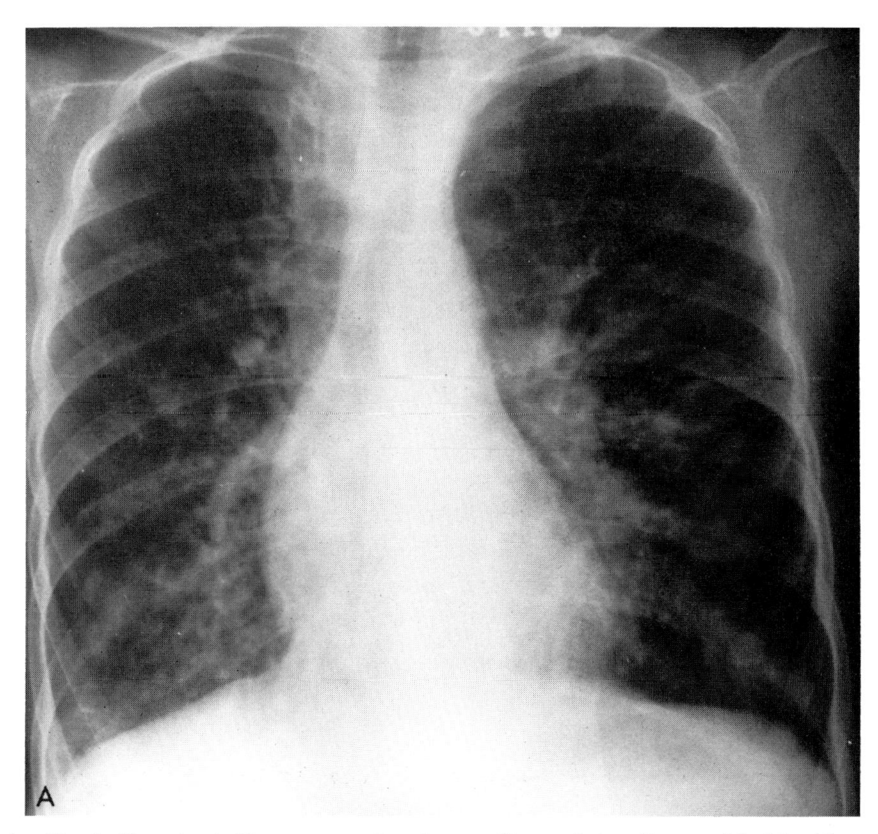

Figure 6–4. Cystic fibrosis. A. Posteroanterior chest radiograph in a 9 year old girl with cystic fibrosis shows diffuse pulmonary infiltrates and hyperinflation.

Legend continued on the opposite page

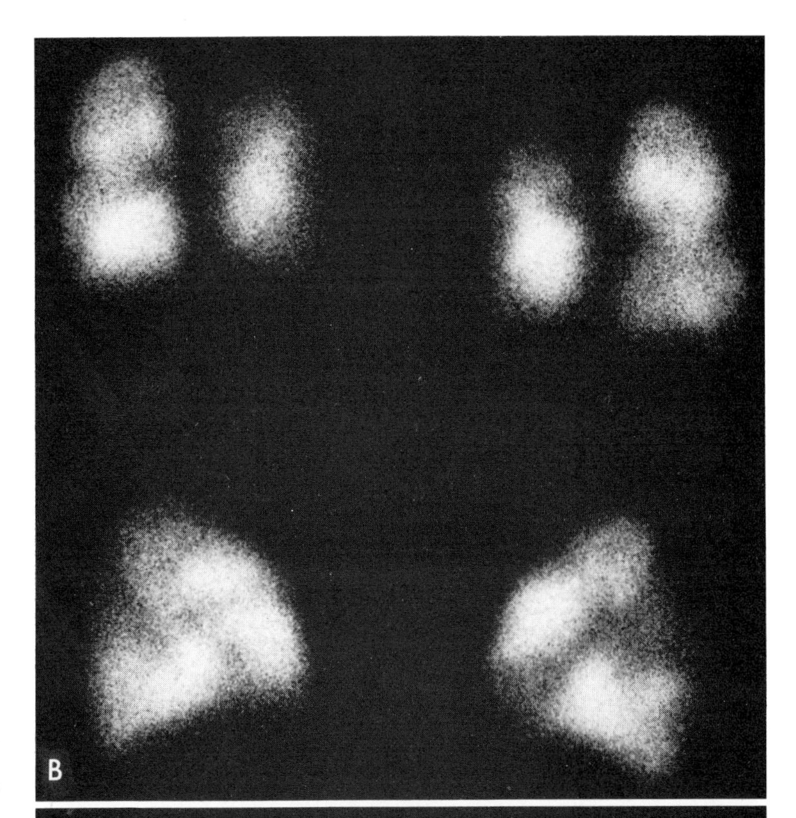

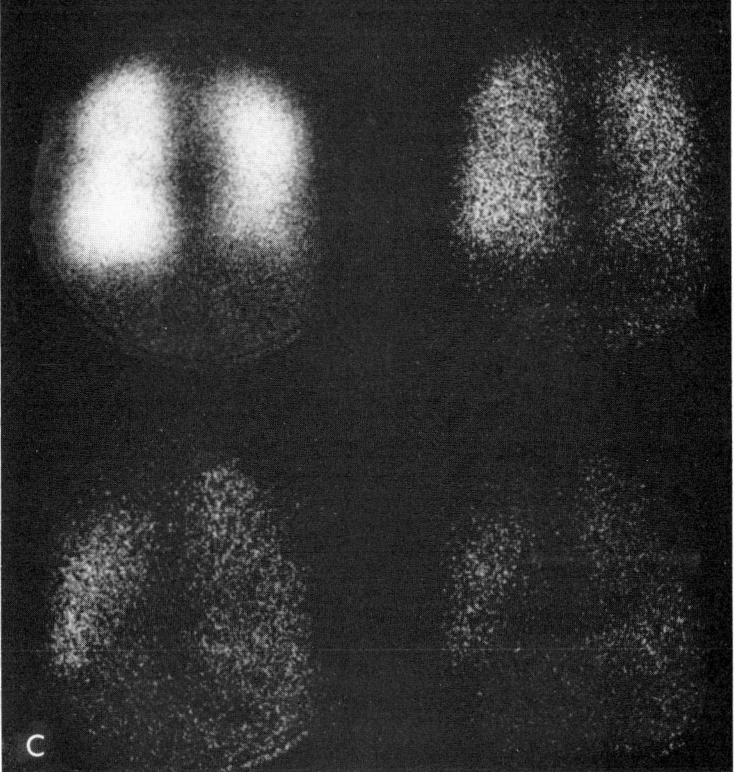

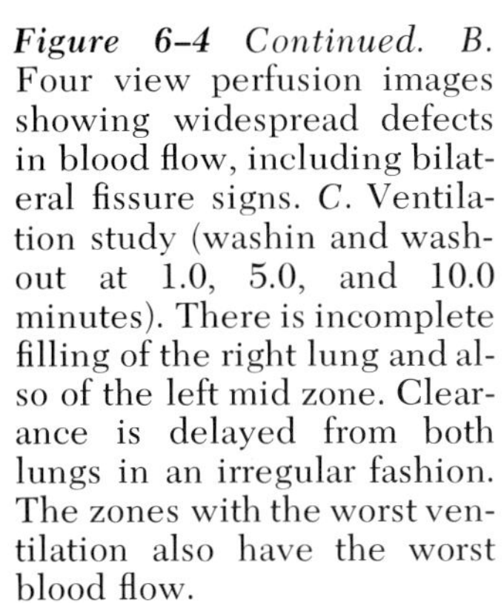

Figure 6–4 *Continued. B.* Four view perfusion images showing widespread defects in blood flow, including bilateral fissure signs. *C.* Ventilation study (washin and washout at 1.0, 5.0, and 10.0 minutes). There is incomplete filling of the right lung and also of the left mid zone. Clearance is delayed from both lungs in an irregular fashion. The zones with the worst ventilation also have the worst blood flow.

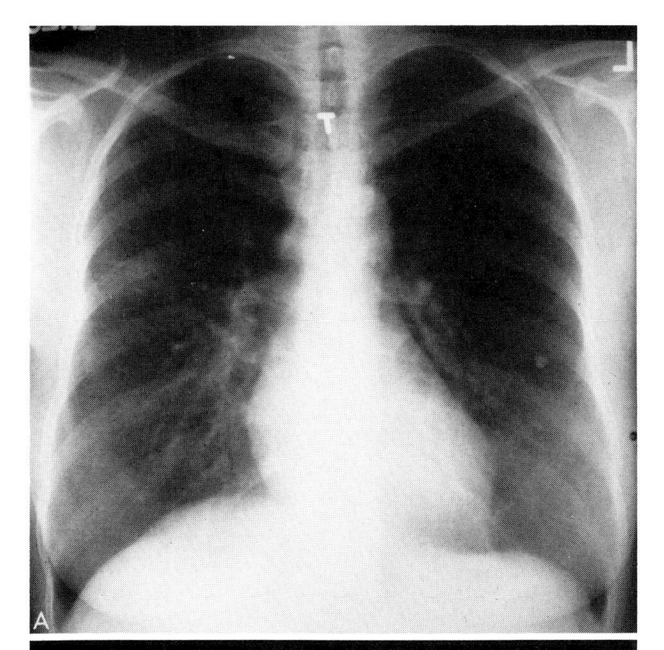

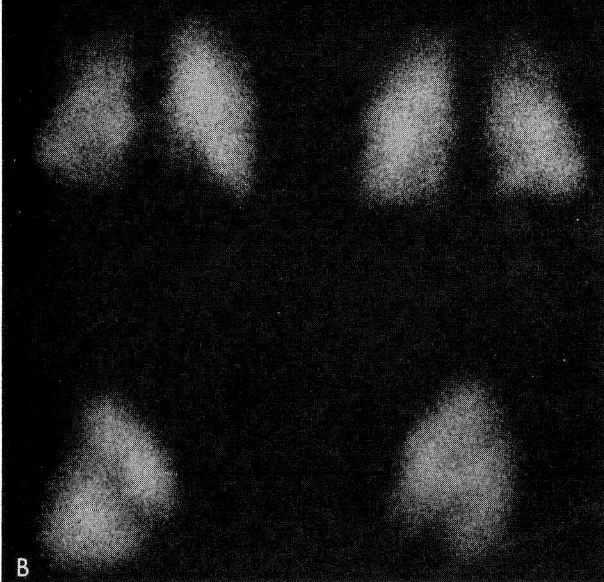

Figure 6–5. Multiple pulmonary embolism. *A*. Posteroanterior chest radiograph of a 46 year old woman who suffered from recurrent pulmonary embolism. There is a small infiltrate in the right mid lung field. *B*. Four view perfusion images showing segmental and subsegmental defects in each lung. A fissure sign is also seen in the right lung.

Legend continued on the opposite page

blood flow (Fig. 6–8). There are few reports documenting the accuracy of ventilation-perfusion studies in this situation.

Perfusion scans are a convenient way to follow the restoration of blood flow as an embolus breaks up or is lysed or absorbed. The time course in any individual is quite variable. Rarely, all signs of an embolus may have vanished within 24 hours. More usually, about 40 per cent of the defect will have resolved in the first 3 to 4 days, to be followed by more gradual improvement over the next 3 to 4 weeks. Some improvement may continue over a period of several months. New defects, which are seen in 30 to 60 per cent of patients, usually occur in the first 2 weeks, while the factors causing the initial thrombus to form are still operative; but they may continue to occur for 1 or 2 months or more. The diagnosis of embolic recurrence based on radioisotopic studies alone should be made with caution,

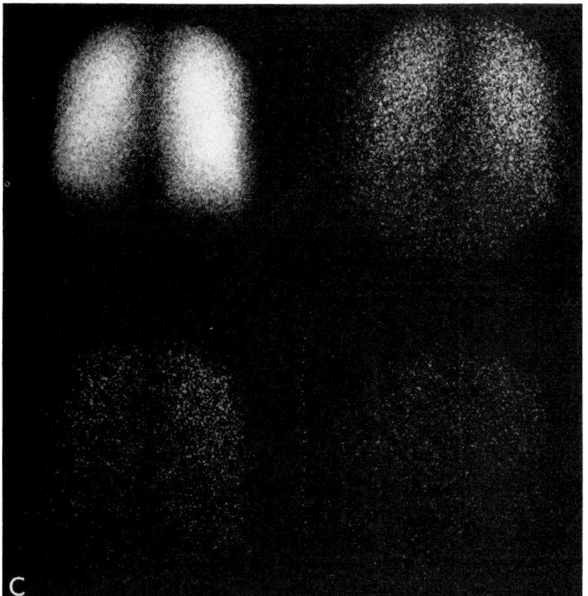

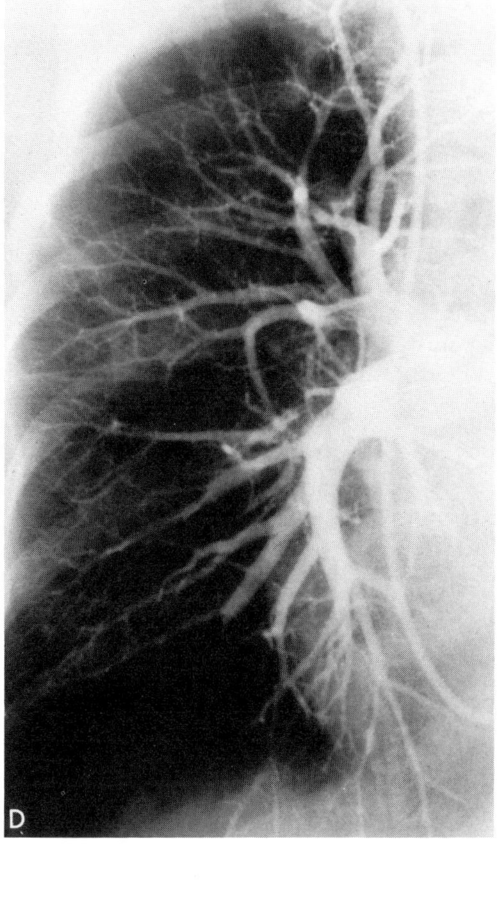

Figure 6–5 Continued. *C.* Ventilation images (washin and washout at 0.5, 1.0, and 2.0 minutes). There is a normal distribution activity at the end of the washin, and rapid clearance during the washout. The lower zones can be seen to clear more rapidly than the upper zones. *D.* Pulmonary angiogram obtained the following day. Selective injection of the right pulmonary artery showing emboli to the right lower lobe. (From Secker-Walker, R. H.: Lung scanning. *In* Gottschalk, A., and Potchen, E. J., editors: Golden's Diagnostic Radiology, Section 20, Diagnostic Nuclear Medicine. © 1975, The Williams & Wilkins Co., Baltimore.)

particularly in patients with multiple emboli and pulmonary hypertension. Spurious scintiphotographic recurrences may be produced by distal migration of emboli or by different rates of embolic resolution.[29] Large defects improve less well than do small ones, and both age and the presence of other cardiorespiratory conditions delay resolution. Probably up to one third of patients with clinically recognizable emboli are left with minor defects in blood flow. Some defects are known to have lasted more than 5 years.

DIAGNOSIS. The clinical diagnosis of pulmonary embolism is fraught with difficulty.[28] Symptoms and signs are mimicked by several other conditions. Blood-gas determinations, biochemical tests, the electrocardiogram, or the plain chest radiograph may be suggestive, but are rarely definitive. In fact, they may all be negative in the presence of serious pulmonary embolic disease.

Blood gases will give an indication of the size of the embolus – but a perfusion defect of at least 10 to 15 per cent (that is, two segments) must be present before P_aO_2 begins to drop. The P_aCO_2 and (H^+) will both fall as hyperventilation ensues. The electrocardiogram may indicate the presence of other pathologic conditions, but the signs of right heart strain appear only with large emboli.

The plain chest radiograph may be helpful, and correlation of it with radioisotopic studies is imperative. It should be emphasized that the majority of pulmonary emboli do not produce any abnormality on plain films.[31] Paradoxically, a normal plain chest radiograph should be thought of as valuable additional information, for such a film is compatible with a diagnosis of pulmonary embolism and can be of considerable help in comparison with the perfusion scan.[37] At times the chest radiograph may show changes consonant with pulmonary infarction or, rarely, some of the classic signs of pulmonary embolism—cut-off vessels, enlargement of a central pulmonary artery, or an elevated hemidiaphram.

But the most valuable, non-invasive procedure available for the diagnosis of pulmonary thromboembolism is the radioisotopic perfusion study. For practical purposes, a normal radioisotopic perfusion study excludes clinically significant pulmonary embolism,[31] although some experimental and angiographic evidence suggests that a few small emboli will be missed.[27] If both ventilation and perfusion are normal, or if the ventilation-perfusion scans show evidence only of obstructive airways disease, then anticoagulant therapy need not be given. If the perfusion image shows defects in blood flow in areas where ventilation is normal (i.e., the pattern of pulmonary embolism), the patient should be treated if there is good clinical substantiation of the diagnosis, with the physician realizing that pulmonary vasculitis or areas of fibrosis can produce a similar pattern.

Pulmonary angiography should be reserved for those patients in whom there is still diagnostic doubt, and for those in whom surgical intervention is being considered either for prevention of further emboli (e.g., by inferior vena cava plication or insertion of an umbrella) or rarely for pulmonary embolectomy. Lung scanning can do no more than show the relative distribution of pulmonary arterial blood flow and ventilation, and the diagnosis of embolism always remains inferential, whereas pulmonary angiography may show conclusive evidence of emboli.

The size of the defects seen on perfusion lung scans corresponds quite well with their size estimated angiographically. In general, lung scans tend to underestimate the size of an embolus when it is larger and lies more centrally, while angiograms tend to underestimate the functional disturbance when the emboli are smaller and situated more peripherally.[27]

CHRONIC OBSTRUCTIVE PULMONARY DISEASE

The prevalence of acute and chronic obstructive airways disease makes an assessment of the distribution of ventilation es-

Text continued on page 168

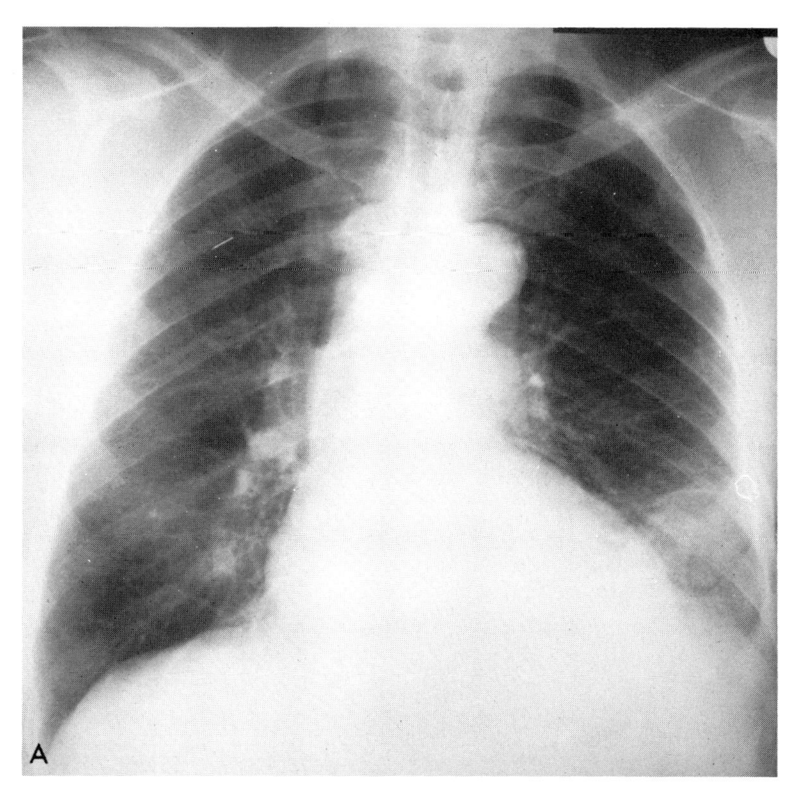

Figure 6–6. Pulmonary embolism and pulmonary infarction. *A.* Posteroanterior chest radiograph of a 51 year old man who presented with left-sided pleuritic chest pain and dyspnea. There is cardiomegaly, elevation of the left hemidiaphragm, and an infiltrate at the left lung base.

Legend continued on the opposite page

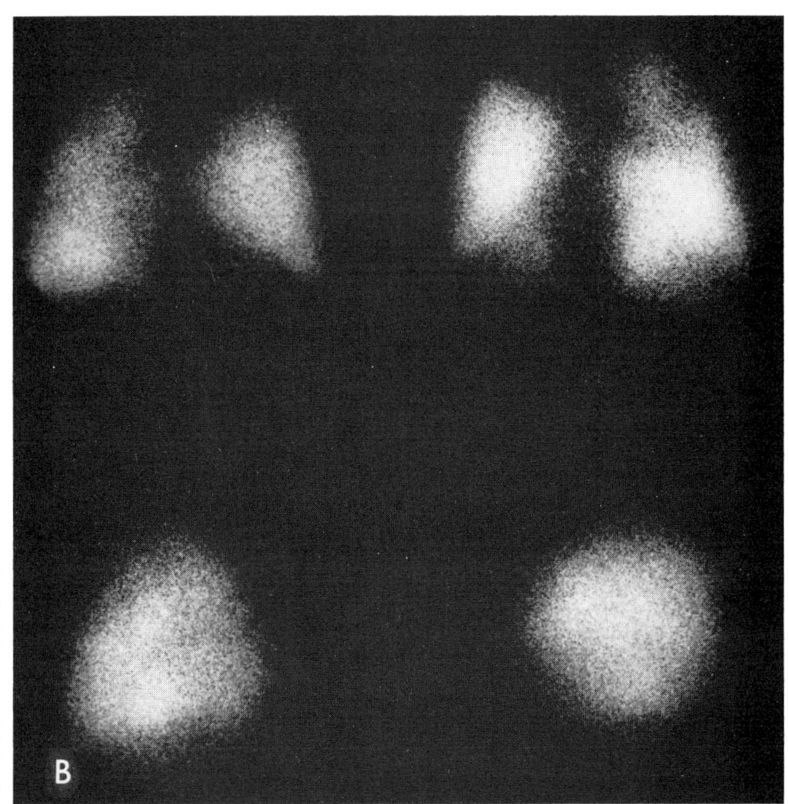

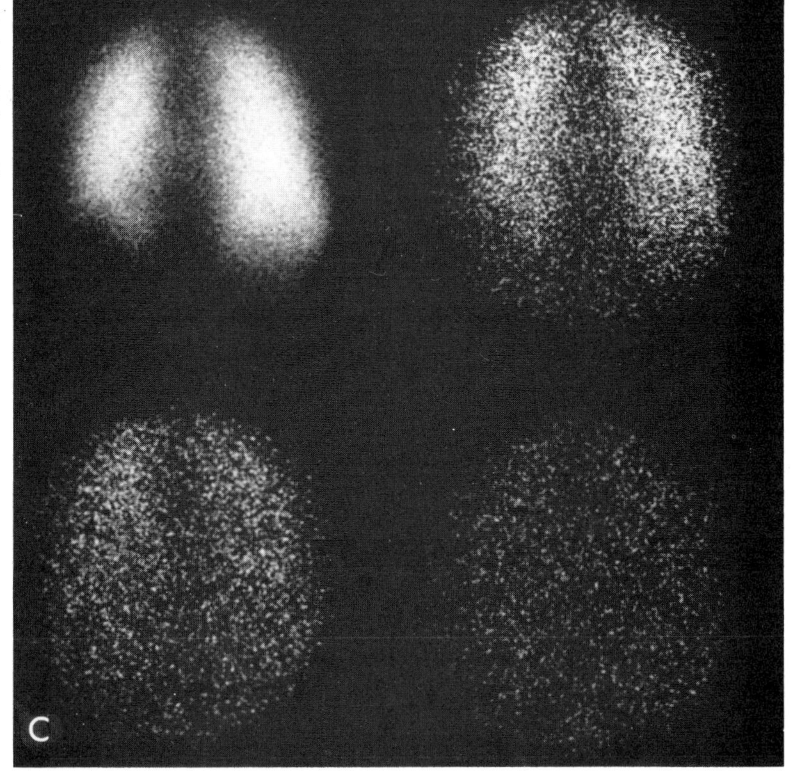

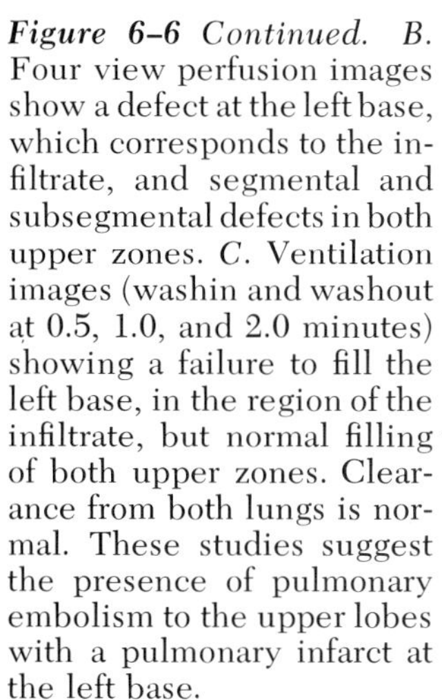
Figure 6–6 *Continued. B.* Four view perfusion images show a defect at the left base, which corresponds to the infiltrate, and segmental and subsegmental defects in both upper zones. *C.* Ventilation images (washin and washout at 0.5, 1.0, and 2.0 minutes) showing a failure to fill the left base, in the region of the infiltrate, but normal filling of both upper zones. Clearance from both lungs is normal. These studies suggest the presence of pulmonary embolism to the upper lobes with a pulmonary infarct at the left base.

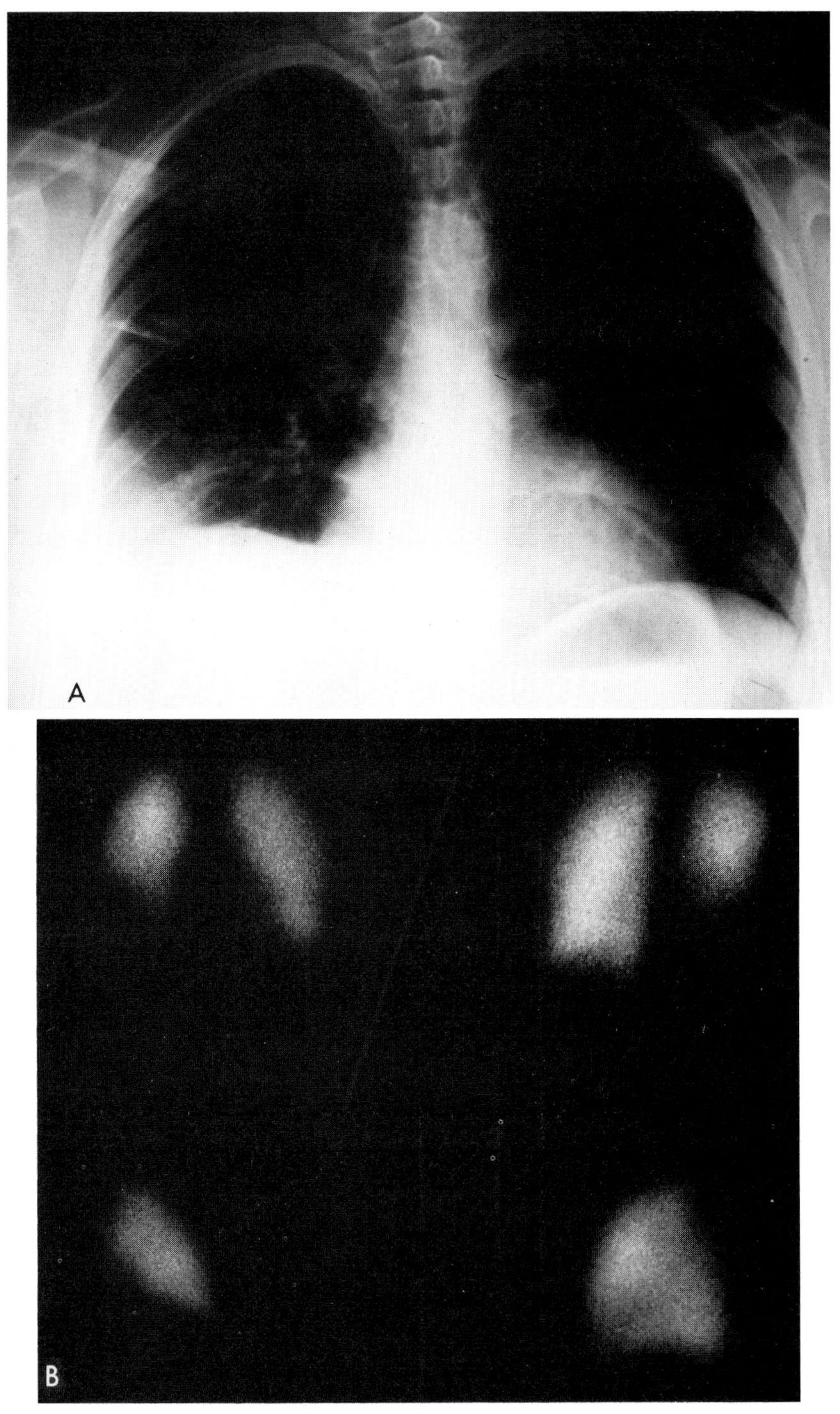

Figure 6–7. Pulmonary embolism, infarction, and a pleural effusion. *A*. Posteroanterior chest radiograph of a 31 year old woman who presented with right-sided pleuritic chest pain and fever. There is an infiltrate at the right base with elevation of the right hemidiaphragm and a right pleural effusion. *B*. Four view perfusion images show a large defect in blood flow to the whole of the right lower lobe and part of the right upper lobe. A fissure sign is seen on the left with a defect in the posterior segment of the left upper lobe. The large defect in blood flow in the right lung, which is more extensive than the radiographic changes, and the small defect in the left lung suggest the diagnosis of pulmonary embolism with infarction. This was confirmed by pulmonary angiography.

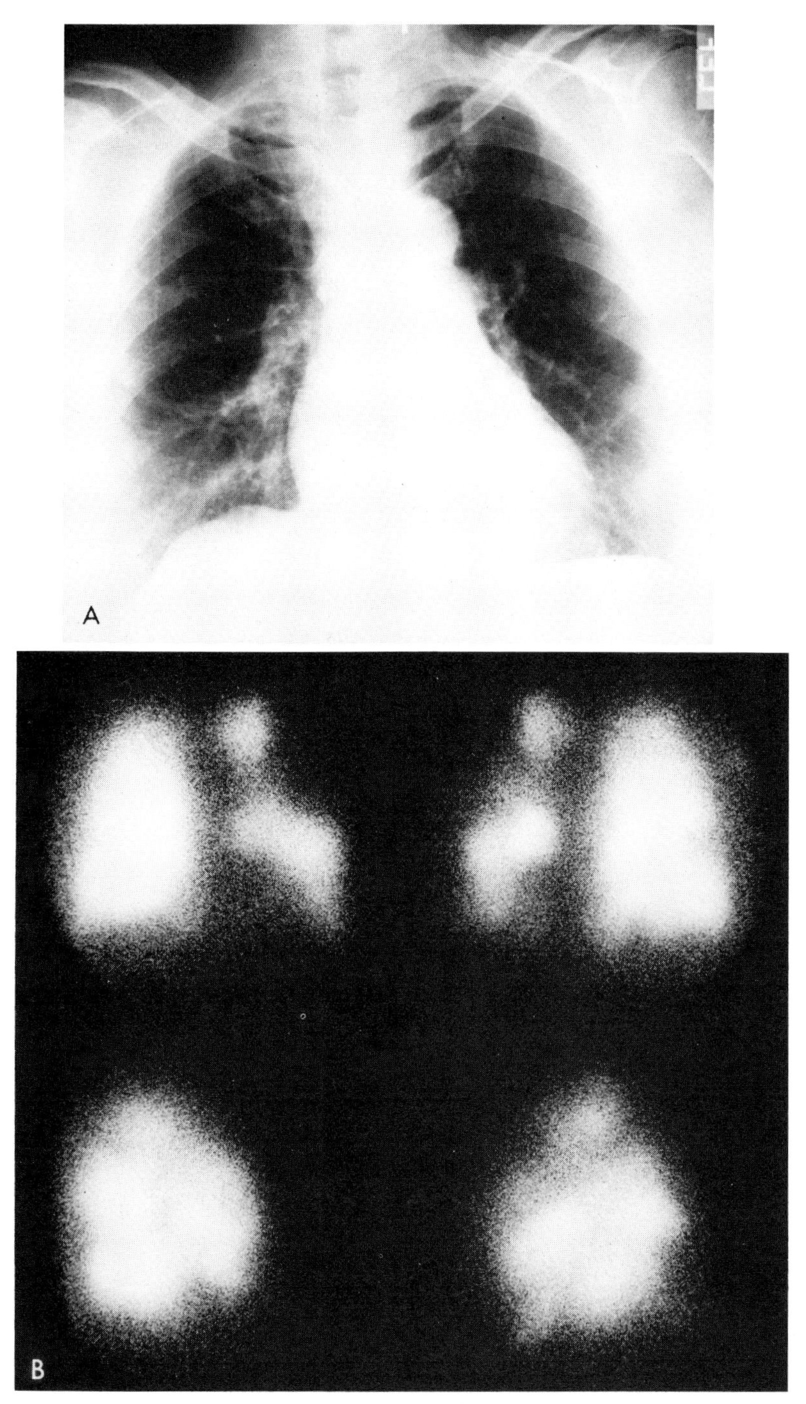

Figure 6–8. Pulmonary embolism and chronic obstructive pulmonary disease. *A*. Anteroposterior chest radiograph of a 79 year old woman, who presented with acute dyspnea and syncope 3 weeks after a hysterectomy for carcinoma of the uterus, demonstrates no definite abnormality. *B*. Four view perfusion images show large defects in blood flow in the left lung, especially in the lower lobe, and smaller defects in blood flow in the right lung.

Legend continued on the following page

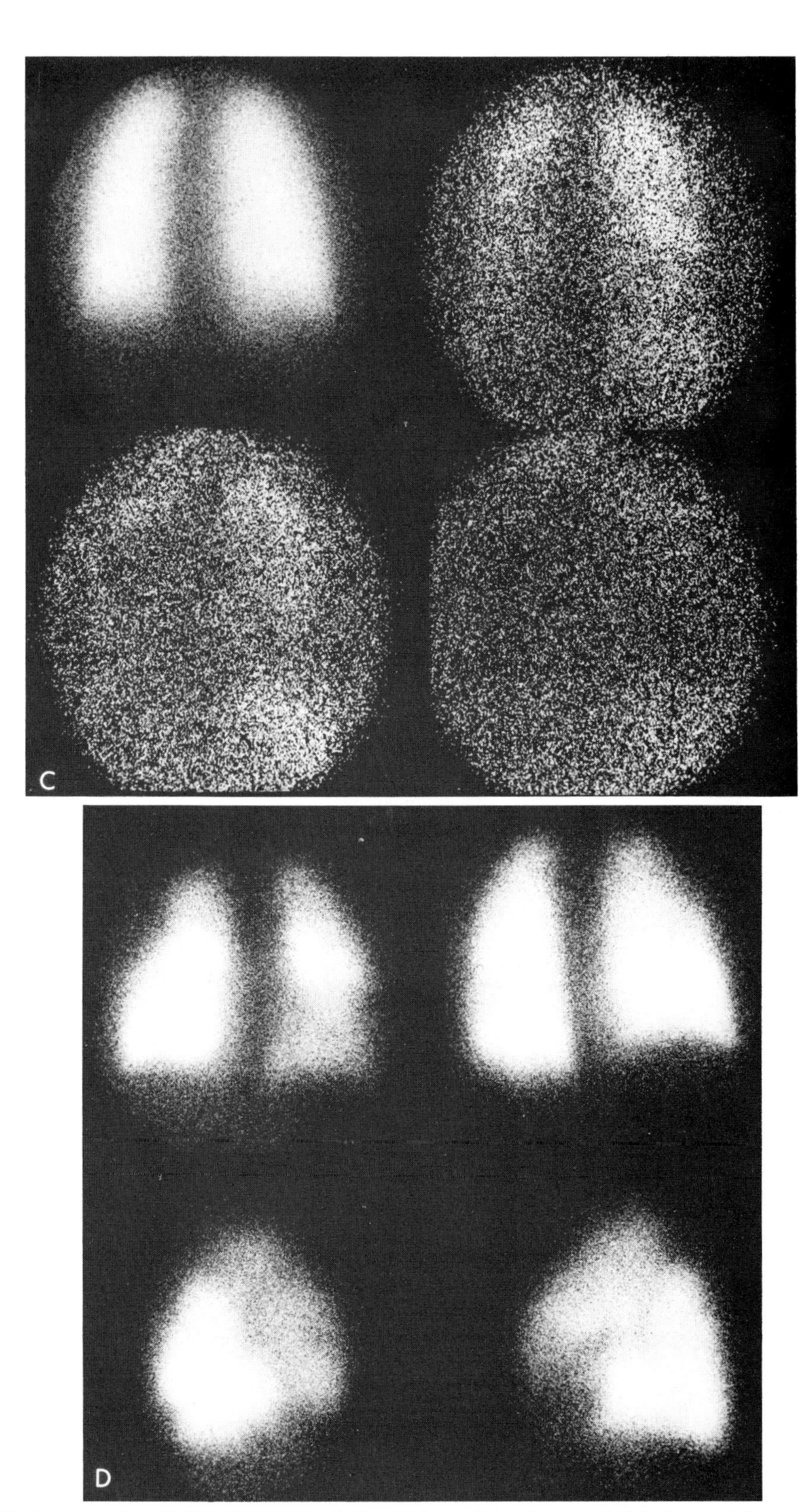

Figure 6–8 *Continued.* *C.* Ventilation study (washin and washout at 1.0, 3.0, and 6.0 minutes). There is normal filling of both lungs at the end of the washin. During the washout there is normal clearance from the left lung, except for the apex, and also from the right mid zone. There is delayed clearance from the right upper zone, right base, and left apex. These studies show evidence of pulmonary embolism in the left lung and right mid zone. In addition, there is evidence of airway obstruction in both upper lobes and probably the right base. She was treated with anticoagulants. *D.* Repeat studies five days later. Four view perfusion images show improvement in blood flow to both lungs. Both upper lobes have diminished blood flow.

Legend continued on the opposite page

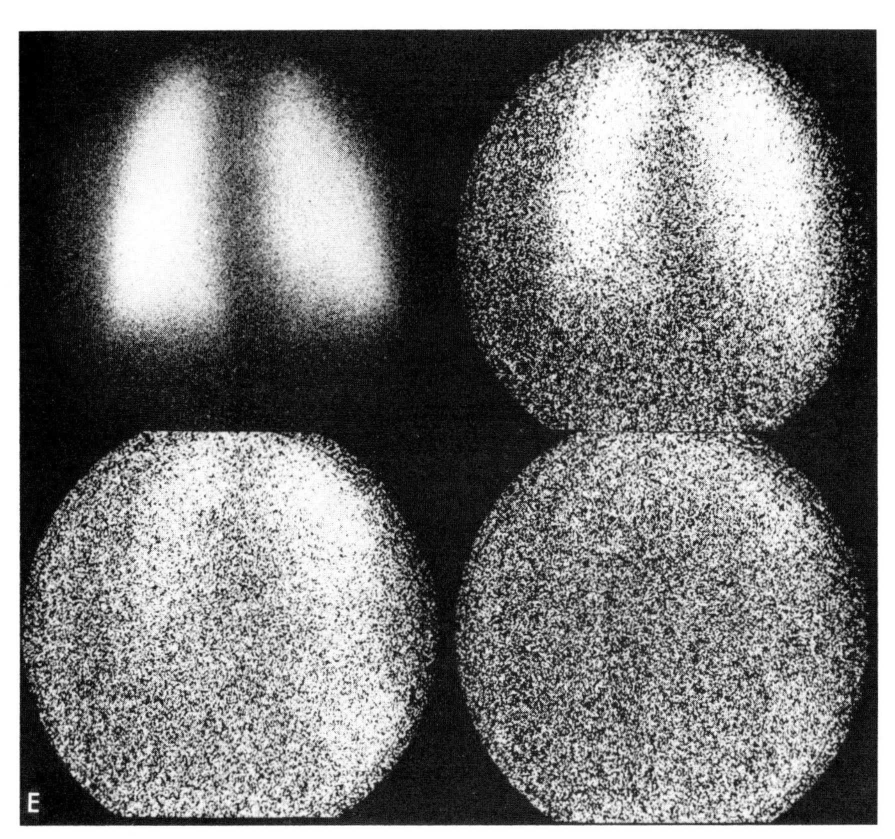

***Figure 6–8** Continued.* *E.* Ventilation study (washin and washout at 1.0, 3.0, and 6.0 minutes). The pattern is virtually unchanged from the earlier study. The improvement in blood flow is in keeping with the resolution of pulmonary embolism. The continued presence of impaired clearance of xenon indicates that the findings on the initial study were not due to the transient bronchoconstriction that may accompany pulmonary embolism, but were due to chronic obstructive pulmonary disease.

sential for the proper interpretation of perfusion lung scans. Chronic bronchitis and emphysema are common diseases in older people, while bronchial asthma may be seen at almost any age. Bronchiectasis is becoming less common. Each of these conditions may not be accompanied by any abnormality on the plain chest radiograph. As a cause of perfusion defects seen in a busy nuclear medicine department, this group of conditions outweighs pulmonary embolism by about 3:1. About half of such a population with airway obstruction will have normal chest radiographs.[2] Although the clinical findings may indicate the presence of airway obstruction, it is still necessary to know whether the defects in blood flow seen on a perfusion scan are associated with a similar degree of impaired ventilation or whether they are accompanied by more normal ventilation. There is little doubt that washout images taken after a 3 to 5 minute rebreathing period provide more reliable evidence of impaired ventilation than either single breath studies or washin sequences. Only severely affected regions or emphysematous bullae can be identified by their lack of filling in the equilibrium image obtained at the end of a washin.

The patterns of disturbed ventilation and perfusion seen in emphysema vary from predominantly upper zone disease through mid zone problems to predominantly basal disease.[7] In general, the pattern of dysfunction is fairly symmetrical, with each lung being involved to a similar, although rarely identical, extent (Fig. 6–9). Occasionally,

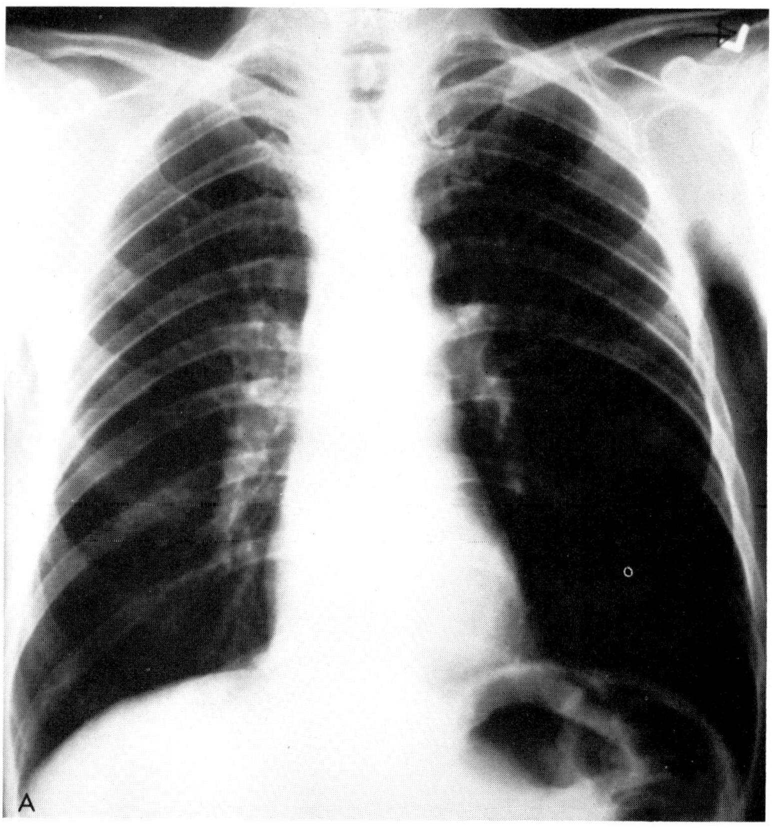

Figure 6–9. Chronic obstructive airways disease. *A*. Posteroanterior chest radiograph of a 57 year old man, with chronic cough and dyspnea and evidence of airways obstruction on pulmonary function testing, demonstrates some hyperinflation. *B*. Four view perfusion images showing numerous defects in blood flow. Some of the defects are segmental while others are more diffuse. The right lung receives less blood flow than the left. *C*. Ventilation study (washin and washout at 1.0, 5.0, and 10.0 minutes). The right lung contains less activity at the end of the washin, especially in the right mid zone, indicative of failure to reach equilibrium here. There is marked delay in clearance from both lungs, with the most severe impairment corresponding to the regions with the greatest defects in blood flow.

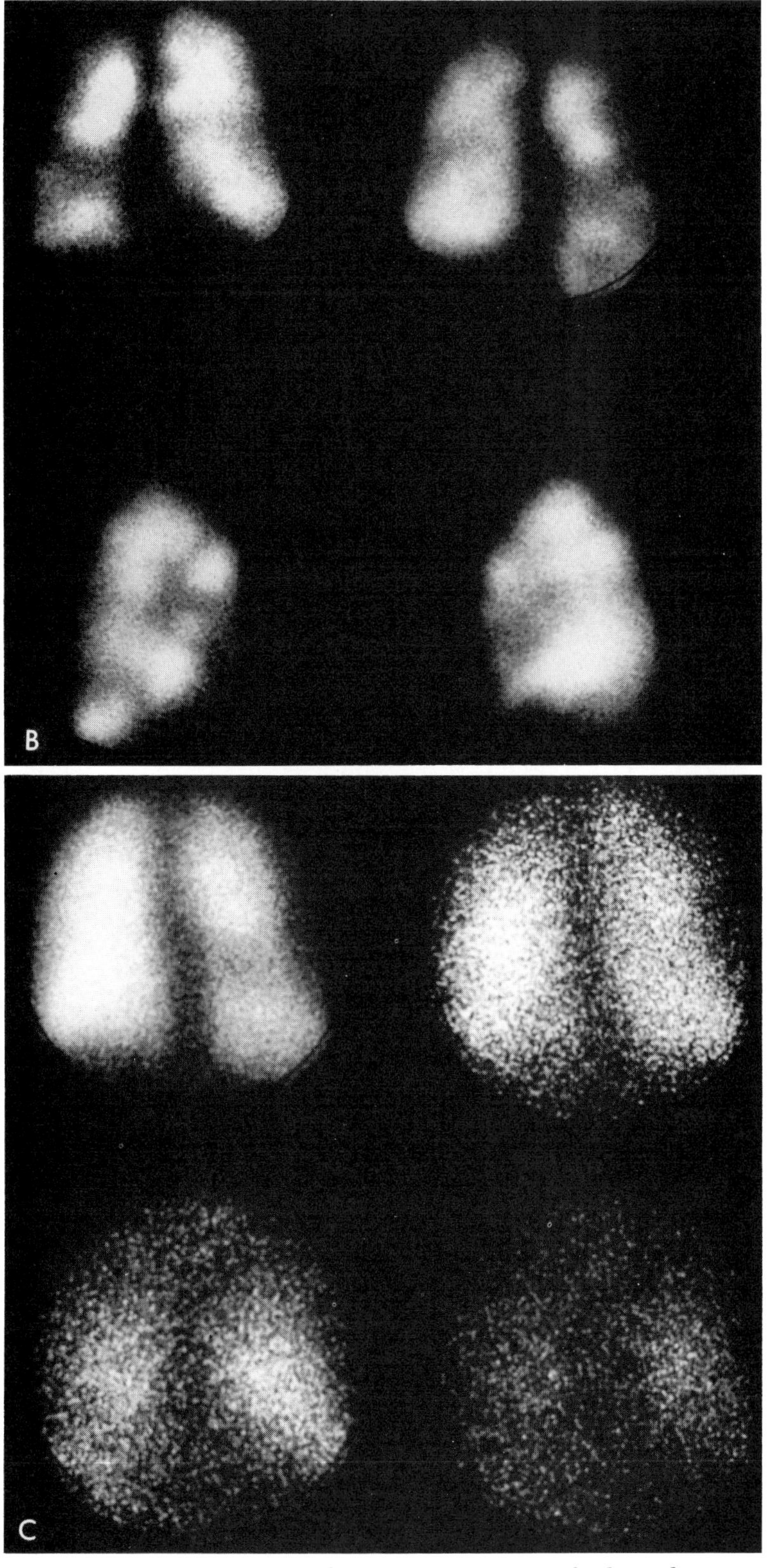

Figure 6–9 *Continued.* *See opposite page for legend.*

one lung is severely involved while its companion has only trivial impairment (Fig. 6–10). The defects in blood flow tend to be non-segmental and overlap both segmental and lobar boundaries. Radiologically visible bullae, or cysts, are always accompanied by defects in blood flow, and such bullae show evidence of grossly impaired or virtually absent gas exchange (Fig. 6–11). The delay in whole lung clearance of xenon-133 has been shown to correlate quite well with other evidence of airway obstruction in both adults and children, so that an assessment of the severity of the disease can be made from the washout images. In emphysema, the defects in blood flow follow the disturbance in ventilation, being either of the same magnitude or else less severe. Only very rarely is the defect in blood flow apparently greater than the defect in ventilation. If the presence of obstructive airways disease can be recognized on the chest radiograph, ventilation and blood flow are always abnormal. The converse is not true. Regions of severe ventilatory impairment may be found in areas that appear radiographically normal.[2] Patients with chronic bronchitis and bronchial asthma tend to show a greater disturbance in ventilation than in blood flow, compared to patients with emphysema.[4] Furthermore, in both conditions – but especially in asthma – the patterns may change as the degree of airway obstruction improves or worsens.[41] The changes in asthma occur within a few moments of the onset of an attack, and will

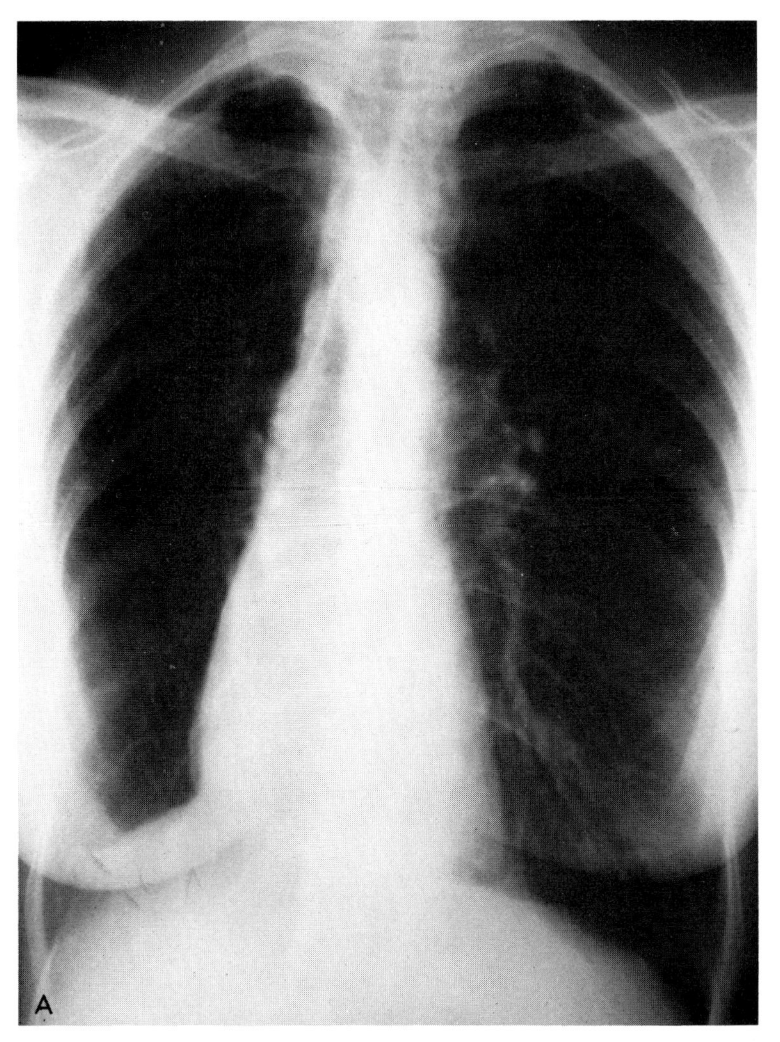

Figure 6–10. Chronic obstructive airways disease – predominantly unilateral. *A.* Posteroanterior radiograph of a 57 year old woman, who had a history of dyspnea, demonstrates hyperlucency of the right lung and deviation of the trachea and mediastinum toward the right.

Legend continued on the opposite page

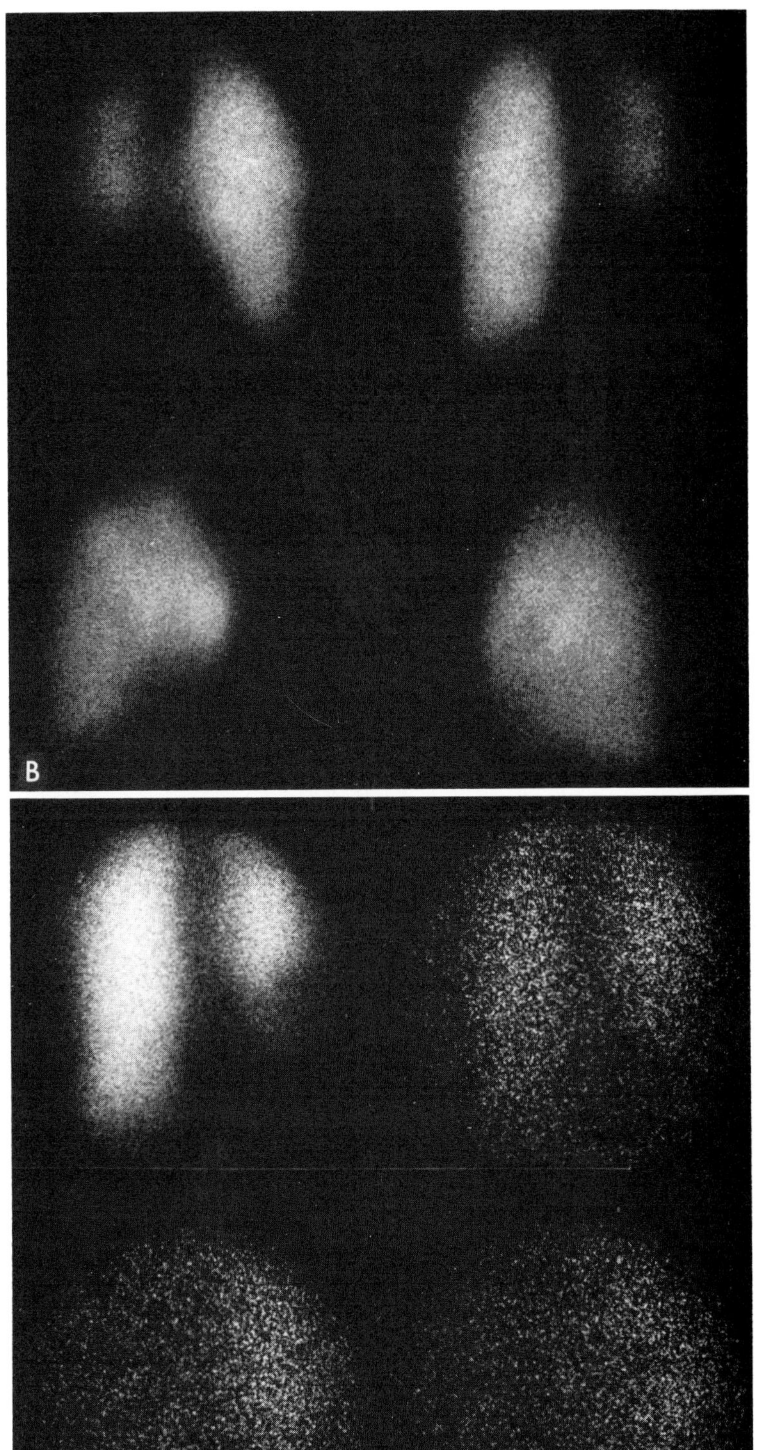

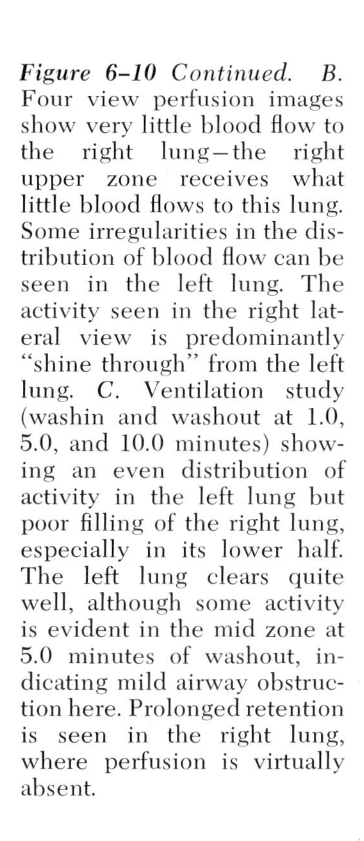

Figure 6–10 Continued. *B.* Four view perfusion images show very little blood flow to the right lung—the right upper zone receives what little blood flows to this lung. Some irregularities in the distribution of blood flow can be seen in the left lung. The activity seen in the right lateral view is predominantly "shine through" from the left lung. *C.* Ventilation study (washin and washout at 1.0, 5.0, and 10.0 minutes) showing an even distribution of activity in the left lung but poor filling of the right lung, especially in its lower half. The left lung clears quite well, although some activity is evident in the mid zone at 5.0 minutes of washout, indicating mild airway obstruction here. Prolonged retention is seen in the right lung, where perfusion is virtually absent.

fade as the attack subsides. However, asymptomatic asthmatics, who are clinically free of wheezes, may still have abnormal studies. The defects in bronchial asthma tend to be more focal than those seen in emphysema, and are often segmental or subsegmental, so that the distinction from pulmonary embolism, in the absence of a ventilation study, can be difficult (Fig. 6–12). Furthermore, the defects in blood flow may disappear at a similar rate, increasing the difficulty of distinguishing between these conditions on the basis of perfusion scans alone.

In children and young adults with cystic fibrosis, the fissure sign is seen in more than half the patients, and may be present in relatively mild disease. As the disease progresses, ventilation becomes more impaired, with defects visible during both washin and washout studies. Widespread patchy non-segmental defects in blood flow also become apparent and correspond closely to the defects in ventilation. The upper lobes are usually most severely affected (Fig. 6–4). The overall lung clearance rate has been shown to correlate with both the forced expiratory volume at 1 second and the peak flow rate in such children.[3]

SURGERY FOR EMPHYSEMATOUS BULLAE. Ventilation and perfusion scans may be used in the preoperative evaluation of patients with emphysematous bullae. Removal or plication of bullae is not indicated when most of the physiologic disturbance is due to associated parenchymal disease. When there is good perfusion of the remainder of the lung around a bullous area, and the bullae have been enlarging as the

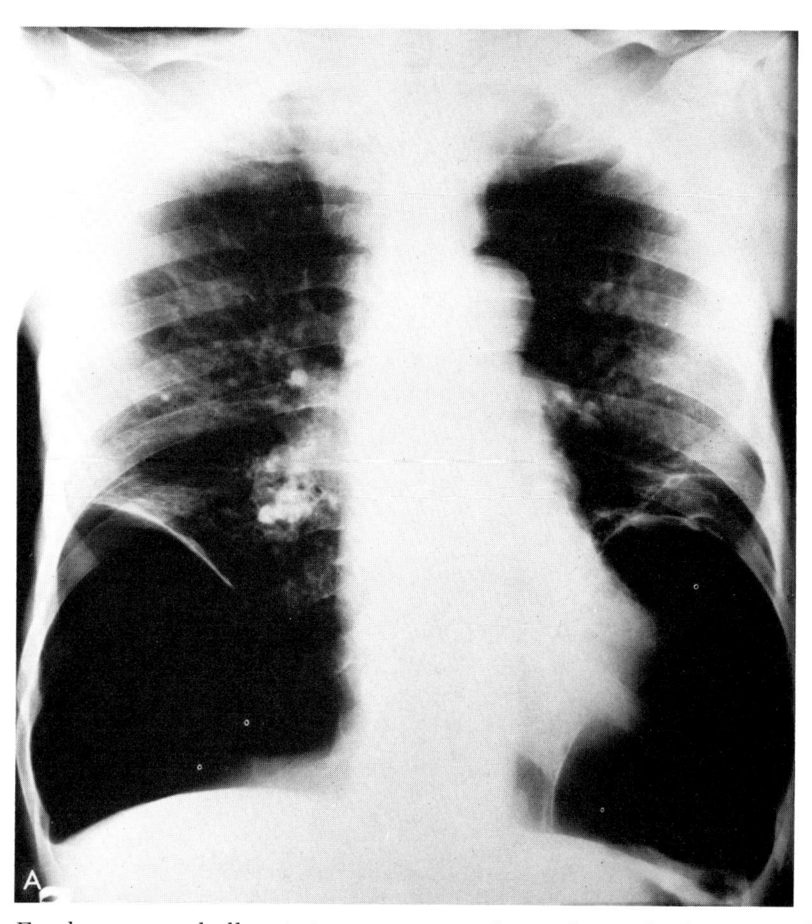

Figure 6–11. Emphysematous bullae. A. Anteroposterior chest radiograph of a 64 year old man shows bullous regions in both bases.

Legend continued on the opposite page

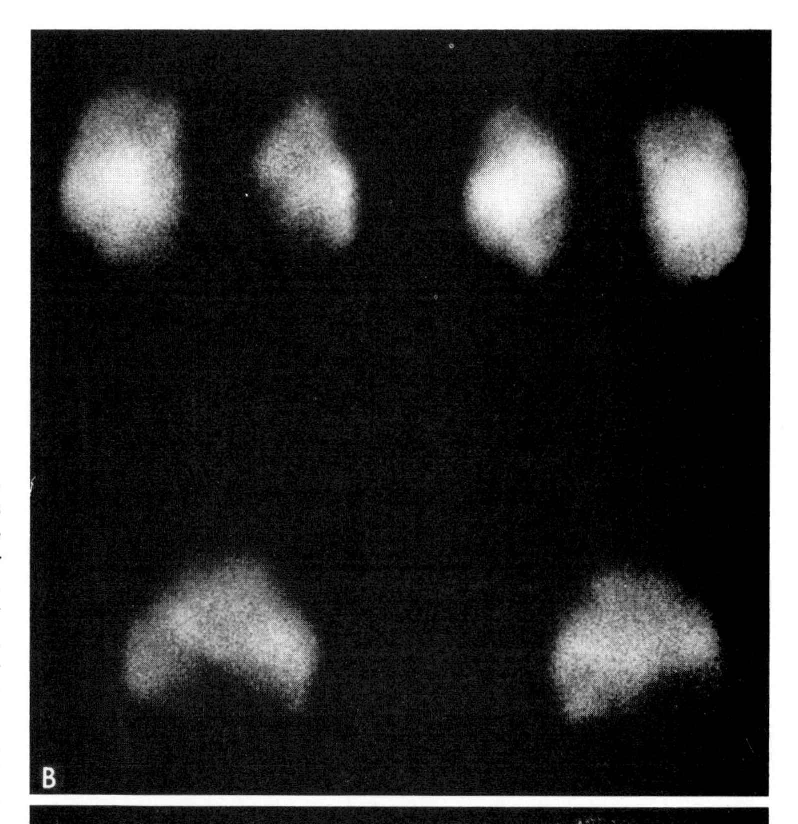

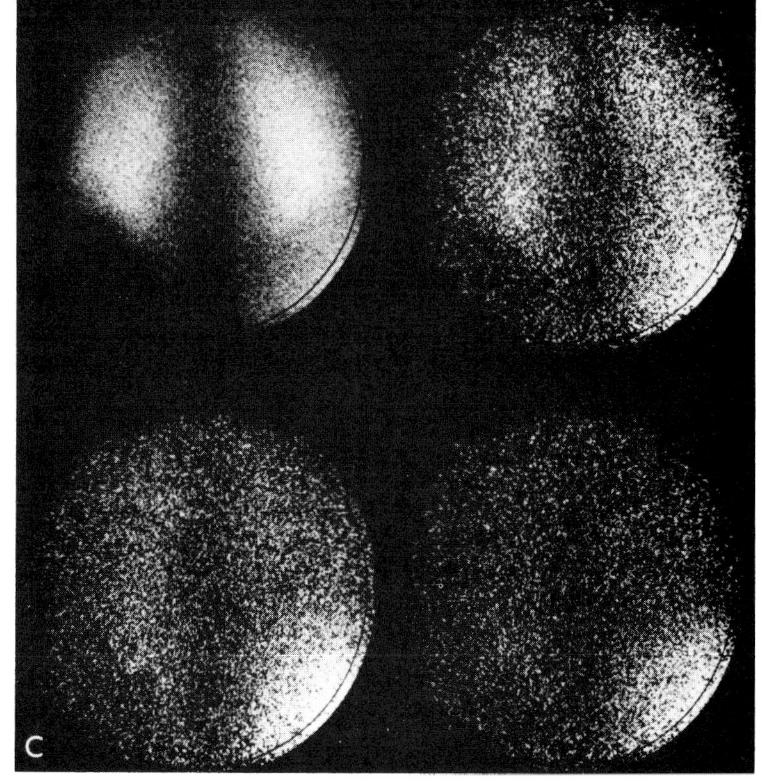

Figure 6–11 *Continued. B.* Four view perfusion images show absent blood flow in the bullous areas and irregular perfusion to the rest of his lungs. *C.* Ventilation study (washin and washout at 1.0, 5.0, and 10.0 minutes). No activity enters the bullous zone at the left base, while there is incomplete filling of the right base and left apex. Clearance is delayed from both lungs through 10 minutes, but especially from the bullous region at the right base. It looks as though the left base takes no part in gas exchange. (From Secker-Walker, R. H.: Lung scanning. *In* Gottschalk, A., and Potchen, E. J., editors: Golden's Diagnostic Radiology, Section 20, Diagnostic Nuclear Medicine. © 1975, The Williams & Wilkins Co., Baltimore.)

patient's symptoms become worse, some improvement in function can be expected from surgery. When blood flow around a bullous region is impaired, it implies more extensive parenchymal disease and surgery is best avoided[13] (Fig. 6–13).

Bronchiectasis. Bronchiectatic regions of the lung are clearly delineated by ventilation-perfusion imaging, for both ventilation and blood flow are grossly impaired. The extent of the defect corresponds to the anatomic segments or lobes that are involved. Usually, the affected region fails to fill with xenon-133 during the washin procedure, and there is a great delay in the clearance of what little gas enters this region. There is nothing diagnostic about these studies – they merely indicate a region of severe ventilatory impairment with equally severely impaired blood flow – but if the diagnosis has not been established, such findings should lead to further investigation of the cause of an apparent bronchial obstruction, via such procedures as bronchoscopy or bronchography (Fig. 6–14).

Bronchial obstruction. Conditions associated with bronchial obstruction, such as tumors, inhaled foreign bodies, or impacted mucus, show varying degrees of impaired ventilation and blood flow depending on both the site and the extent of the obstructing lesion. The more severe the obstruction, the greater the diminution in gas exchange; this causes localized hypoxia and reflex constriction of pulmonary arterioles. The associated defect in blood flow corresponds to the anatomic distribution of the affected bronchus. As a lobar bronchus becomes obstructed, the affected lobe will usually collapse because there is no collateral ventilation between lobes.

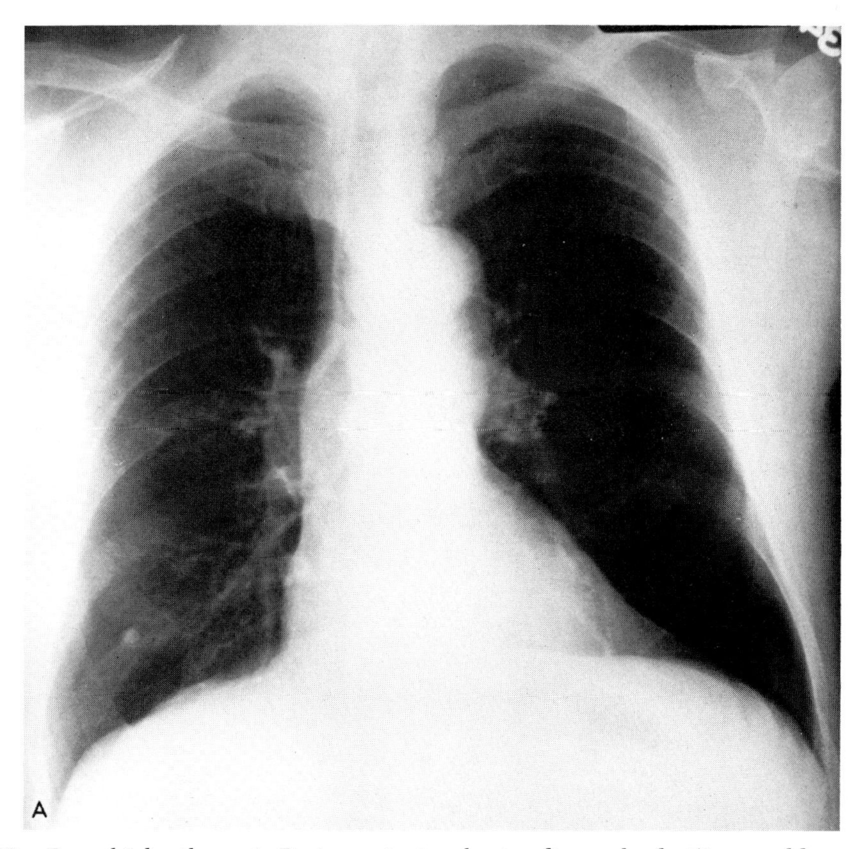

Figure 6–12. Bronchial asthma. *A.* Posteroanterior chest radiograph of a 71 year old man with bronchial asthma demonstrates some hyperinflation of the left mid and lower lung field.

Legend continued on the opposite page

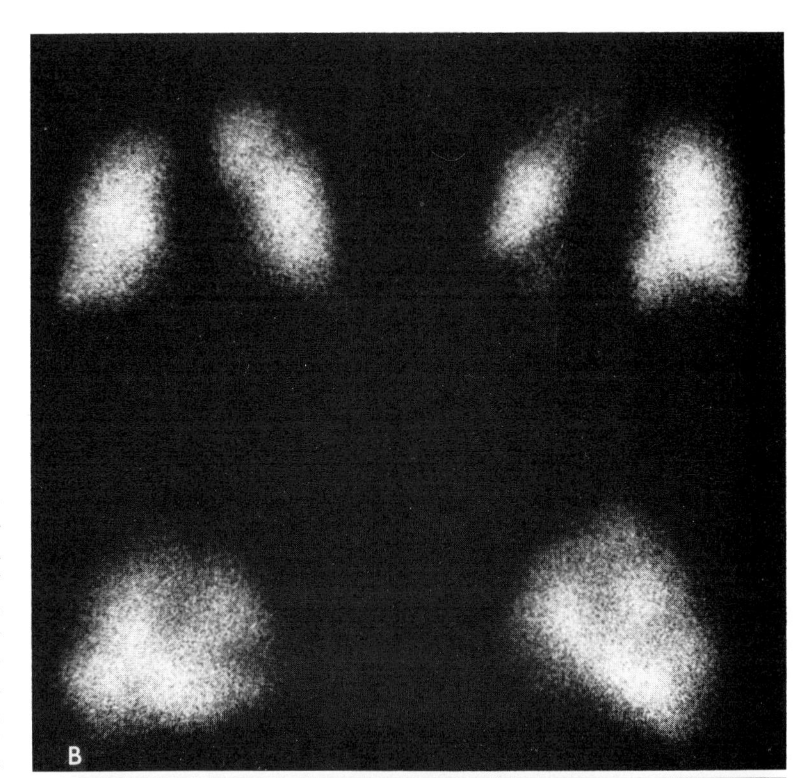

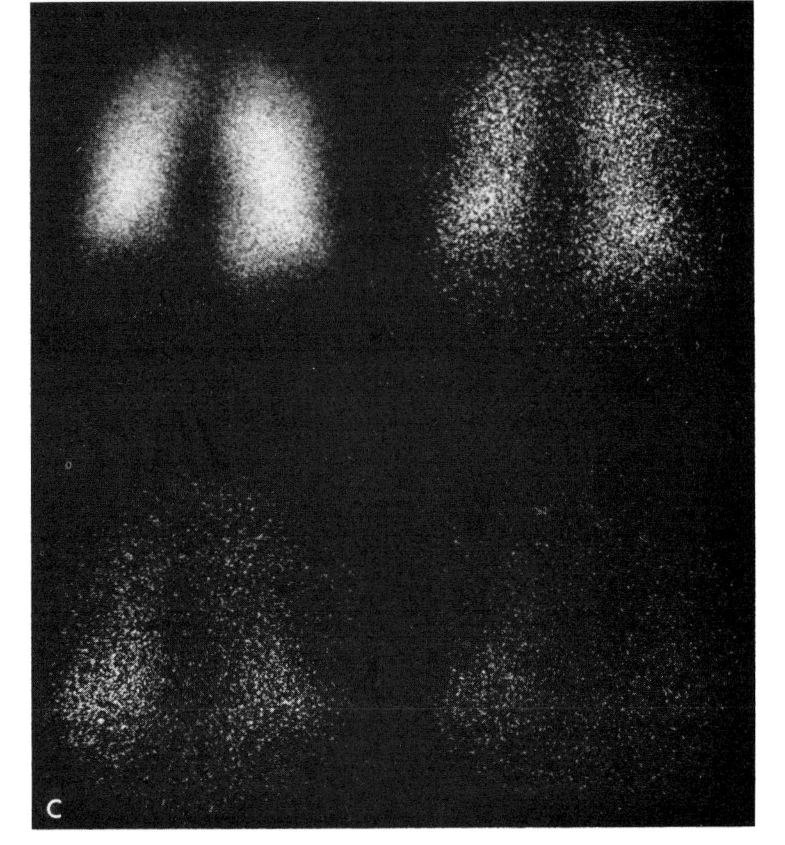

Figure 6–12 *Continued.* *B.* Four view perfusion images showing segmental and subsegmental defects in blood flow. *C.* Ventilation study (washin and washout at 1.0, 5.0, and 10.0 minutes) showing partial failure to fill the left lower zone and delayed clearance from both lungs, but especially the bases. The areas of most severe impairment of ventilation correspond to those with the worst blood flow. (From Secker-Walker, R. H.: Lung scanning. *In* Gottschalk, A., and Potchen. E. J., editors: Golden's Diagnostic Radiology, Section 20, Diagnostic Nuclear Medicine. © 1975, The Williams & Wilkins Co., Baltimore.)

However, segmental or subsegmental lesions may cause complete obstruction without collapse; air reaches the alveoli beyond the obstruction through the pores of Kohn and the channels of Lambert. Such ventilation is considerably less efficient than normal, and the affected segment is usually readily identified during a ventilation study (Fig. 6–15).

Following removal of foreign bodies, blood flow returns over the course of several days. When there is evidence of localized bronchial obstruction, but the defect in blood flow is greater than the defect in ventilation, a tumor that has spread to involve the pulmonary vessels should be considered.

CARCINOMA OF THE BRONCHUS

Carcinoma of the bronchus may present with a variety of functional disturbances. These tumors derive their blood supply from the bronchial arteries, so that they appear as defects in blood flow on a perfusion scan. Small tumors, less than 2 or 3 cm. in diameter, are unlikely to be seen unless they already involve the hilar vessels. Larger tumors produce defects in blood flow that may correspond to the size of the tumor or may involve a segment, a lobe, or the whole lung. Defects in ventilation correspond to the anatomical distribution of the affected bronchus (Fig. 6–16).

The size of the defect in blood flow is closely related to the extent of tumor involvement of the pulmonary vessels, either by compression or by distortion, or less commonly by direct invasion of either the pulmonary veins or arteries. Bronchial obstruction plays a smaller part in reducing blood flow, for it is not uncommon to find diminished blood flow in neighboring segments or lobes, whose bronchi are fully patent and whose ventilation is unimpaired (Fig. 6–17).

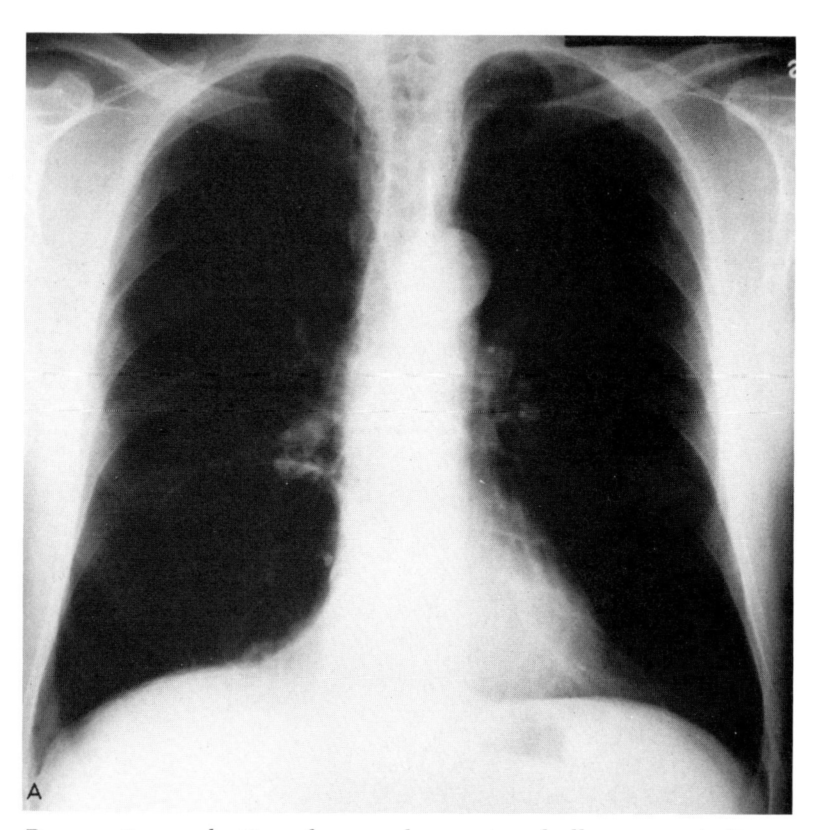

Figure 6–13. Preoperative evaluation of an emphysematous bullous area. *A.* Posteroanterior chest radiograph of a 62 year old man demonstrates a bullous region at the right base.

Legend continued on the opposite page

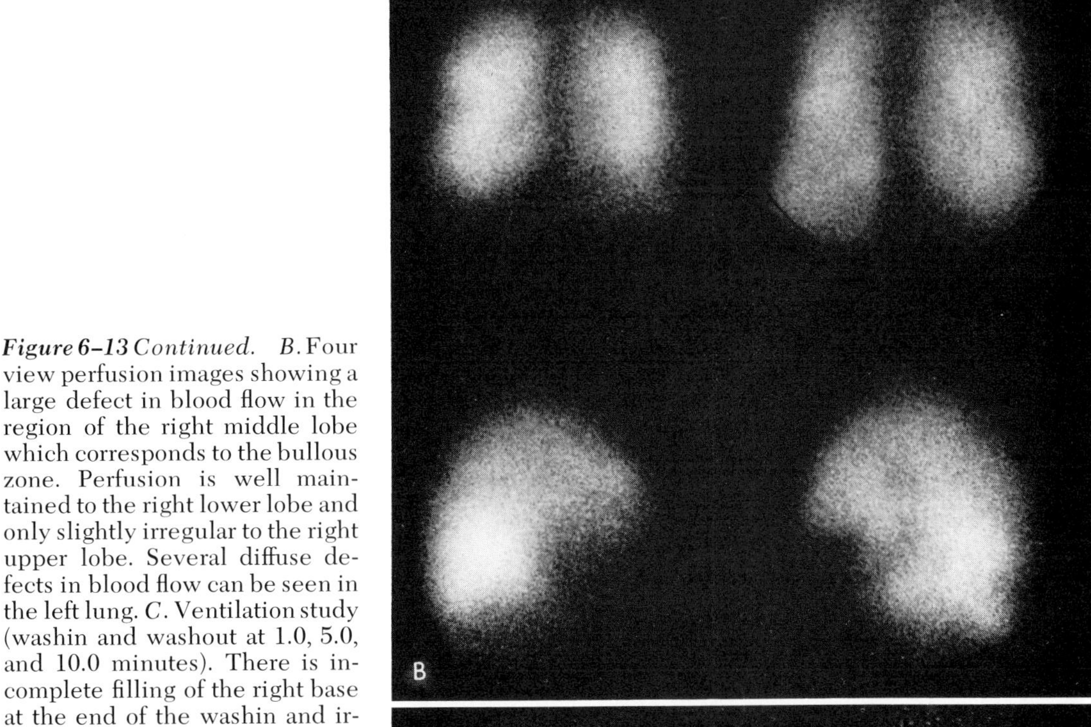

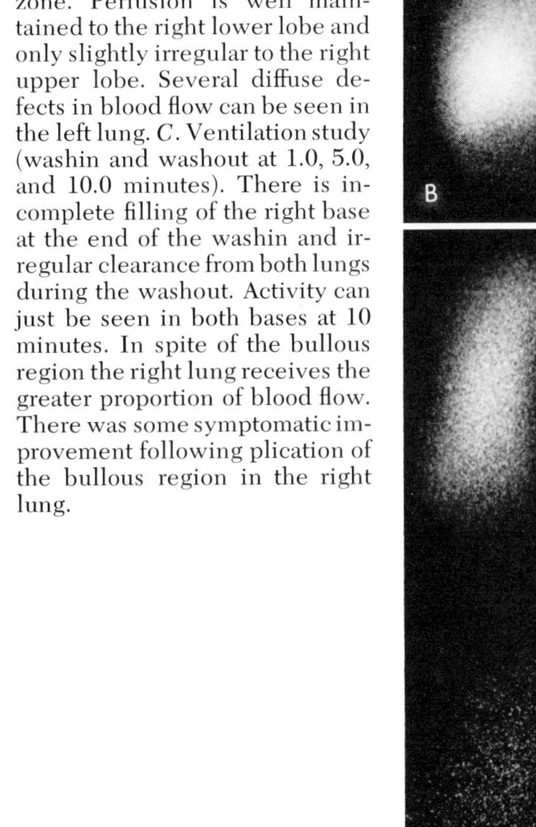

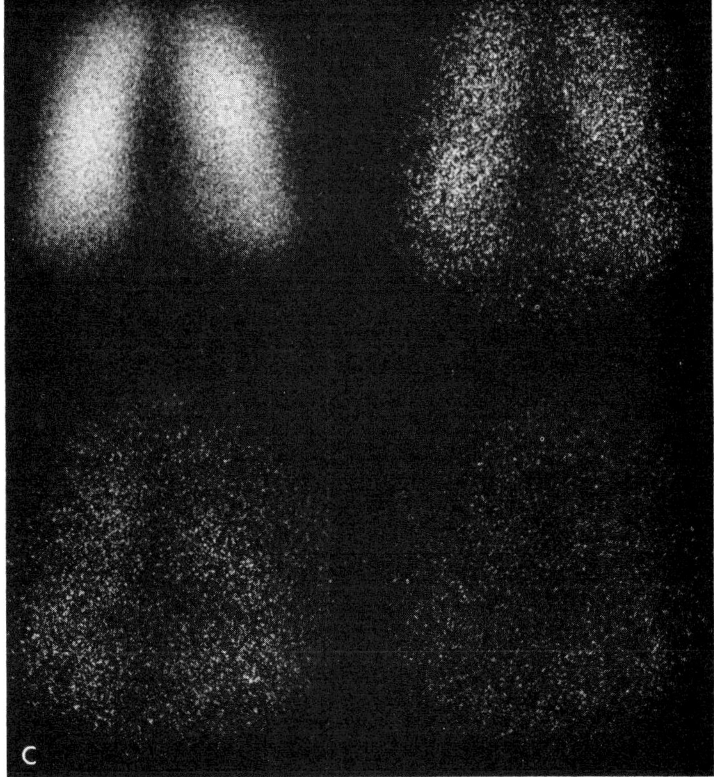

Figure 6–13 *Continued.* *B.* Four view perfusion images showing a large defect in blood flow in the region of the right middle lobe which corresponds to the bullous zone. Perfusion is well maintained to the right lower lobe and only slightly irregular to the right upper lobe. Several diffuse defects in blood flow can be seen in the left lung. *C.* Ventilation study (washin and washout at 1.0, 5.0, and 10.0 minutes). There is incomplete filling of the right base at the end of the washin and irregular clearance from both lungs during the washout. Activity can just be seen in both bases at 10 minutes. In spite of the bullous region the right lung receives the greater proportion of blood flow. There was some symptomatic improvement following plication of the bullous region in the right lung.

A number of indications for ventilation-perfusion studies in patients with carcinoma of the bronchus have been suggested.[33] First, the combined studies provide an excellent indication of the functional integrity of each lung and of the regions within each lung. More than half the patients with carcinoma of the bronchus have defects in blood flow in the opposite lung, and at least three quarters of them have defects in ventilation as well. These figures merely reflect the high incidence of chronic obstructive airways disease in patients with lung cancer. In 10 to 15 per cent of patients, unexpectedly large defects in blood flow may be found in the non-tumor-bearing lung. These may be so large as to lead to a more conservative procedure or contraindicate any surgical approach at all.

Second, whether ventilation-perfusion studies can be used to predict resectability remains debatable. There is some evidence to suggest that if the relative blood flow to the tumor-bearing lung is less than one third of the total blood flow, then the chances of a successful resection are less than 5 per cent. What is clear is that the closer the tumor is to the hilum, the more extensive is the reduction in blood flow to that lung, because the vessels in the hilum are surrounded, compressed, or invaded by tumor tissue. Blood flow is usually more severely affected than is ventilation because there is more tumor spreading outside the bronchus than into its lumen.[6]

A third application of ventilation-perfusion scanning in carcinoma of the bronchus is its use to localize the site of an otherwise occult carcinoma, whose presence has been found by cytology but whose position cannot be seen radiographically or broncho-

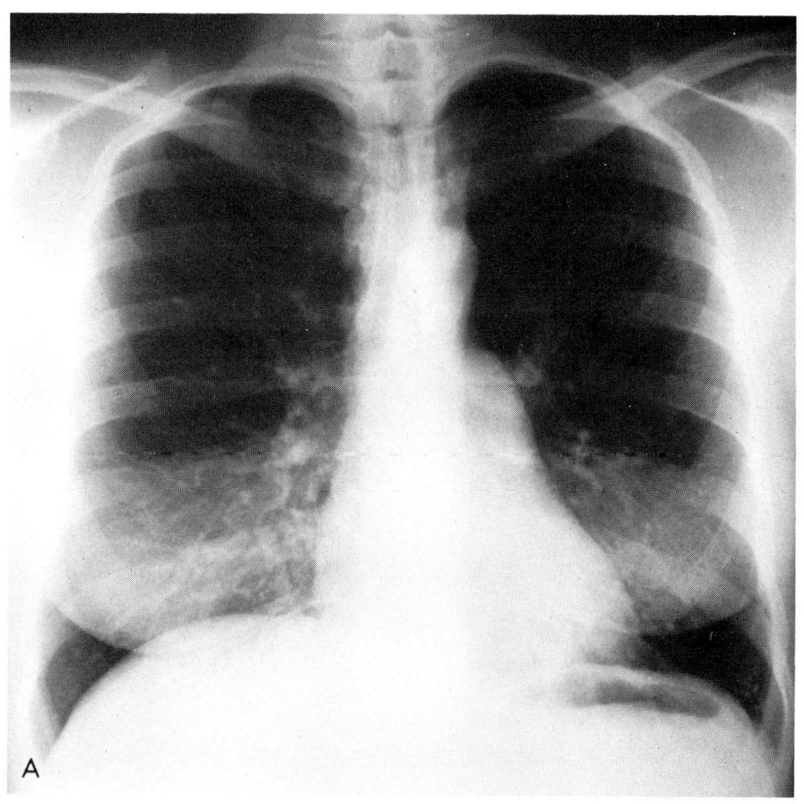

Figure 6–14. Bronchiectasis. *A*. Posteroanterior chest radiograph of a 21 year old woman demonstrates a slight increase in density in the left lower lobe. *B*. Four view perfusion images showing absence of blood flow to the left lower lobe. The right lung is normal. *C*. Ventilation study (washin and washout at 1.0, 5.0, and 10.0 minutes). The left lower lobe does not fill during the washin, and there is prolonged retention in this region during the washout. The right lung clears normally. A bronchogram demonstrated tubular bronchiectasis in the left lower lobe.

Legend continued on the opposite page

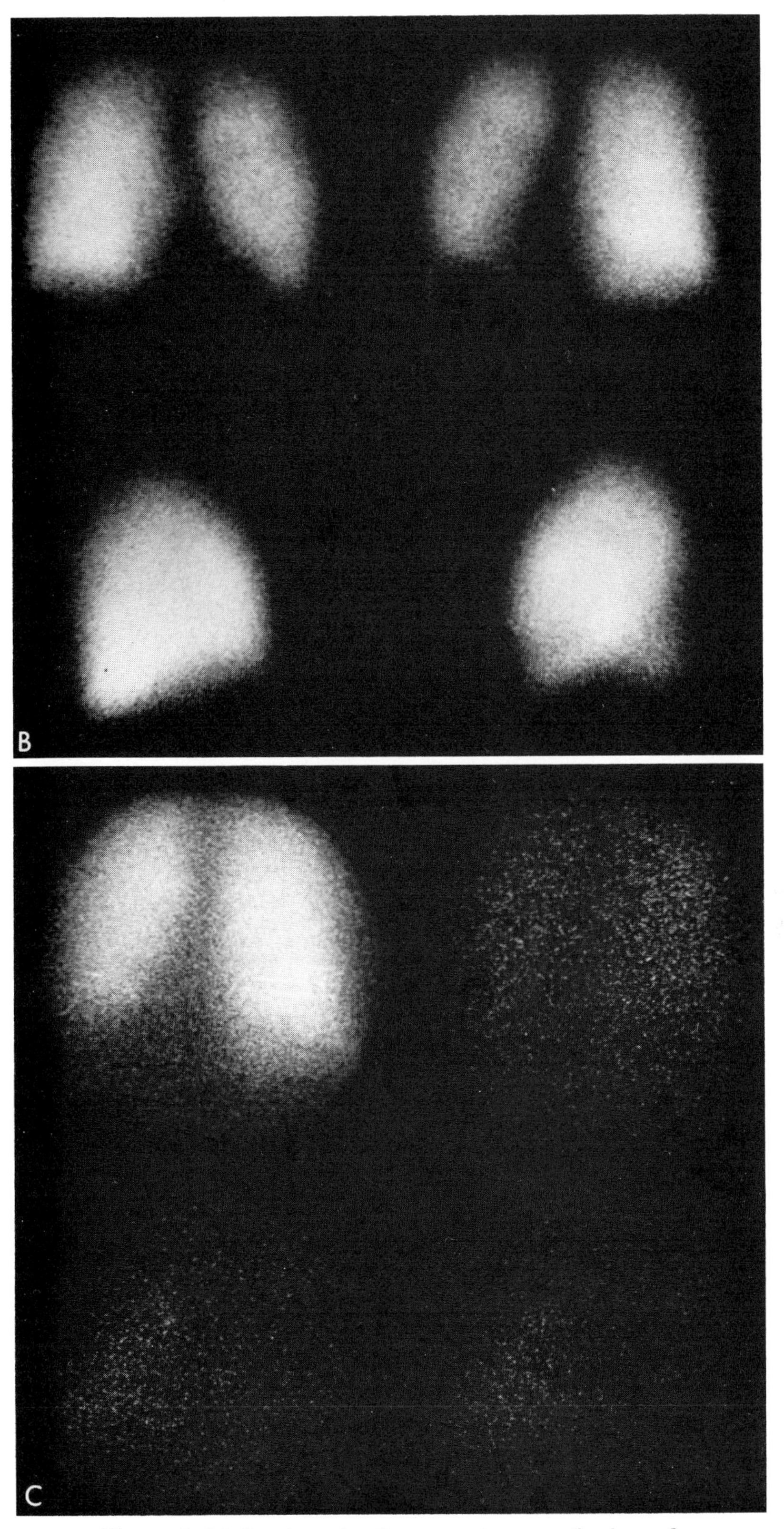

Figure 6–14 *Continued.* *See opposite page for legend.*

scopically. The frequent coexistence of carcinoma of the bronchus and chronic obstructive lung disease means that often it will not be possible to determine which defect in blood flow corresponds to tumor. If there is a region with a higher ventilation-perfusion ratio than normal, this is the one most likely to contain the tumor (Fig. 6–18).

Ventilation-perfusion studies after radiation treatment for carcinoma of the lung show some return of blood flow in about 40 per cent of subjects. Ventilation returns more quickly and often more fully. No correlation has been found between the return of blood flow and length of survival.[19]

Defects in blood flow in relation to hilar node enlargement are certainly not indicative of malignant invasion of these nodes. Sarcoidosis and other chronic granulomatous conditions are usually accompanied by defects in blood flow in both lungs when there is hilar node enlargement. The mechanism is not clear but is probably similar to that proposed for carcinoma of the bronchus, that is, distortion or compression of the pulmonary vessels in the hilum. Additional defects are seen when there is parenchymal disease.

MISCELLANEOUS CONDITIONS

Blood flow is diminished to regions of pneumonic infiltration, and the size of the defects on the scan corresponds closely to the infiltrate seen radiographically. No ventilation takes place in the pneumonic area, so that defects are present on single breath and washin studies. No retention of xenon-133 is seen during the washout procedure, unless there is associated obstructive lung disease. The findings on ventilation-perfusion studies are similar in pneumonia and pulmonary infarction, and it may not be

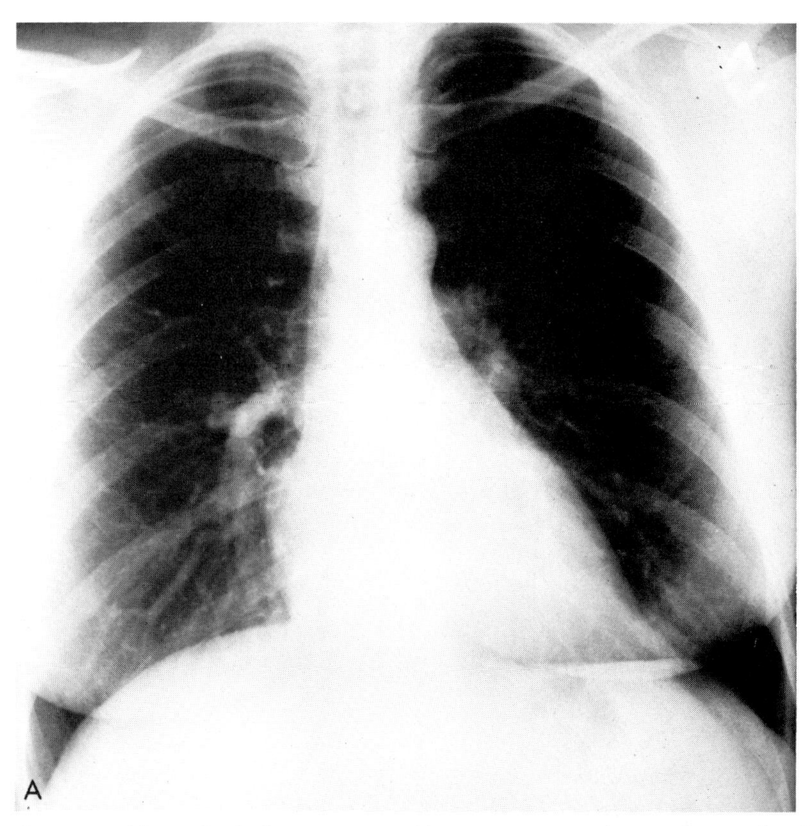

Figure 6–15. Segmental bronchial obstruction. *A.* Posteroanterior chest radiograph of a 45 year old asymptomatic woman. There is a small finger-like density protruding from the right hilum.

Legend continued on the opposite page

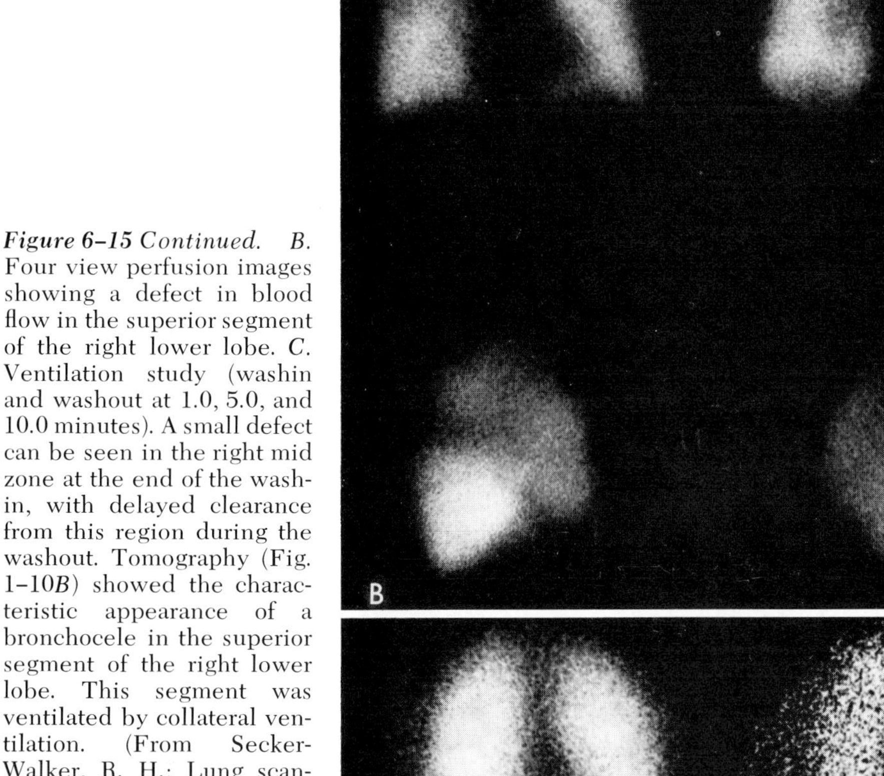

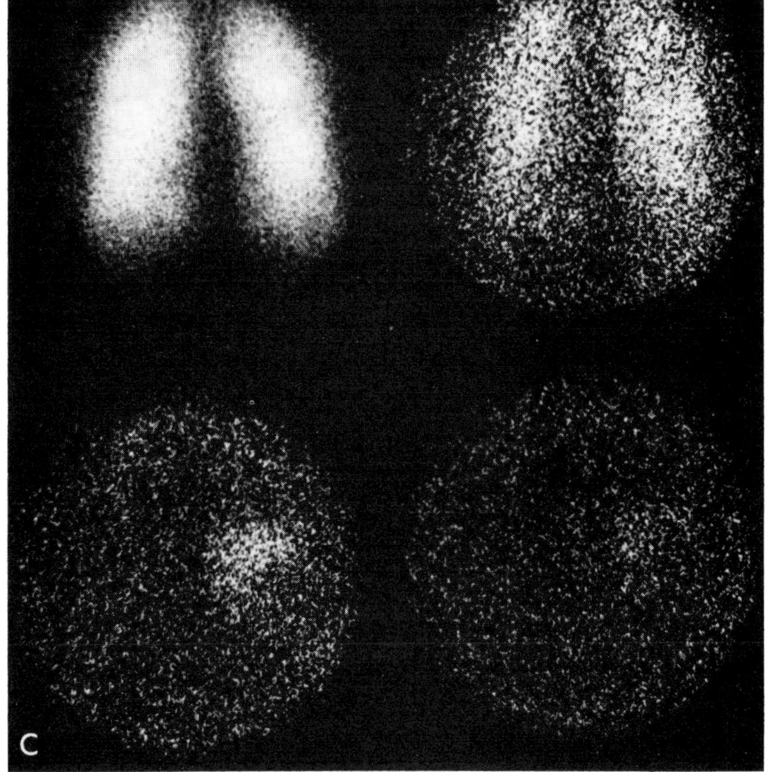

Figure 6–15 *Continued.* *B.* Four view perfusion images showing a defect in blood flow in the superior segment of the right lower lobe. *C.* Ventilation study (washin and washout at 1.0, 5.0, and 10.0 minutes). A small defect can be seen in the right mid zone at the end of the washin, with delayed clearance from this region during the washout. Tomography (Fig. 1–10*B*) showed the characteristic appearance of a bronchocele in the superior segment of the right lower lobe. This segment was ventilated by collateral ventilation. (From Secker-Walker, R. H.: Lung scanning. *In* Gottschalk, A., and Potchen, E. J., editors: Golden's Diagnostic Radiology, Section 20, Diagnostic Nuclear Medicine. © 1975, The Willians & Wilkins Co., Baltimore.)

possible to distinguish these conditions by this method. However, the defects in blood flow in pulmonary infarction are usually more marked and sometimes more extensive than those seen in pneumonia.

In pulmonary tuberculosis and other chronic granulomatous conditions, blood flow is reduced to the involved regions of the lung, and the defects are sometimes larger than the radiological extent of the disease. The defects remain when the disease heals by fibrosis. If perfusion scans have any role in the management of patients with pulmonary tuberculosis, it may lie in aiding decisions regarding the extent of pulmonary resection—but such treatment is rarely undertaken today (Fig. 6–19).

In diseases characterized by diffuse interstitial fibrosis or widespread vasculitis of the pulmonary vessels, perfusion scans show patchy defects in blood flow. Ventilation may appear normal, although the clearance of xenon-133 is usually more rapid than normal, for these diseases are often accompanied by increased minute ventilation. The ventilation-perfusion studies mimic those of multiple small emboli, but the clinical findings and chest radiographs and other measurements of lung function will usually resolve the problem (Fig. 6–20).

Congestive cardiac failure. Perfusion scans are often requested on patients with congestive heart failure, in an effort to determine whether thromboembolic disease is a cause of the heart failure or a significant contributing factor to the patient's

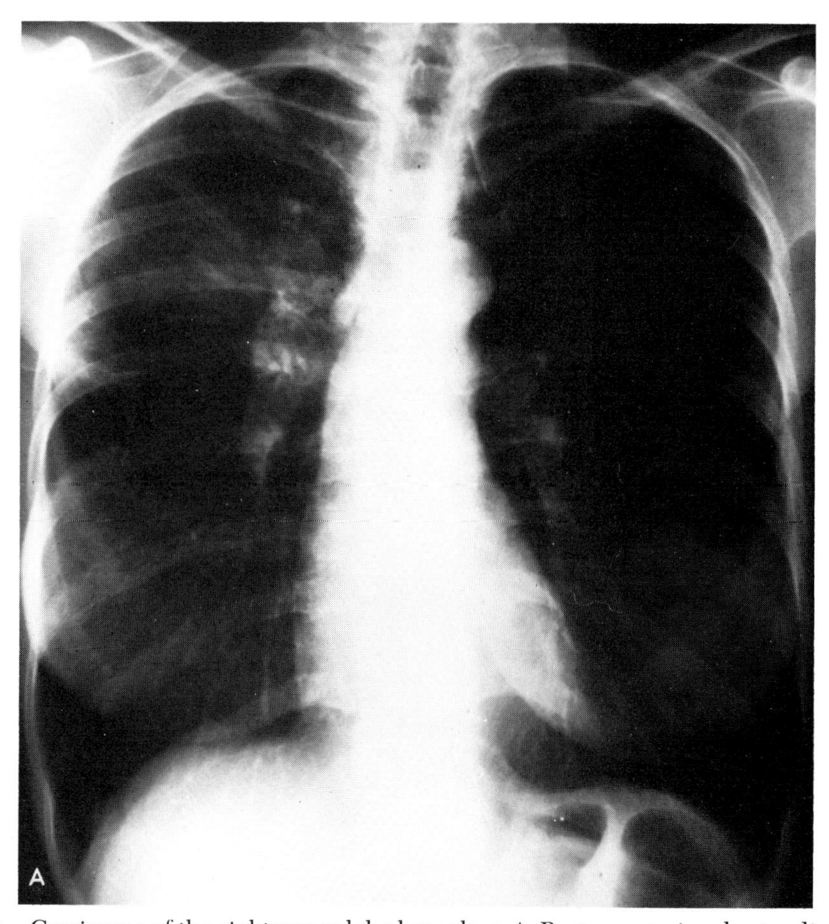

Figure 6–16. Carcinoma of the right upper lobe bronchus. *A.* Posteroanterior chest radiograph of a 50 year old woman demonstrates a right upper lobe mass and a right hilar lymph node enlargement. On bronchoscopy, a squamous cell carcinoma was found obstructing the right upper lobe bronchus.

Legend continued on the opposite page

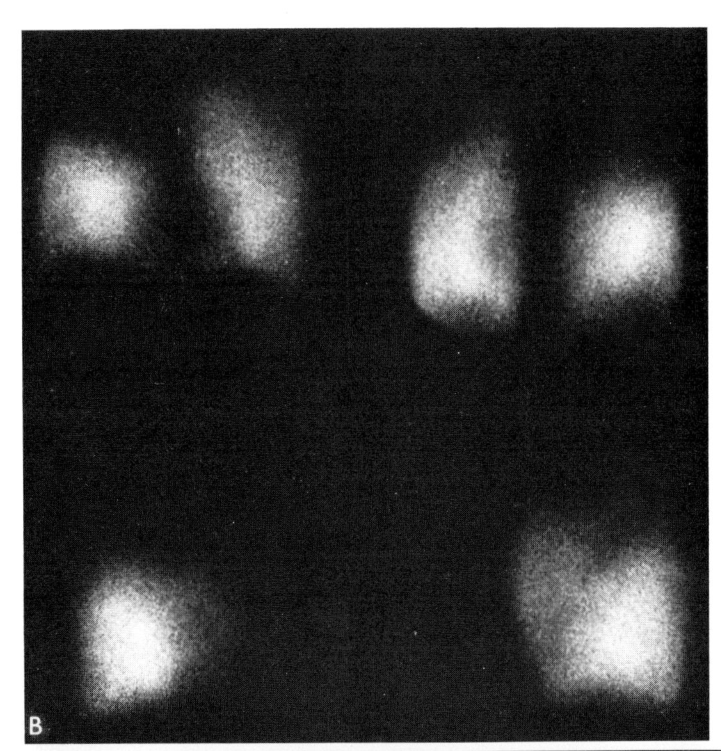

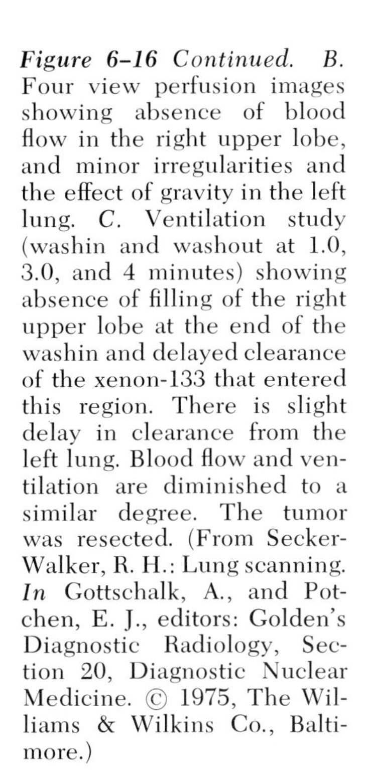

Figure 6–16 *Continued.* *B.* Four view perfusion images showing absence of blood flow in the right upper lobe, and minor irregularities and the effect of gravity in the left lung. *C.* Ventilation study (washin and washout at 1.0, 3.0, and 4 minutes) showing absence of filling of the right upper lobe at the end of the washin and delayed clearance of the xenon-133 that entered this region. There is slight delay in clearance from the left lung. Blood flow and ventilation are diminished to a similar degree. The tumor was resected. (From Secker-Walker, R. H.: Lung scanning. *In* Gottschalk, A., and Potchen, E. J., editors: Golden's Diagnostic Radiology, Section 20, Diagnostic Nuclear Medicine. © 1975, The Williams & Wilkins Co., Baltimore.)

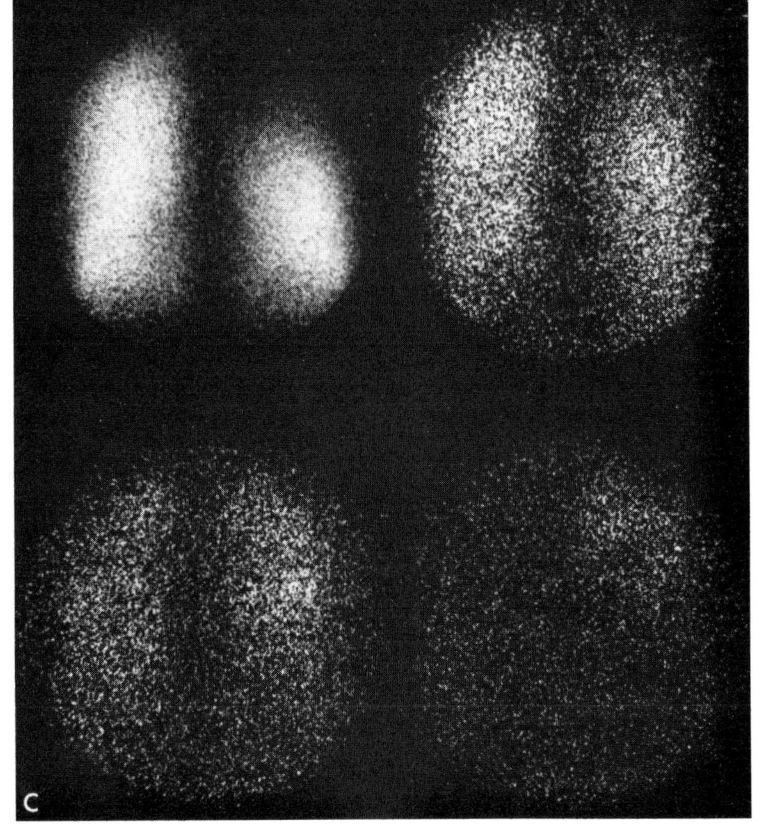

illness. Minor patchy defects in blood flow are usually seen in patients with congestive heart failure, and these are more common in the bases. If the injection of the labeled particles is given with the patient lying supine, symmetrical concave defects in blood flow are frequently seen along the posterior borders of the lateral scans (Fig. 6–21). When areas of pulmonary edema are visible on the chest radiograph, they are accompanied by corresponding defects in blood flow. The presence of a pleural effusion is associated with blunting of the costophrenic angles, or larger defects, depending on the size of the effusion, and also with the fissure sign. The reversal of the normal distribution of blood flow that accompanies left ventricular failure may be seen in about two thirds of patients, but its recognition is not always accompanied by radiologic evidence of a reversal of blood flow.[18] In mitral valve disease, the elevation of left atrial pressure is closely related to the redistribution of blood flow in the lungs, with a greater proportion flowing to the upper zones in the upright position as the pressure increases. This redistribution can often be recognized on perfusion scans, which show diminished activity toward the bases and increased activity in the mid and upper zones, along with normal lung contours. The ratio of upper zone to lower zone blood flow has been shown to correlate well with left atrial pressure and pulmonary arterial pressure.[16]

Regional ventilation shows no clear pattern. In the absence of chronic bronchitis or emphysema, the lungs usually clear rapidly because minute ventilation is often increased. Areas with frank pulmonary edema and pleural effusion show no filling during a washin procedure. With a large

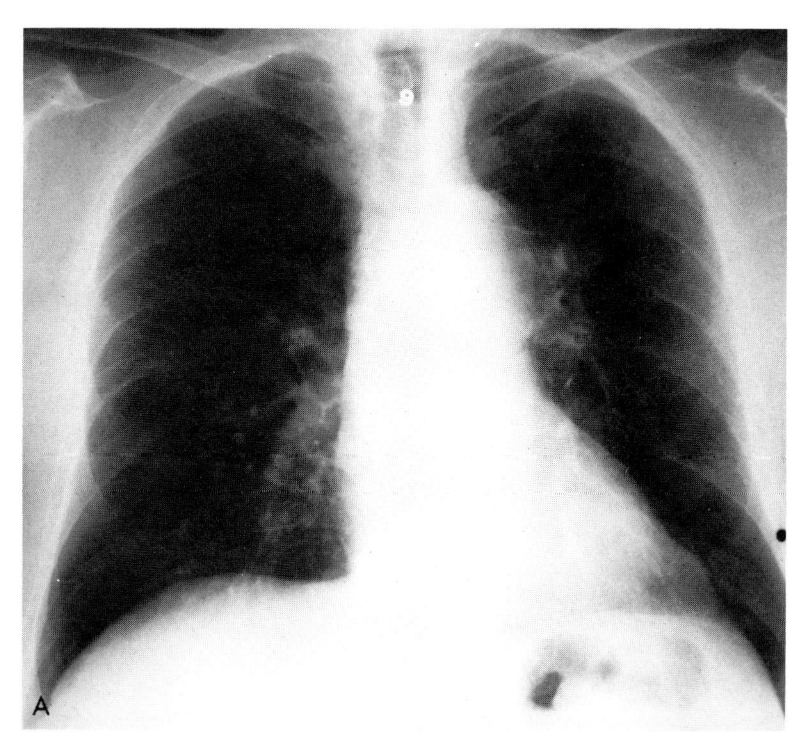

Figure 6–17. Carcinoma of the bronchus with extensive involvement of the vessels in the hilum. *A*. Posteroanterior chest radiograph of a 69 year old man showing a tumor at the upper pole of the left hilum. *B*. Four view perfusion images showing markedly reduced blood flow to the left lung. The activity seen in the left lateral view is largely "shine through" from the right lung. *C*. Ventilation study (washin and washout at 1.0, 5.0, and 10.0 minutes) showing incomplete filling of the left lung at the end of the washin, especially at the left apex, and delayed clearance from this lung during the washout. Clearance from the right lung is normal. On bronchoscopy, the tumor was seen partially obstructing the left upper lobe bronchus. A left vocal cord palsy precluded surgical removal, indicating spread to the mediastinum.

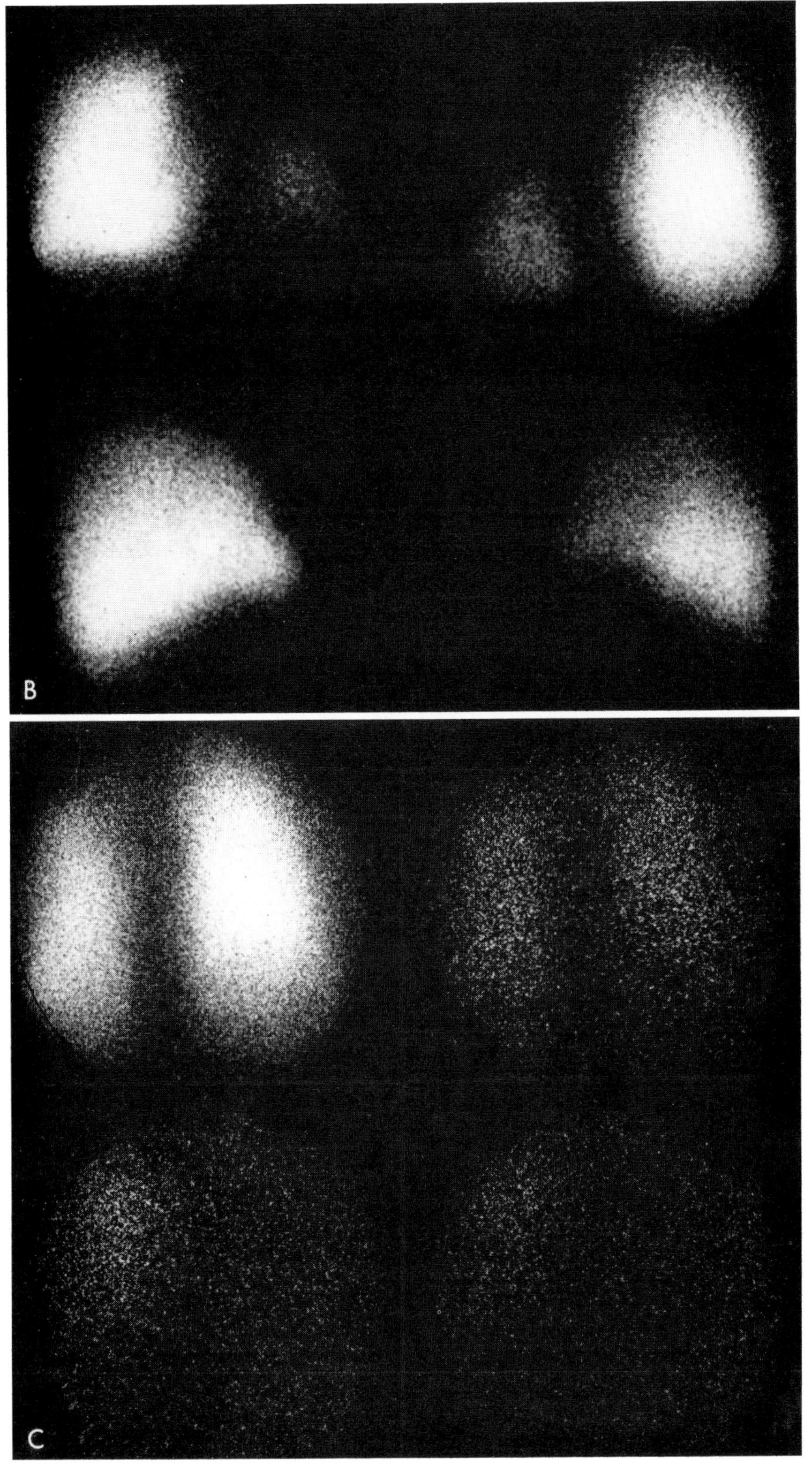

Figure 6–17 *Continued.* *See legend on the opposite page.*

heart, clearance from the left lung as a whole may be slightly delayed. The distribution of ventilation in mitral valve disease may be normal, although some studies have shown a shift toward the upper zones that matches the change in blood flow.

In myocardial infarction and to a lesser extent in angina pectoris, blood flow is diminished toward the bases. This change reflects the increasing extraalveolar vascular resistance resulting from perivascular edema. In the few studies of ventilation in these conditions, there have been no consistent changes.

CONGENITAL HEART DISEASE. Perfusion scans in patients with congenital heart disease often show a redistribution of blood flow within the lungs. Vascular anomalies, such as an anomalous origin of the pulmonary artery, may be accompanied by a profound reduction in blood flow to the affected lung with normal ventilation. Reduction of blood flow to the whole lung may be seen after the repair of anomalous venous return, when the anastomic channel becomes stenosed. Ventilation remains normal. Pulmonary arteriovenous malformations, when large enough (that is, greater than 2 to 3 cm. in diameter), are accompanied by localized defects in perfusion which correspond in size to the lesion seen radiographically. Small malformations cause no perfusion defect.

Perfusion scans cannot distinguish between hyperemic lungs and oligemic lungs, because they show only the relative distribution of blood flow. The presence of right-to-left shunts, of more than 10 to 15 per cent, is usually readily appreciated because activity will be visualized in the kidneys on the posterior and lateral scans. Activity will also be found within the brain and spleen and to a lesser extent in the heart and liver. Several patients with right-to-left shunts have suffered transient ischemic episodes following the injection of

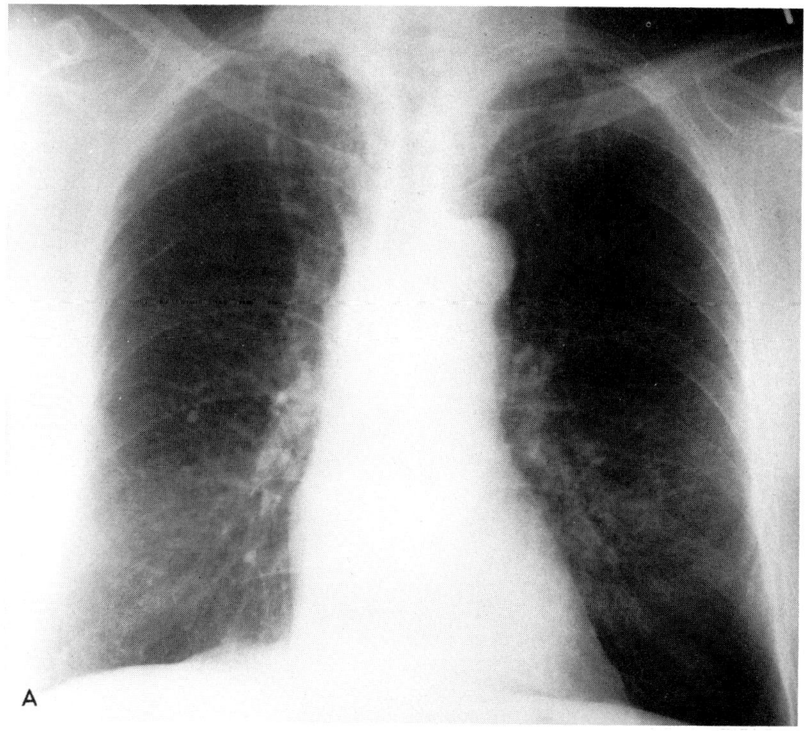

Figure 6–18. Occult carcinoma. *A.* Posteroanterior chest radiograph of a 69 year old man, with cells considered characteristic of squamous cell carcinoma in his sputum. There are ill-defined infiltrates in both upper zones.

Legend continued on the opposite page

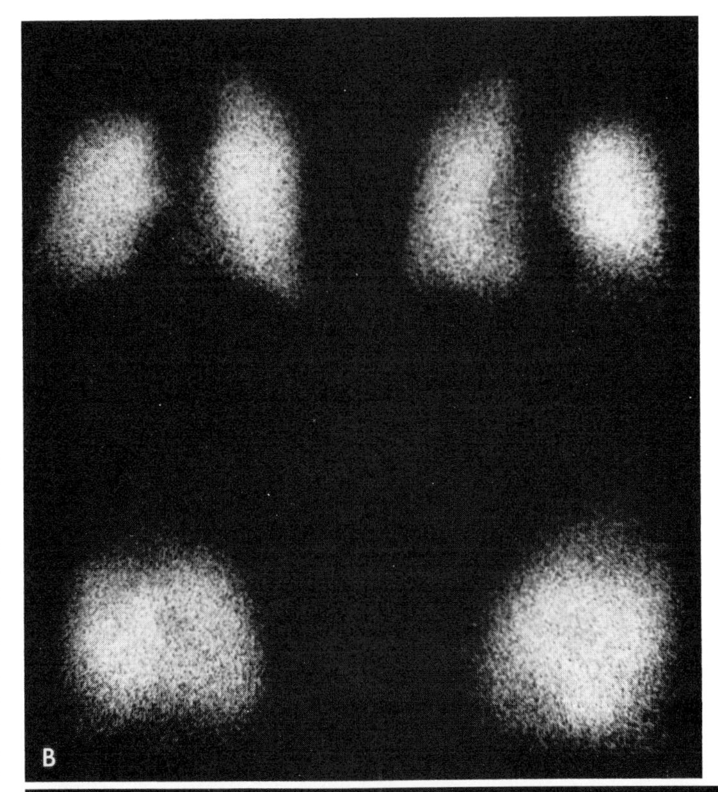

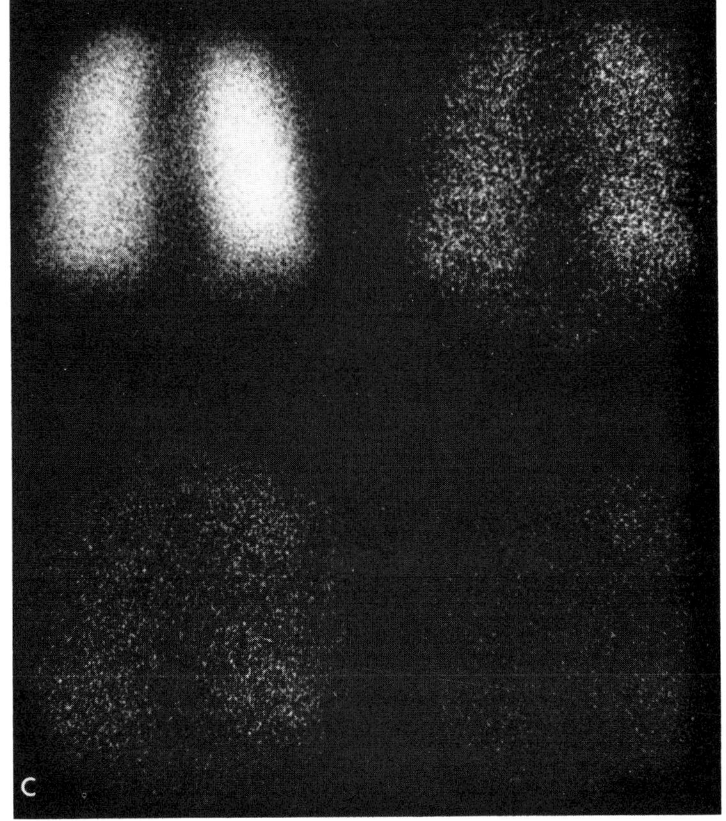

Figure 6–18 *Continued.* *B.* Four view perfusion images showing absence of blood flow to the right upper zone. *C.* Ventilation study (washin and washout at 1.0, 4.0, and 7.0 minutes) showing a normal distribution at the end of the washin and impaired clearance from the right upper and lower zones and the left lower zone. Bronchoscopy was normal. The greater reduction of blood flow than ventilation in the right upper zone suggested that the tumor was in the right upper lobe. Thoracotomy showed an unresectable tumor in the right upper lobe which had spread to encircle the superior vena cava. (From Secker-Walker, R. H.: Lung scanning. *In* Gottschalk, A., and Potchen, E. J., editors: Golden's Diagnostic Radiology, Section 20, Diagnostic Nuclear Medicine. © 1975, The Williams & Wilkins Co., Baltimore.)

labeled macroaggregates, and for this reason such studies are best avoided. Labeled microspheres have a better reputation.

QUANTITATIVE ASPECTS OF VENTILATION-PERFUSION STUDIES

Much interest has developed in the quantitative information that can be obtained from ventilation-perfusion studies. With multiple probe systems, the numerical information can be obtained from the graphical output from each probe. For gamma camera studies, the images must be stored on video tape, magnetic tape, or magnetic disc if any mathematical treatment is to be undertaken. There is at present no universally accepted way of analyzing such studies, but two rather different types of analysis have been undertaken.

QUASI-STATIC METHODS. In such studies the distribution of a single breath of xenon-133 is compared to the distribution of xenon-133 after a period of rebreathing the gas to equilibrium, to give figures for the regional distribution of ventilation per unit lung volume. The equilibrium image represents the distribution of lung volume. The distribution of intravenously injected xenon-133 in saline during breath holding is used to determine the distribution of blood flow and is compared with the equilibrium image to give regional perfusion per unit lung volume. Ventilation and perfusion indices may be derived using the concentration of xenon-133 in the spirometer, the quantity of xenon-133 injected, and the measured inspired volume and

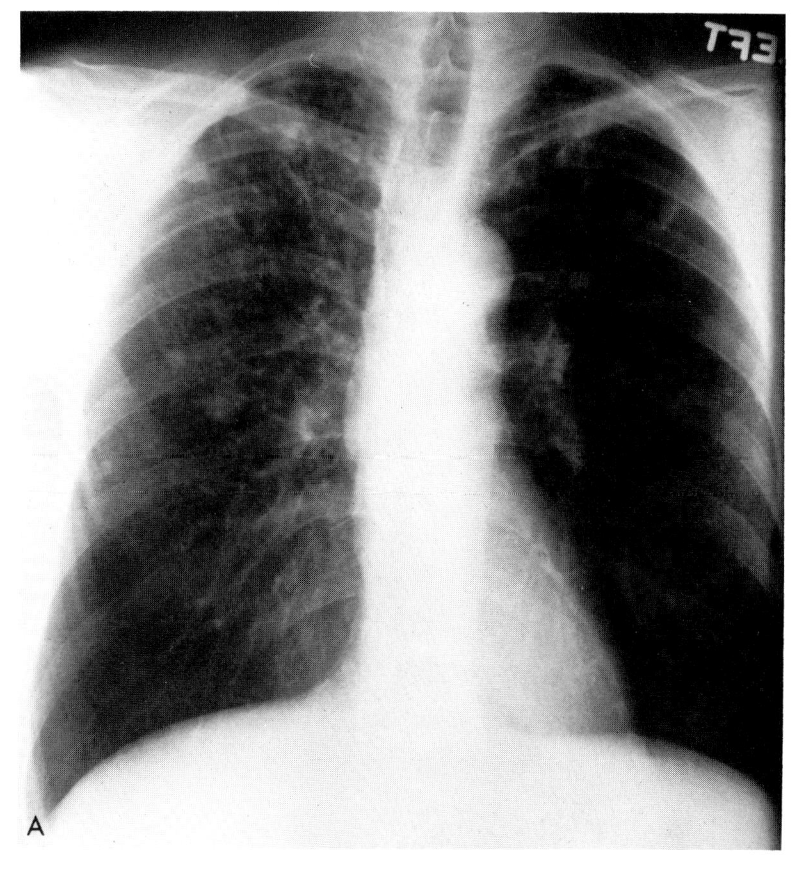

Figure 6–19. Inactive pulmonary tuberculosis. *A.* Posteroanterior chest radiograph of a 50 year old man who had been treated for pulmonary tuberculosis ten years previously. Streaky infiltrates are seen in the right upper lobe with some calcification and other nodular densities. Old scarring is also present in the left upper lobe.

Legend continued on the opposite page

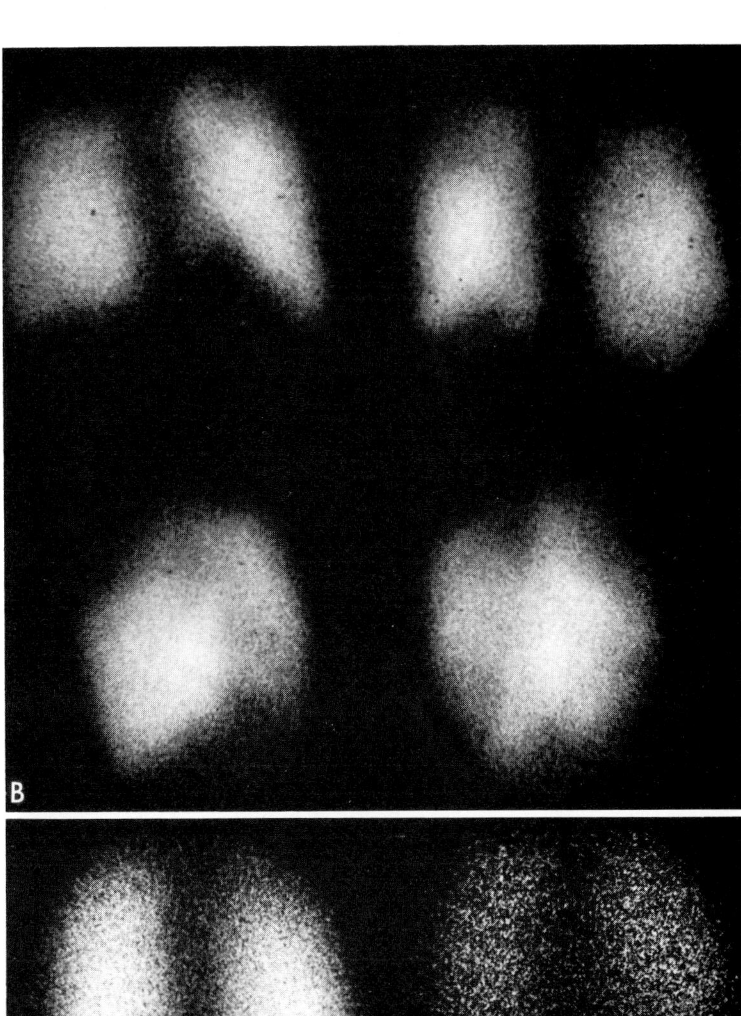

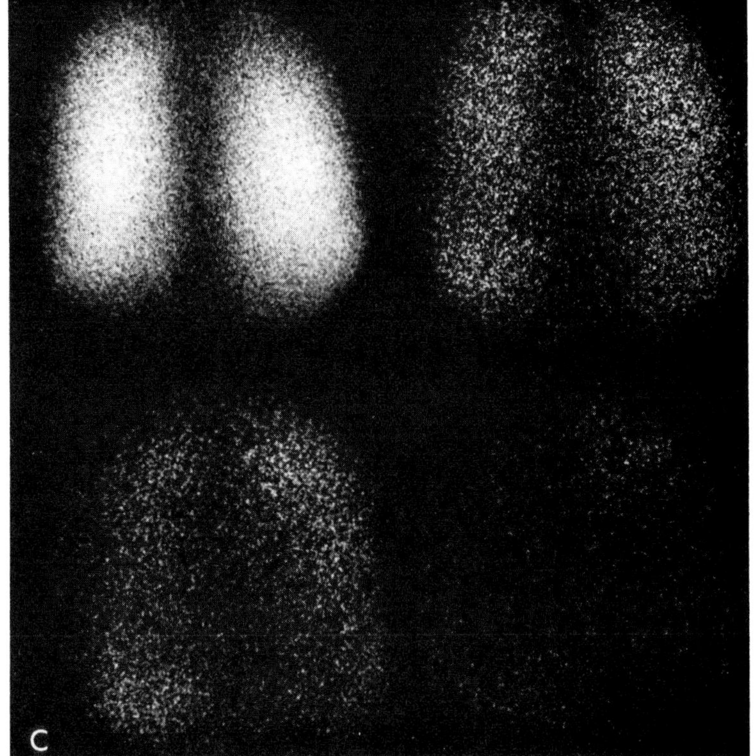

Figure 6–19 *Continued.* *B.* Four view perfusion images show defects in blood flow in both upper lobes which are more extensive on the right. Additional diffuse defects are present in the middle lobe and both lower lobes. *C.* Ventilation study (washin and washout at 1.0, 5.0, and 10.0 minutes) shows even filling of both lungs at the end of the washin except for some diminution at the right apex. During the washout there is impaired clearance from both lungs in an irregular fashion. The right upper zone and left base have the least efficient ventilation.

total lung capacity. These indices have the advantage of allowing comparisons between subjects.

However, it is more usual to normalize the regional values in each image (single breath, perfusion, and equilibrium), expressing the regional counts as a fraction of the total counts in each image, and to use these figures for ventilation per unit volume and perfusion per unit volume. Ventilation-perfusion ratios are then derived by dividing the regional values for ventilation by those for perfusion.

These quasi-static indices provide information on how much air enters a region in relation to the volume of that region. In healthy lungs this corresponds closely to the efficiency of gas exchange, but in patients with chronic obstructive airways disease this is not necessarily so. In this same group of subjects, equilibrium is rarely reached, so that the distribution of lung volume is underestimated in the poorly ventilated regions, giving falsely elevated values for both ventilation and blood flow per unit volume in these regions. Ventilation-perfusion ratios are unaffected because the volume determination cancels out.

DYNAMIC METHODS. In these methods, an indication of ventilation is derived during the washin or washout of xenon-133. The time required for 50 or 90 per cent of the equilibrium count rate to be reached during the washin has been used. However, figures derived from the washout of xenon-133, following a rebreathing period, are more widely used. A variety of analyses have been tried, from the time to reach 50

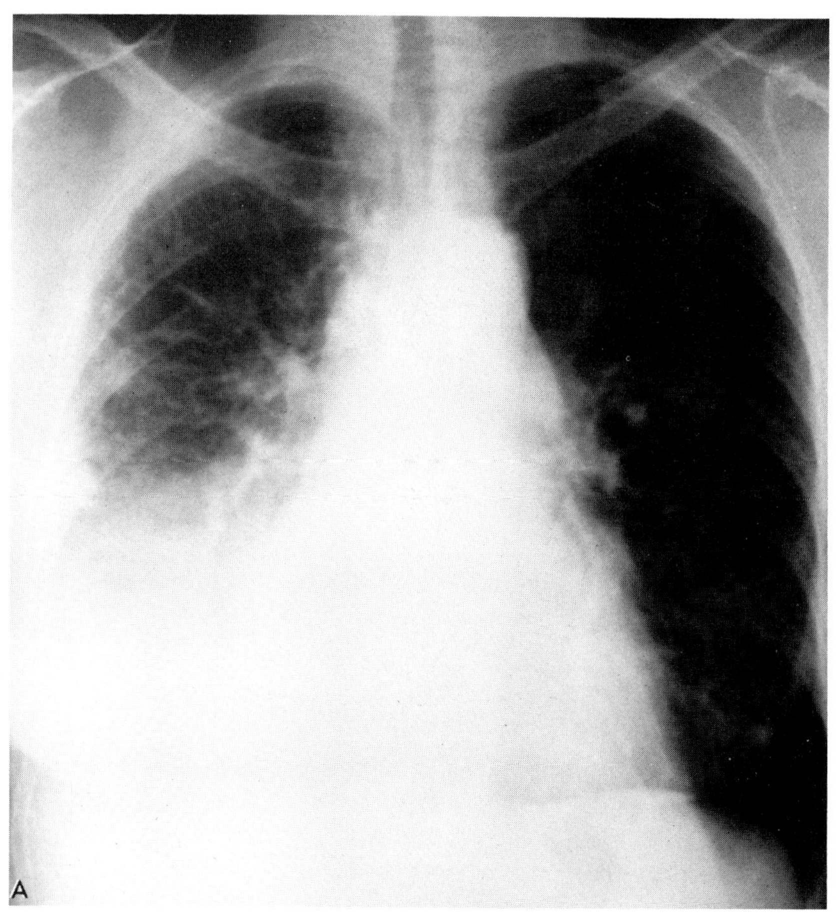

Figure 6–20. Pulmonary fibrosis. A. Posteroanterior chest radiograph of a 53 year old woman with severe granulomatous disease in the right lung with extensive fibrosis.

Legend continued on the opposite page

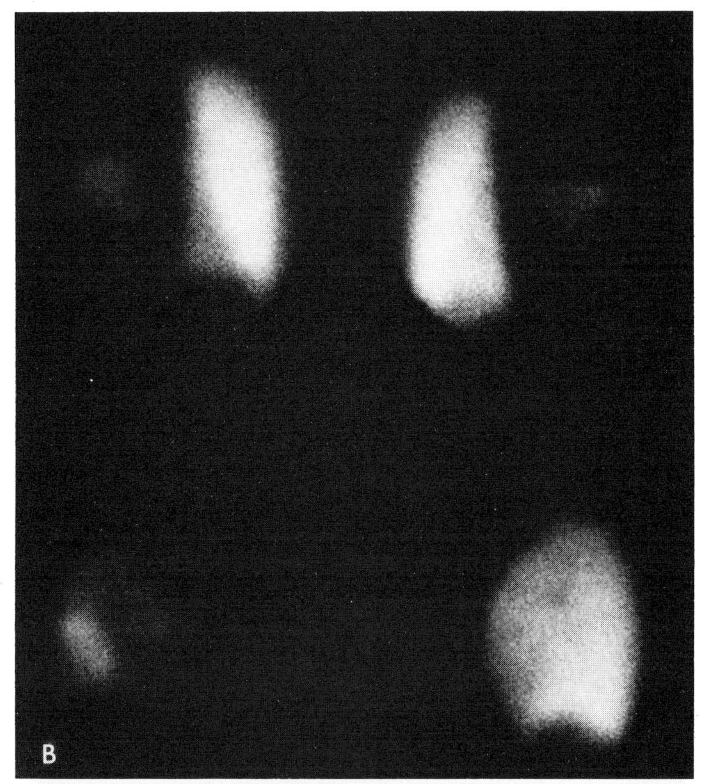

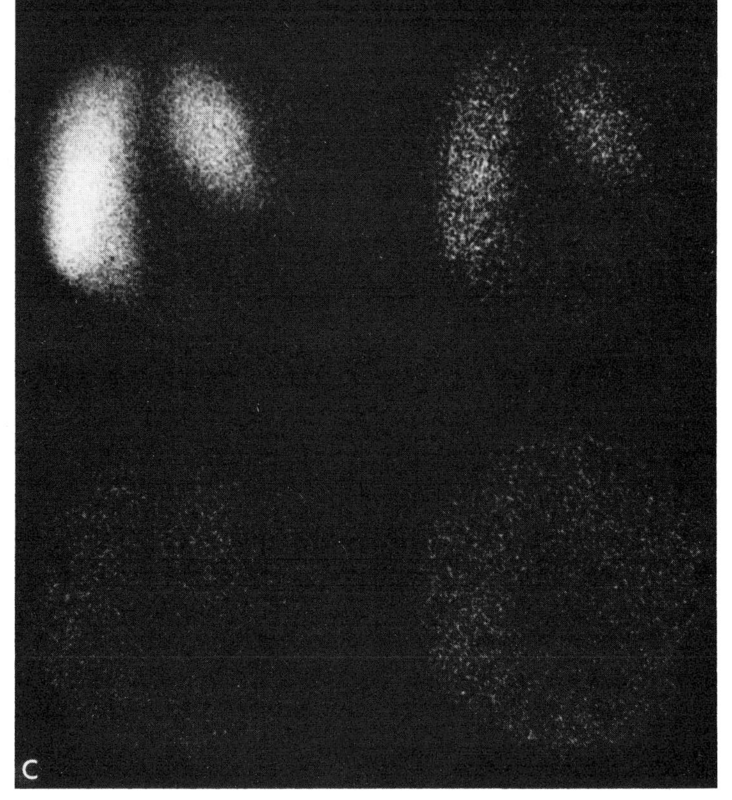

Figure 6–20 *Continued.* *B.* Four view perfusion images showing a small region of perfusion in the right mid zone. Perfusion on the left is normal. *C.* Ventilation study (washin and washout at 0.5, 1.0, and 2.0 minutes) shows normal filling of the left lung, but only partial filling of the right upper lobe. Clearance from both lungs is normal. The granulomatous and fibrotic reaction have caused a much greater disturbance of blood flow than of ventilation. The findings mimic pulmonary embolism. (From Secker-Walker, R. H.: Lung scanning. *In* Gottschalk, A., and Potchen, E. J., editors: Golden's Diagnostic Radiology, Section 20, Diagnostic Nuclear Medicine. © 1975, The Williams & Wilkins Co., Baltimore.)

per cent or 10 per cent of equilibrium value, or the fall in count rate at 3 minutes, to more elaborate calculations of the regional rate constants.[24]

Several problems surround the washout calculations. First, the "equilibrium image" at the end of a 3 to 5 minute washin does not represent lung volume in patients with chronic obstructive lung disease, because the poorly ventilated regions have not reached equilibrium. Second, xenon-133 dissolves in the blood and tissues during the washin and contributes to the washout curves, becoming a larger proportion of these as the washout continues. Third, the counting statistics become less and less reliable as the washout continues because the counts in any region become smaller and smaller. Fourth, the rate of clearance depends on tidal volume and respiratory frequency.

Rate constants have been derived from the first 50 or 60 per cent of the washout curves, assuming that this part can be fitted to a single exponential process. Such calculations tend to favor the better ventilated regions at the expense of the poorly ventilated ones, which contribute more to the tails of the washout curves. In any small region of the lungs the poor counting statistics preclude any compartmental analysis; but if upper, mid, or lower zone figures are considered, then fast and slow components can be derived, with a third, much slower

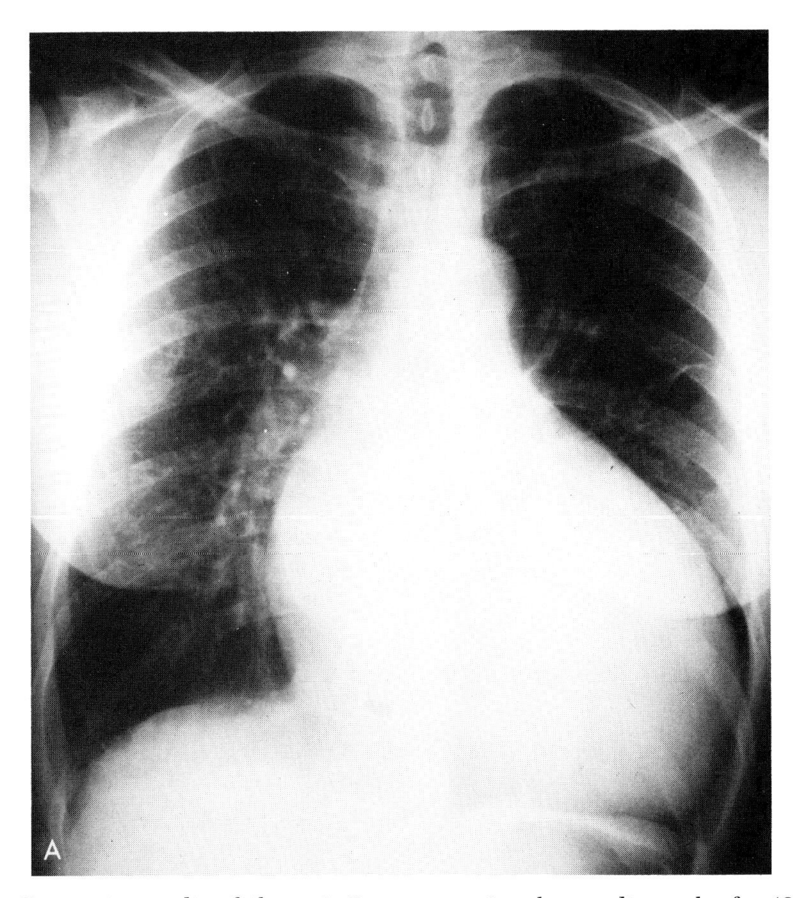

Figure 6–21. Congestive cardiac failure. *A.* Posteroanterior chest radiograph of a 48 year old man with congestive heart failure. There is marked cardiomegaly and dilatation of the upper lobe vessels. *B.* Four view perfusion images show the large heart and concave defects along the posterior margin of both lungs on the lateral views. *C.* Ventilation study (washin and washout at 0.5, 1.0, and 2.0 minutes) shows diminished filling of the left base at the end of the washin due to the large heart, but rapid clearance from both lungs during the washout.

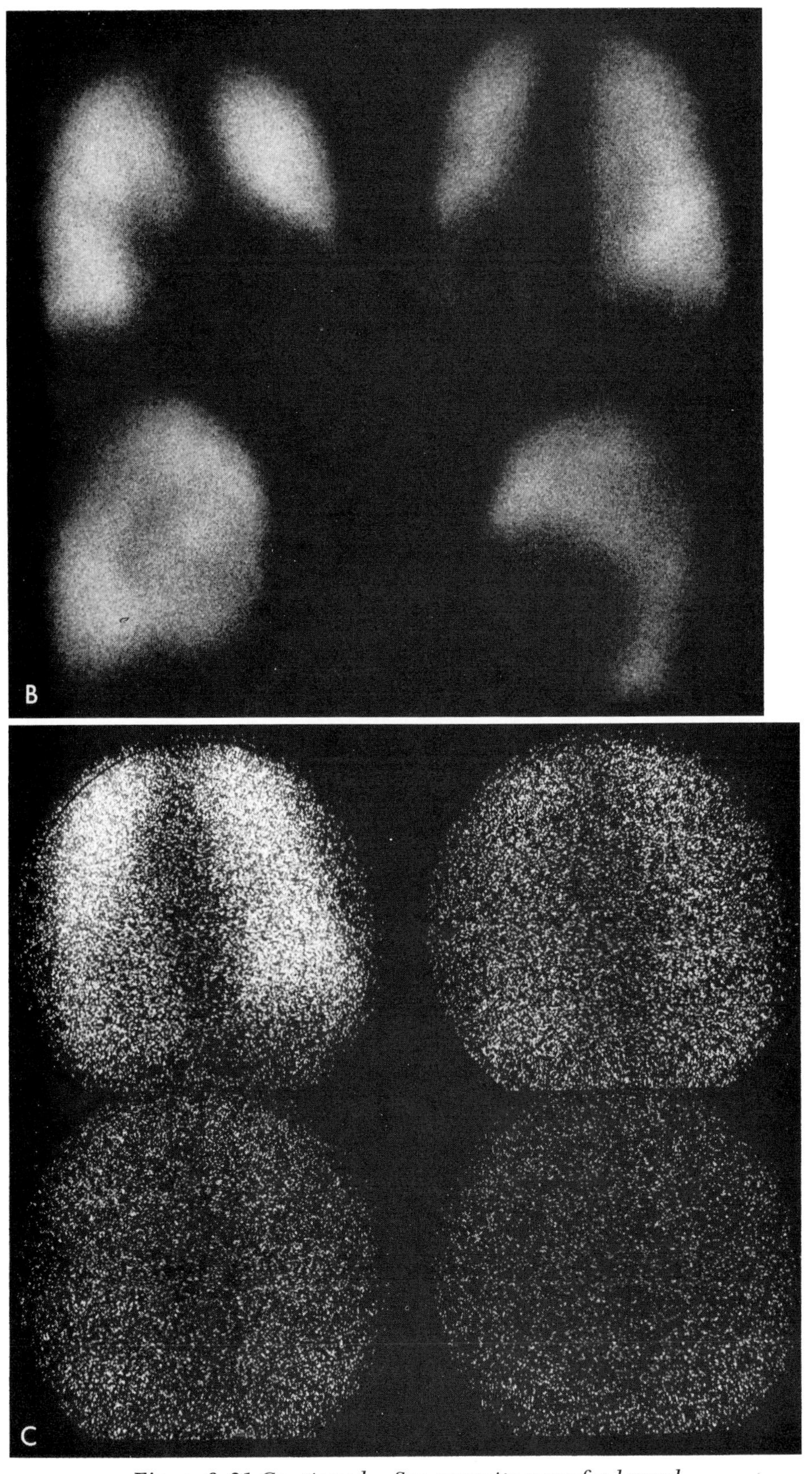

Figure 6–21 Continued. *See opposite page for legend.*

component representing the tissue and blood contributions. The tissue background may also be subtracted from the curves, using an area beneath the lungs as a representative of the tissue over the lungs and the blood within them. Figures for the regional fractional exchange of air have been derived in this way using the Stewart-Hamilton equation, or Height/Area approach, which requires very little mathematical manipulation of the data.[34]

The singular advantage of calculating the fractional exchange of air is that it provides a measure of the efficiency of ventilation—i.e., what proportion of regional lung volume is actually exchanged. Corrections for tidal volume and respiratory frequency should probably be included. The figures for whole lung fractional exchange have been shown to correlate with tidal volume and minute volume in normal subjects and with forced expiratory volume at 1 second, forced vital capacity, peak flow, and maximum mid-expiratory flow rate in patients with chronic obstructive airways disease.

The results of these studies may be presented as numerical values for various zones or else as functional images. These latter, which may be shown as contour images, three-dimensional images, color scans, or grey scale images, have the advantage of showing the functional relationship of all parts of the lung in a readily assimilated form.[9, 23, 24, 34] It is possible to obtain images of the distribution of pulmonary arterial blood flow, of ventilation, of lung volume, of perfusion or ventilation indices, of ventilation-perfusion ratios, of the fractional exchange of air, and of regional area gas exchange (Fig. 6–22).

A critical evaluation of the use of such figures, or the function images, in patient care, in addition to the original ventilation and perfusion studies, has not been undertaken. They may prove of some value in the preoperative assessment of patients in whom pulmonary resection is being considered, such as carcinoma of the bronchus or emphysematous bullae. They can give a numerical value to the regional severity of obstructive airways disease and could be used in the assessment of bronchodilator therapy, radiation therapy for carcinoma of the lung, or anticoagulant therapy in pulmonary embolism. Such figures, or images, may also help in those patients who have obstructive airways disease but in whom pulmonary embolism is also being considered; but their value has yet to be established in this situation.

THE USE OF AEROSOLS

Studies of the lungs after the inhalation of labeled aerosols have been used in two ways, first as an indication of the distribution of ventilation, and second as an indication of mucociliary clearance. Technetium-99m labeled human serum albumin or sulfur colloid and neutralized indium-113m chloride are suitable agents.

The aerosols may be produced with positive pressure nebulizers or ultrasonic nebulizers. Such devices produce a polydisperse aerosol with particles of many sizes. A large proportion of the administered dose is deposited in the tubing. Approximately 35 per cent reaches the patient, and most of this is deposited in the mouth and pharynx. Less than 10 per cent of the original material actually reaches the lungs. Particles less than 2 μ in diameter may reach the alveoli. Large particles are deposited in the larger airways, and very small particles, less than 0.5 μ, may enter and leave the alveoli.

Radioaerosol inhalation scintiphotography is not generally used because of the difficulty in producing small particles of a uniform size which will readily pass to distal portions of the lungs. In addition, extreme care must be used to prevent significant radioactive contamination in the immediate environment from exhaled aerosol. An exhaust system to remove the exhaled aerosol particles is mandatory.

The deposition of the aerosol particles also depends on air flow rates and turbulence. Increased deposition is seen in regions of partial obstruction where there is greater turbulence. With complete obstruction, no deposition takes place.

In normal subjects who are breathing quietly, the deposition and accumulation of the aerosol proceeds in a linear fashion. A four view scan at the end of the inhalation period resembles a perfusion scan, although activity is often seen in the pharynx, esophagus, stomach, and sometimes the main bronchi. In smokers and in normal subjects breathing more rapidly

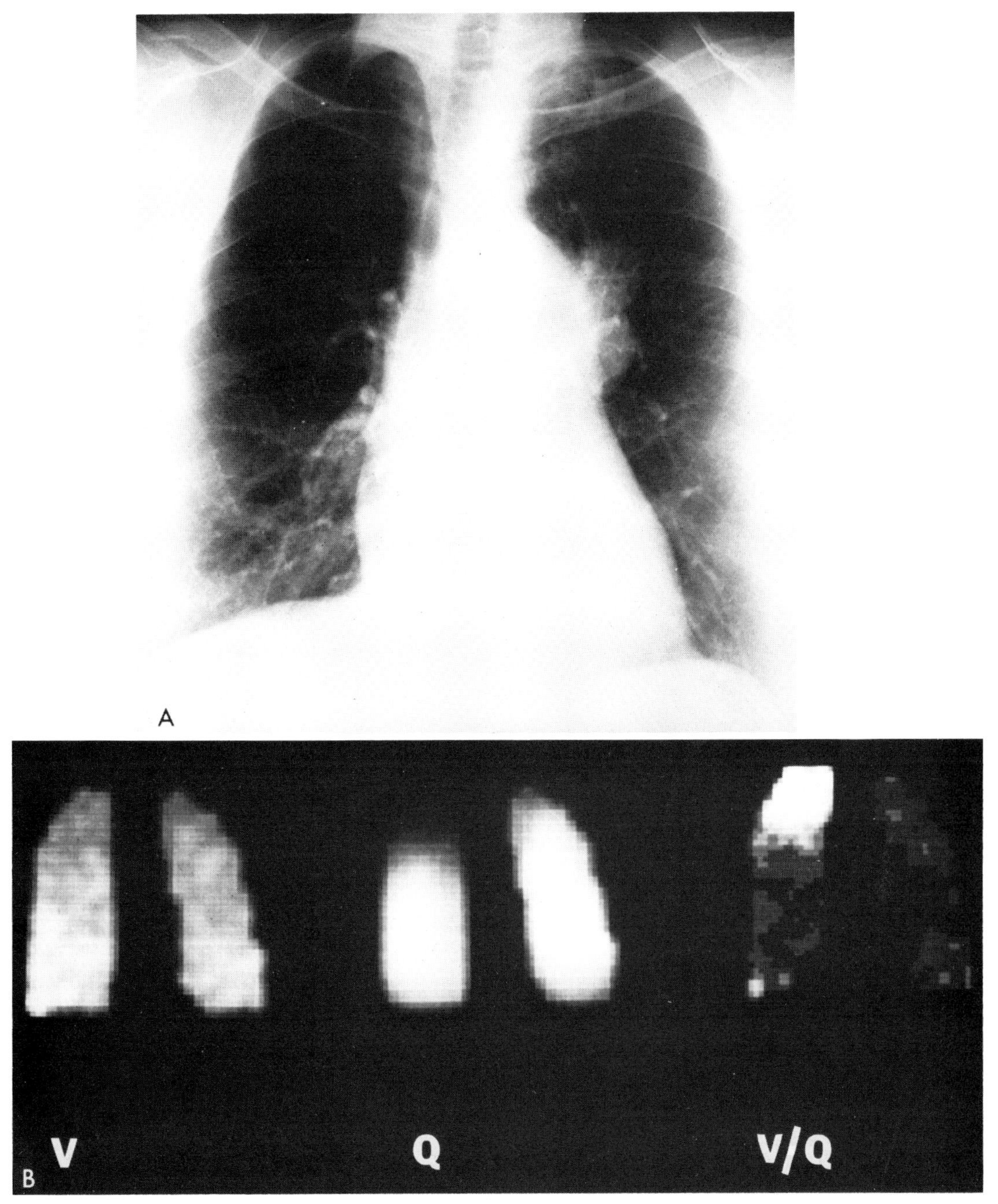

Figure 6–22. Functional images. *A.* Posteroanterior chest radiograph of a 54 year old woman who presented with a left vocal cord palsy. A mass is visible at the left hilum. Bronchoscopy was normal, but the sputum contained cells characteristic of squamous cell carcinoma. *B.* Functional images generated by a small digital computer. V represents the distribution of the fractional exchange of air per second and gives an indication of the regional efficiency of ventilation. There is a normal gradient from the apex to the base, although some unevenness is apparent in each lung. Q represents blood flow per unit volume. There is no blood flow to the left upper zone. V/Q represents the ventilation-perfusion "ratio." This is very high in the left upper zone, but the pattern is normal in the rest of this lung and in the right lung, for a patient breathing at functional residual capacity. Regions of abnormally elevated ventilation-perfusion ratio indicate extensive vascular involvement, and tumors producing such a disturbance are often unresectable.

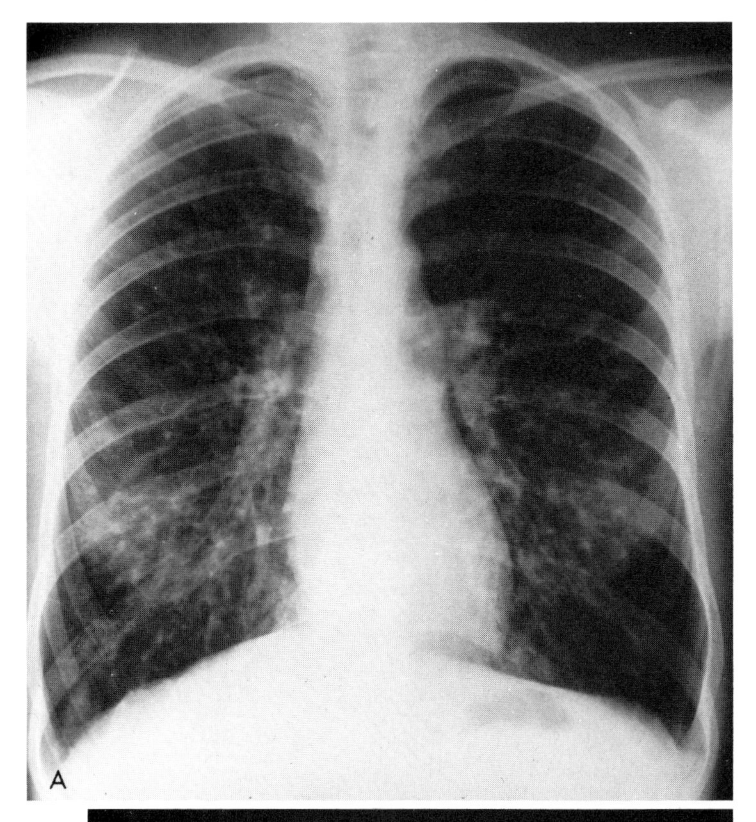

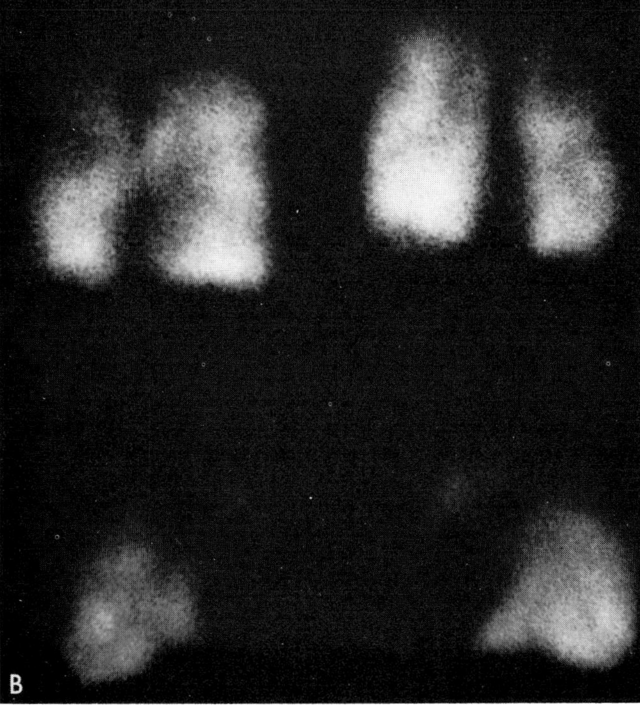

Figure 6–23. Aerosol deposition. *A.* Posteroanterior chest radiograph of a 16 year old girl with cystic fibrosis demonstrates diffuse cystic lung changes and hyperinflation. *B.* Four view perfusion study showing widespread defects in blood flow. Fissure signs can be seen on both sides. The disturbance in blood flow is more severe in the upper zones, but no part of either lung is spared.

Legend continued on the opposite page

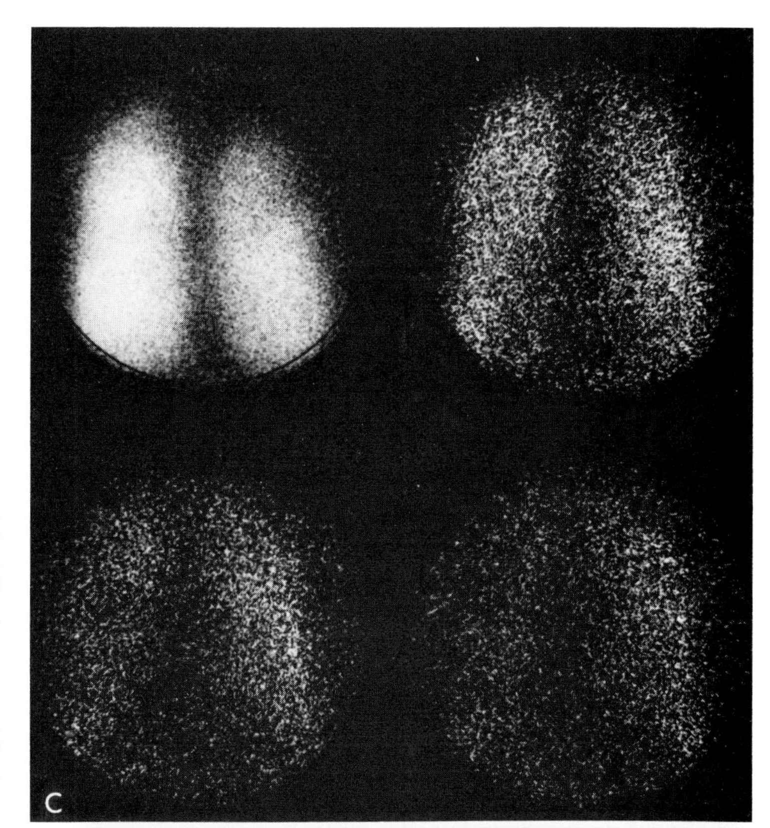

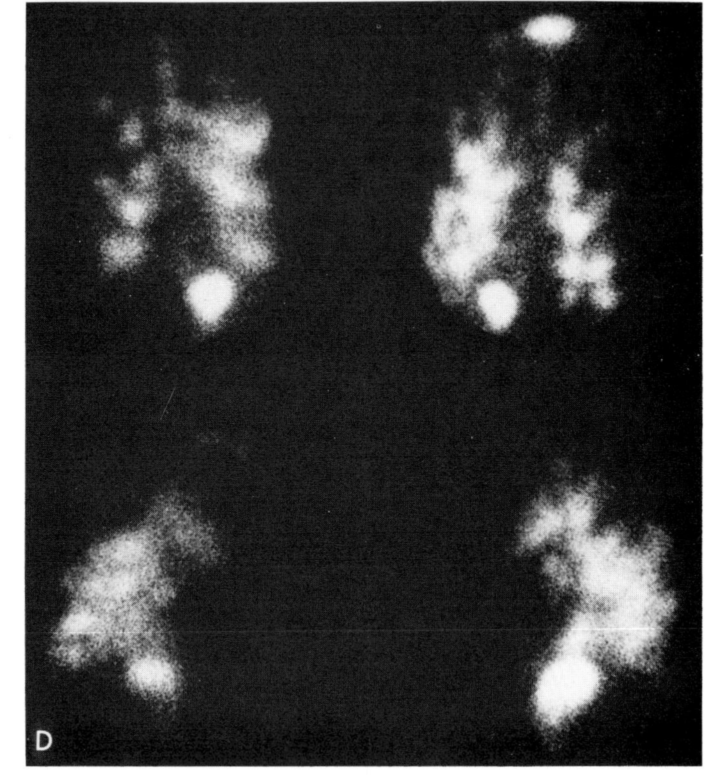

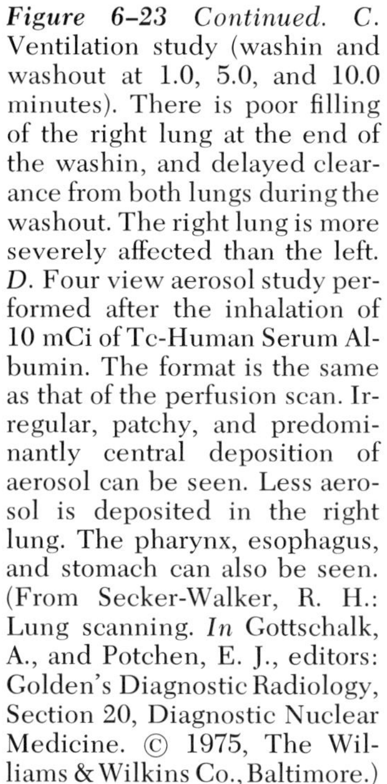
Figure 6–23 *Continued. C.* Ventilation study (washin and washout at 1.0, 5.0, and 10.0 minutes). There is poor filling of the right lung at the end of the washin, and delayed clearance from both lungs during the washout. The right lung is more severely affected than the left. *D.* Four view aerosol study performed after the inhalation of 10 mCi of Tc-Human Serum Albumin. The format is the same as that of the perfusion scan. Irregular, patchy, and predominantly central deposition of aerosol can be seen. Less aerosol is deposited in the right lung. The pharynx, esophagus, and stomach can also be seen. (From Secker-Walker, R. H.: Lung scanning. *In* Gottschalk, A., and Potchen, E. J., editors: Golden's Diagnostic Radiology, Section 20, Diagnostic Nuclear Medicine. © 1975, The Williams & Wilkins Co., Baltimore.)

than normal, a rather more patchy deposition is seen, especially centrally around the larger bronchi. In pulmonary embolism, aerosol can be seen to enter regions where perfusion is diminished or absent, implying better ventilation than blood flow.

In patients with emphysema, less aerosol reaches the more severely affected regions (Fig. 6–23). There is often considerable central deposition in the larger airways and poor peripheral filling. The resulting aerosol scans rarely match the perfusion scans, so that it can be difficult to decide whether a defect in blood flow corresponds to a defect in ventilation. Scans in which the defects in aerosol deposition are more peripheral, without the central increase, tend to be found in patients with symptoms of chronic bronchitis.

Aerosol scans depict abnormalities of air flow and cannot be used to measure ventilation.[36]

The inhalation of radioactive aerosols with subsequent monitoring to determine lung retention provides some information on mucociliary transport. Mucociliary clearance can be studied by serial images after the inhalation of labeled aerosol. Such studies have been carried out in non-smoking normal subjects, smokers, and patients with chronic obstructive lung disease, and also to study the effects of mucolytic agents.[32] The ability to obtain quantitative information is limited.[1]

THE USE OF "TUMOR-SEEKING" RADIONUCLIDES

A number of radiopharmaceuticals have been used in an attempt to identify malignant tissue. 197-Hg chlormerodrin, 197-$HgCl_2$, 75-Se selenomethionine, 75-Se selenite, and more recently gallium-67 and

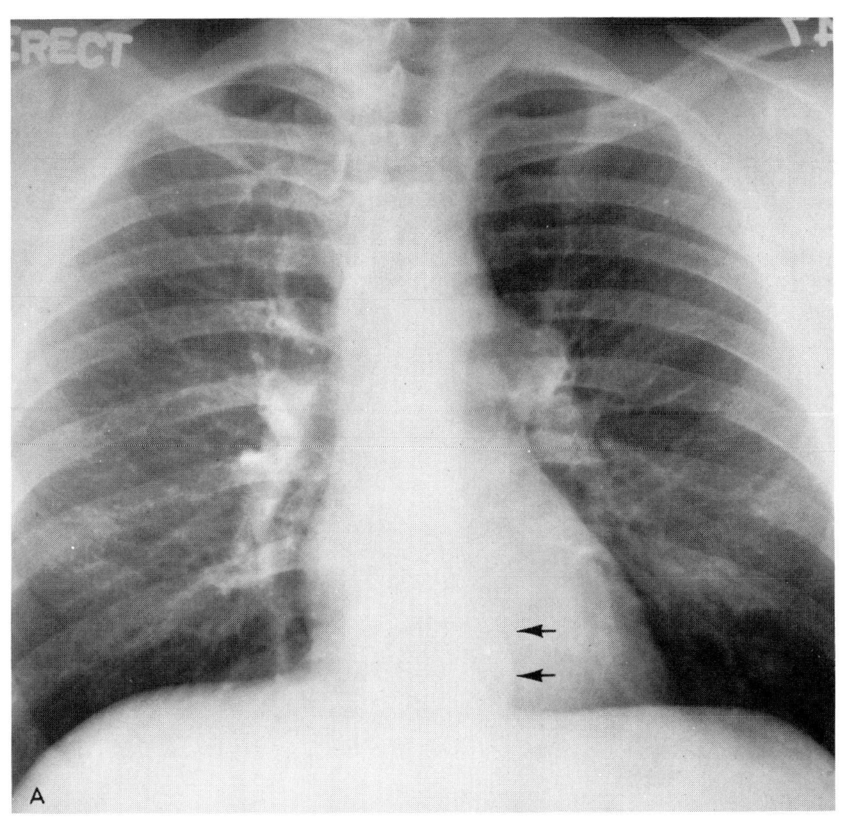

Figure 6–24. Locating occult disease with gallium. *A.* Posteroanterior chest roentgenogram in a 32 year old man with fever and pruritus demonstrates left hilar lymph node enlargement and a left paraspinal mass (arrows). Presumptive diagnosis was Hodgkin's disease. No peripheral lymph nodes were palpable, and thoracotomy was contemplated for definitive diagnosis.

Legend continued on the opposite page

labeled bleomycin have all been used. Each of these substances is incorporated into malignant tissue, but each is also concentrated in inflammatory tissue. The underlying mechanisms are obscure, but part of the increase in activity found in such lesions can be ascribed to the increased capillary permeability of the new vessels that grow in malignant or inflammatory tissue.

GALLIUM-67. 67-Ga citrate has been found to accumulate in both tumors and inflammatory conditions. Its place in the investigation and management of patients with disease of the chest is not yet established.

Gallium-67 scans are best performed 48 to 72 hours after the intravenous injection of 2.0 to 3.0 mCi of carrier-free 67-Ga citrate. The tissue levels of gallium are lower at this time and regions of abnormal uptake are more readily discerned. If whole body scans are being done, it is advisable to give laxatives prior to scanning, in order to clear

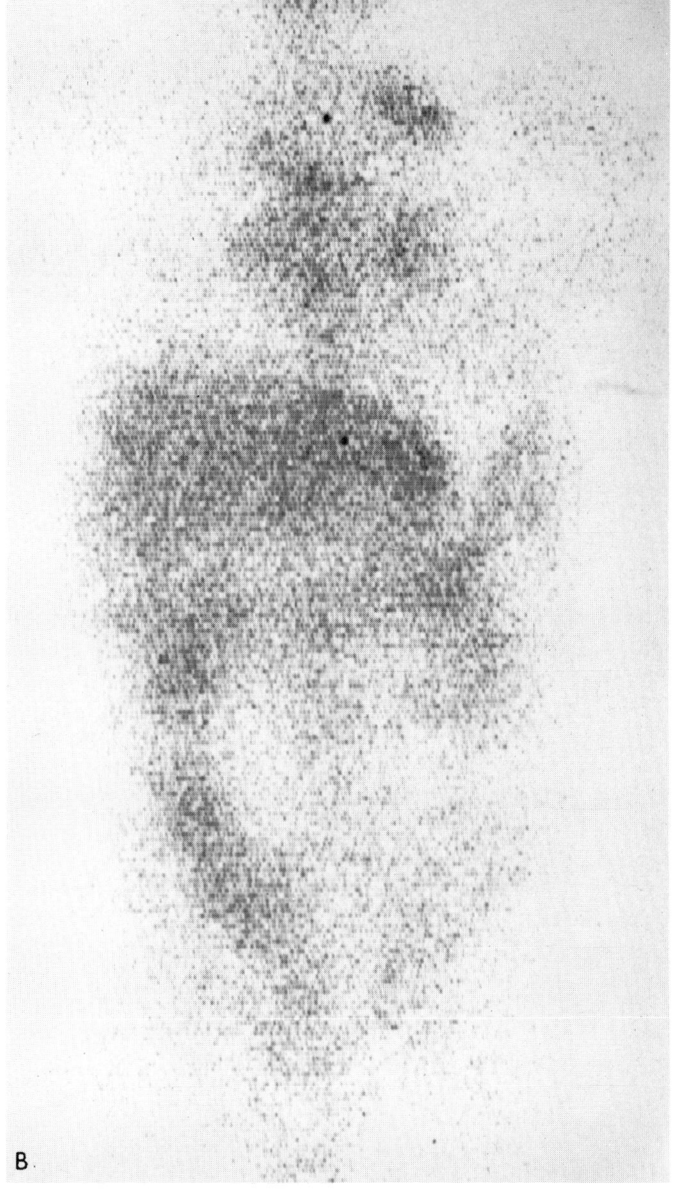

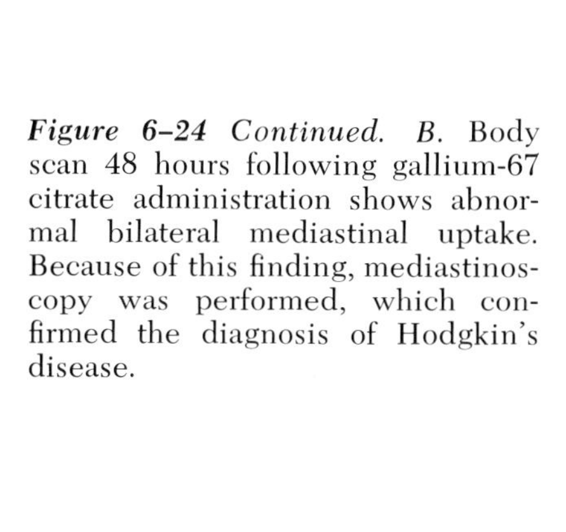

Figure 6–24 *Continued. B.* Body scan 48 hours following gallium-67 citrate administration shows abnormal bilateral mediastinal uptake. Because of this finding, mediastinoscopy was performed, which confirmed the diagnosis of Hodgkin's disease.

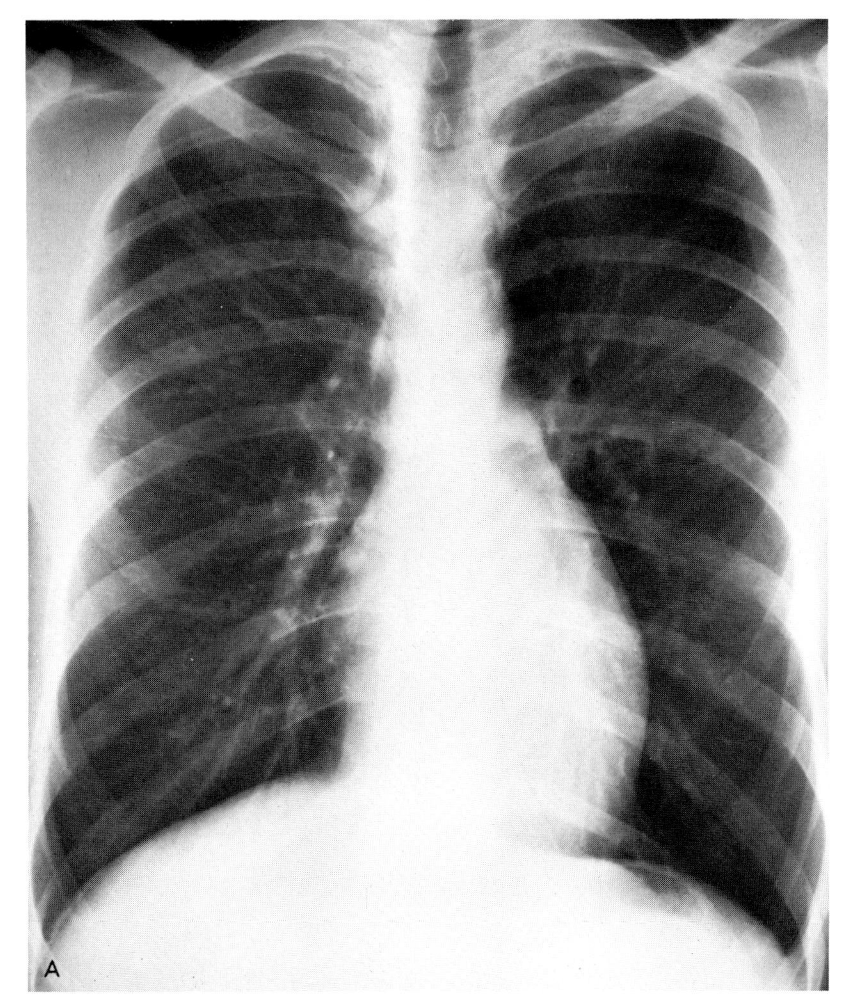

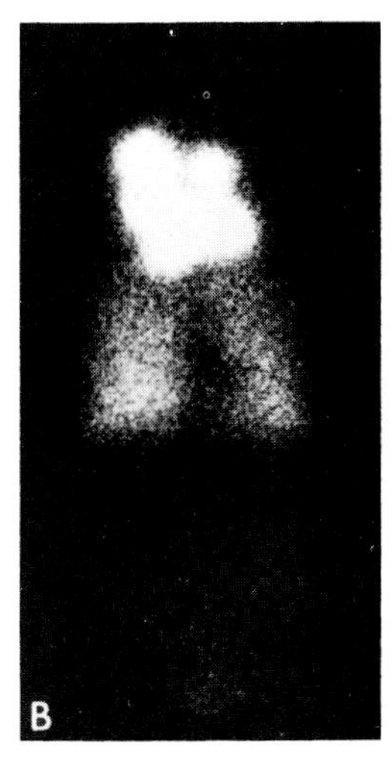

Figure 6–25. Metastatic thyroid carcinoma. *A.* Posteroanterior chest radiograph in a 28 year old man, with dyspnea and a large neck mass, is normal except for a slight indentation along the right side of the cervical trachea. Biopsy of the mass demonstrated mixed papillary-follicular thyroid carcinoma. *B.* Scintiphoto utilizing pin-hole collimator following administration of 150 mCi iodine-131 demonstrates uptake in the large neck mass, and diffusely throughout both lungs, consistent with widespread pulmonary metastases. The dyspnea improved markedly following the iodine-131 therapy.

the colon of 67-Ga that is excreted into the bowel. This is particularly important if an attempt is being made to stage lymphoma in the abdomen. Uptake is normally seen in the liver, the sternum, the thoracic spine, and the angles of the scapula. In women, uptake may also be seen in the breast.

In patients with carcinoma of the bronchus, the tumor can be visualized in more than 90 per cent of cases. Lesions as small as 1.5 cm. in diameter have been seen. In patients in whom the diagnosis of carcinoma of the lung has been established, 67-Ga citrate scanning of the thorax may help define the extent of spread in the mediastinum and hence provide additional information on which to base a decision for or against a thoracotomy. If a whole body scan is done, then distant metastases may also be revealed.

Likewise, in patients with suspected lymphoma, 67-Ga citrate may be of value in selecting a site for biopsy (Fig. 6–24), or in proven disease it can be used to determine the distribution of lymphomatous tissue within the body.

Although gallium-67 is a sensitive agent

for tumor localization in the lung, it is not specific. Active inflammatory lesions including acute pneumonia, chronic pneumonia, bronchiectasis, lung abscesses, tuberculous lesions, and fungal infections have all been visualized with this radionuclide. The uptake in acute inflammatory processes is even greater than in tumors, and decreases as the inflammatory process resolves. Inactive pulmonary tuberculosis is usually negative. Sarcoidosis is associated with obvious hilar node uptake when these lymph glands are involved by granulomata. Benign tumors may occasionally concentrate gallium-67.[12, 21]

OTHER RADIONUCLIDES. Radioactive iodine is a more specific scanning agent. When metastases from carcinoma of the thyroid concentrate radioactive iodine, they are readily visualized by scanning, after the administration of 1.0 to 5.0 mCi of iodine-131. Profuse uptake of 131-I has been seen throughout the lungs in patients with widespread but radiologically invisible pulmonary metastases from thyroid cancer[8] (Fig. 6–25). Retrosternal goiters can also be recognized from their uptake of 131-I, although this is usually a patchy and irregular uptake in keeping with the histologic degeneration found in such goiters.

Pulmonary metastases from osteogenic sarcoma have been shown to concentrate bone scanning agents such as strontium-85 or 99m-Tc labeled polyphosphate. Pulmonary calcification has also been visualized in this way in patients with renal failure and secondary hyperparathyroidism and in patients with hypercalcemia due to malignant disease.[14]

BIBLIOGRAPHY

1. Albert, R. E., Lippman, M., Peterson, H. T., Jr., Berger, J., Sanborn, K., and Bohming, D.: Bronchial deposition and clearance of aerosols. Arch. Intern Med., 131:115–127, 1973.
2. Alderson, P. O., Secker-Walker, R. H., and Forrest, J. V.: Detection of obstructive pulmonary disease. Radiology, 112:643–648, 1974.
3. Alderson, P. O., Secker-Walker, R. H., Strominger, D. B., McAlister, W. H., Hill, R. L., and Markham, J.: Quantitative assessment of regional ventilation and perfusion in children with cystic fibrosis. Radiology, 111:151–155, 1974.
4. Anthonisen, N. R., Bass, H., Oriel, A., Place, R. E. G., and Bates, D. V.: Regional lung function in patients with chronic bronchitis. Clin. Sci., 35:495–511, 1968.
5. Arborelius, M., and Lilja, B.: Effect of sitting, hypoxia, and breath-holding on the distribution of pulmonary blood flow in man. Scand. J. Clin. Lab. Invest., 24:261–269, 1969.
6. Arborelius, M., Kristersson, S., Lindell, S. E., Miorner, G., and Svanberg, L.: 133 Xe-radiospirometry and extension of lung cancer. Scand. J. Resp. Dis., 52:145–152, 1971.
7. Ball, W. C., Stewart, P. B., Newsham, L. G. S., and Bates, D. V.: Regional pulmonary function studied with Xenon-133. J. Clin. Invest. 41:519–531, 1962.
8. Bonte, F. J., and McConnell, R. W.: Pulmonary metastases from differentiated thyroid carcinoma demonstrable only by nuclear imaging. Radiology, 107:585–590, 1973.
9. Burdine, J. A., Murphy, P. H., Alazarsamy, V., Ryder, L. A., and Car, W. N.: Functional pulmonary imaging. J. Nuc. Med., 12:933–938, 1972.
10. DeNardo, G. L., Goodwin, D., Ravasini, R., and Dietrich, P. A.: The ventilatory lung scan in the diagnosis of pulmonary embolism. N. Engl. J. Med., 282:1334–1336, 1970.
11. Dollery, C. T., and Gillam, P. M. S.: The distribution of blood and gas within the lungs measured by scanning after administration of 133 Xe. Thorax, 18:316–325, 1963.
12. Fogh, J., Bertelsen, S. V., and Schmidt, A.: Diagnostic value of 67 Ga-scintigraphy in chest surgery. Thorax, 29:26–31, 1974.
13. Foreman, S., Weill, H., Duke, R., George, R., and Ziskind, M.: Bullous disease of the lung. Ann. Int. Med., 69:757–767, 1968.
14. Grames, G. M., Sauser, D. D., Jansen, C., Soderblom, R. E., Hodgkin, J. E., and Stilson, M. S.: Radionuclide detection of diffuse interstitial pulmonary calcification. JAMA, 230:992–995, 1974.
15. Harding, L. K., Horsfield, K., Singhal, S. S., and Cumming, G.: The proportion of lung vessels blocked by albumin microspheres. J. Nuc. Med., 14:579–581, 1973.
16. Hughes, J. M. B., Glazier, J. B., Rosenzweig, D. Y., and West, J. B.: Factors determining the distribution of pulmonary blood flow in patients with raised pulmonary venous pressure. Clin. Sci., 37:847–858, 1969.
17. Isawa, T., Taplin, G. V., Beazell, J., and Criley, J. M.: Experimental unilateral pulmonary artery occlusion: Acute and chronic effects on relative inhalation and perfusion. Radiology, 102:101–109, 1972.
18. James, A. E., Cooper, M., White, R. I., and Wagner, H. H.: Perfusion changes on lung scans in patients with congestive heart failure. Radiology, 100:99–106, 1971.
19. Johnson, P. M., Sagerman, R. H., and Jacos, H. W.: Changes in pulmonary arterial perfusion due to intrathoracic neoplasia and irradiation of the lung. Amer. J. Roentgen., 102:637–644, 1968.
20. Kessler, R. M., and McNeil, B. J.: Impaired ventilation in a patient with angiographically demonstrated pulmonary emboli. Radiology, 114:111–112, 1975.

21. Kinoshita, F., Ushio, T., Mackawa, A., Ariwa, R., and Kubo, A.: Scintiscanning of pulmonary disease with 67-Ga citrate. J. Nuc. Med., 15:227–233, 1974.
22. Kronenburg, R. S., L'Heureux, P., Ponto, R. A., Drage, C. W., and Loken, M. K.: The effect of aging on lung perfusion. Ann. Intern. Med., 76:413–421, 1972.
23. Loken, M. K.: Camera studies of lung ventilation and perfusion. Sem. Nuc. Med., 1:229–245, 1971.
24. MacIntyre, W. J., Inkley, S. R., Roth, E., Drescher, W. P., and Ishii, Y.: Spatial recording of disappearance constants of xenon-133 washout from the lung. J. Lab. Clin. Med., 76:701–712, 1970.
25. Macklem, P. T.: Airway obstruction and collateral ventilation. Physiol. Rev., 51:368–436, 1971.
26. Mansell, A., Bryan, C., and Levinson, H.: Airway closure in children. J. Appl. Physiol., 33:711–714, 1972.
27. McIntyre, K. M., and Sasahara, A. A.: Angiography, scanning, and hemodynamics in pulmonary embolism; critical review and correlations. CRC Crit. Rev. in Rad. Sci., 3:489–521, 1972.
28. Modan, B., Sharon, E., and Jelin, N.: Factors contributing to the incorrect diagnosis of pulmonary embolic disease. Chest, 62:388–393, 1972.
29. Moser, K. M., Longo, A. M., Ashburn, W. L., and Guisan, M.: Spurious scintiphotographic recurrence of pulmonary emboli. Amer. J. Med., 55:434–443, 1973.
30. Milic-Emili, J.: Radioactive xenon in the evaluation of regional lung function. Sem. Nuc. Med., 1:246–262, 1971.
31. Poulose, K. F., Reba, R. C., Gilday, D. L., Deland, F. H., and Wagner, H. N.: Diagnosis of pulmonary embolism. A correlative study of the clinical, scan, and angiographic findings. Brit. Med. J., 3:67–71, 1970.
32. Sanchis, J., Dolovich, M., Chalmers, R., and Newhouse, M. T.: Quantitation of regional aerosol clearance in the normal human lung. J. Appl. Physiol., 33:757–762, 1972.
33. Secker-Walker, R. H., Alderson, P. O., Wilhelm, J., Hill, R. L., Markham, J., and Kinzie, J.: Ventilation-perfusion scanning in carcinoma of the bronchus. Chest, 65:660–663, 1974.
34. Secker-Walker, R. H., Hill, R. L., Markham, J., Baker, J., Wilhelm, J., Alderson, P. O., and Potchen, E. J.: The measurement of regional ventilation in man. A new method of quantitation. J. Nuc. Med., 14:725–732, 1973.
35. Secker-Walker, R. H., and Siegel, B. A.: The use of nuclear medicine in the diagnosis of lung disease. Radiol. Clin. North Amer., 11:215–241, 1973.
36. Shibel, E. M., Landis, G. A., and Moser, K. M.: Inhalation lung scanning evaluation—Radioaerosol versus radioxenon techniques. Dis. Chest., 56:284–289, 1969.
37. Shoop, J. D.: Why do a lung scan? JAMA, 229: 567–570, 1974.
38. Taplin, G. V., and MacDonald, N. S.: Radiochemistry of macroaggregated albumin and new lung scanning agents. Sem. Nuc. Med., 1:132–152, 1971.
39. Treves, S., Ahnberg, D. S., Laguardo, R., and Strieder, D. J.: Radionuclide evaluation of regional lung function in children. J. Nuc. Med., 15:582–587, 1974.
40. West, J. B.: Respiratory Physiology—The Essentials. Chaps. 2, 4, 5, and 7. Baltimore, Williams & Wilkins Company, 1974.
41. Wilson, A. F., Suprenant, E. L., Beall, G. N., Siegel, S. C., Simmons, D. H., and Bennett, L. R.: The significance of regional pulmonary function changes in bronchial asthma. Amer. J. Med., 48:416–423, 1970.

Chapter 7

PEDIATRIC PULMONARY TECHNIQUES

by Gary D. Shackelford, M.D.

BRONCHOGRAPHY

There are very few valid indications for bronchography in the pediatric patient. A recent commentary on this subject provides a challenge for all radiologists and clinicians who deal with pediatric pulmonary disease to reassess the role of bronchography in various clinical situations.[2] Bronchography must be restricted to conditions in which the results may indicate the need for specific therapeutic measures, usually surgical.[4] Utilization should be limited to circumstances in which other studies—including plain roentgenograms, fluoroscopy, tomography, and isotopic imaging procedures—do not provide sufficient information.

INDICATIONS. Suspected or known bronchiectasis is probably the most common indication for the procedure. Preoperative localization of involved portions of the lung is vital in planning the extent of resection. While occasional asthmatic patients have shown significant clinical improvement after resection of localized bronchiectasis,[7] bronchography is still rarely indicated in childhood asthma.[13] In required cases, bronchography can provide preoperative segmental localization of suspected lung cysts and can allow differentiation between a cyst and bronchiectasis.[4]

While nonradiopaque foreign bodies and other endobronchial masses at times can be demonstrated by bronchography, plain roentgenograms and fluoroscopy usually provide sufficient prebronchoscopic or preoperative information. In cases of recurrent or unremitting pneumonia or atelectasis involving the same lobe or segment, bronchography may be of value in demonstrating extrinsic or intrinsic bronchial obstruction (Fig. 7–1). But surgical management is almost always dictated by refractoriness to medical therapy, regardless of the bronchographic findings.

Bronchography is the most accurate method of delineating congenital anomalies of the tracheobronchial tree, but is not indicated unless surgery is contemplated. In conditions such as congenital bronchobiliary fistula—an anomaly of foregut development whose predominant clinical features are recurrent pneumonia and bile-tinged sputum—bronchography can confirm the diagnosis and demonstrate the site of the fistula.[5]

Bronchography can occasionally distinguish an intrapulmonary mass from a mass located outside the lung, such as an extralobar sequestration (Fig. 7–2). Draping of peripheral bronchi around an intrapulmonary sequestration is a characteristic feature. In some cases bronchography may demonstrate communication between normal bronchi and cystic spaces, even in the absence of infection.[17] But diagnosis of this condition can be accomplished more simply and definitively by aortography.

Persistent unequal aeration of the two lungs or of different lobes of the same lung can be evaluated by bronchography (Fig. 7–3). However, radioisotopic procedures or pulmonary arteriography are usually the procedures of choice in evaluating these conditions *(vide infra)*.

TECHNIQUE. Bronchography is performed under general anesthesia for chil-

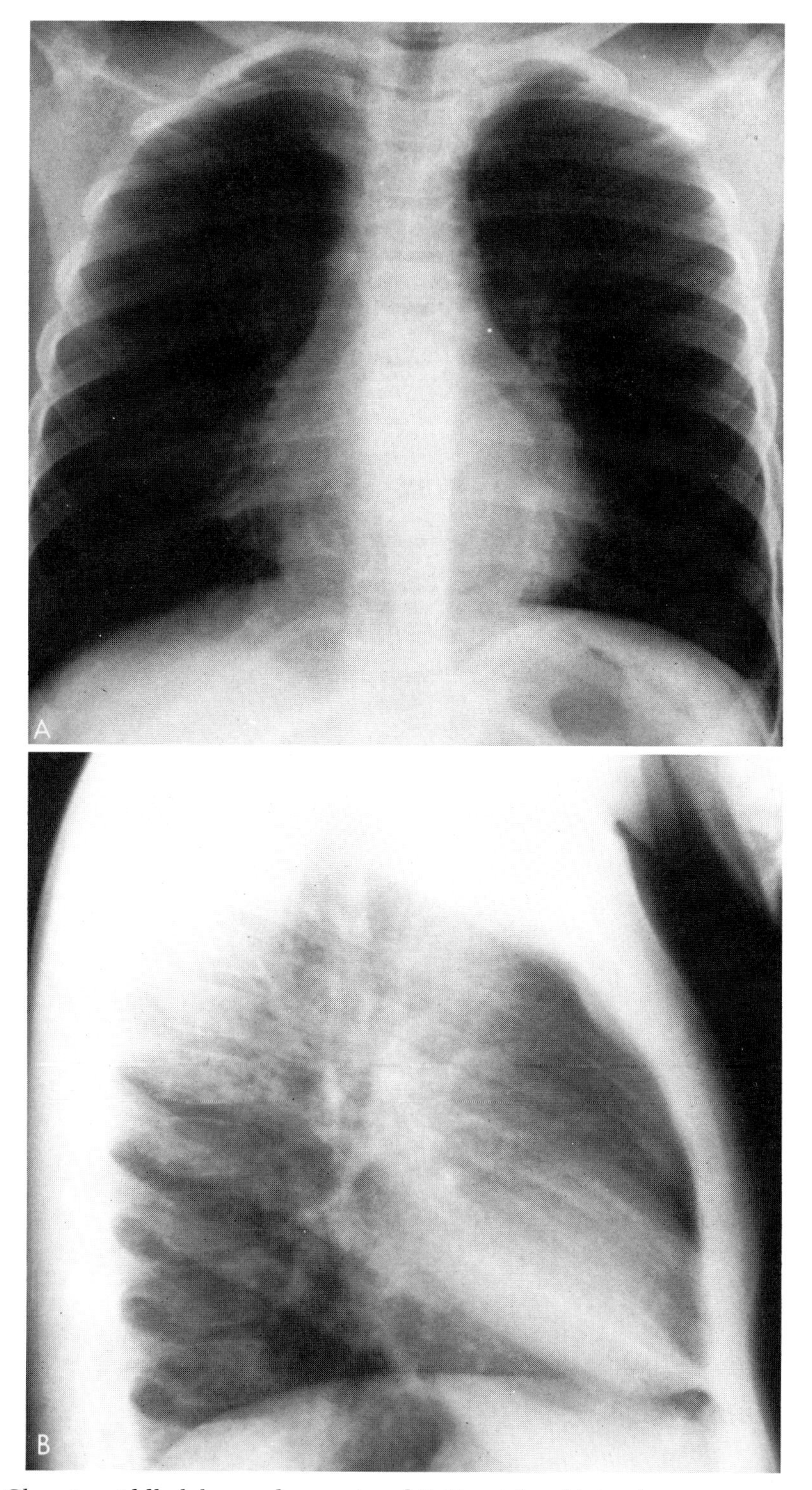

Figure 7–1. Chronic middle lobe syndrome. *A* and *B*. Frontal and lateral roentgenograms in a 10 year old child show right middle lobe atelectasis.

Legend continued on the opposite page

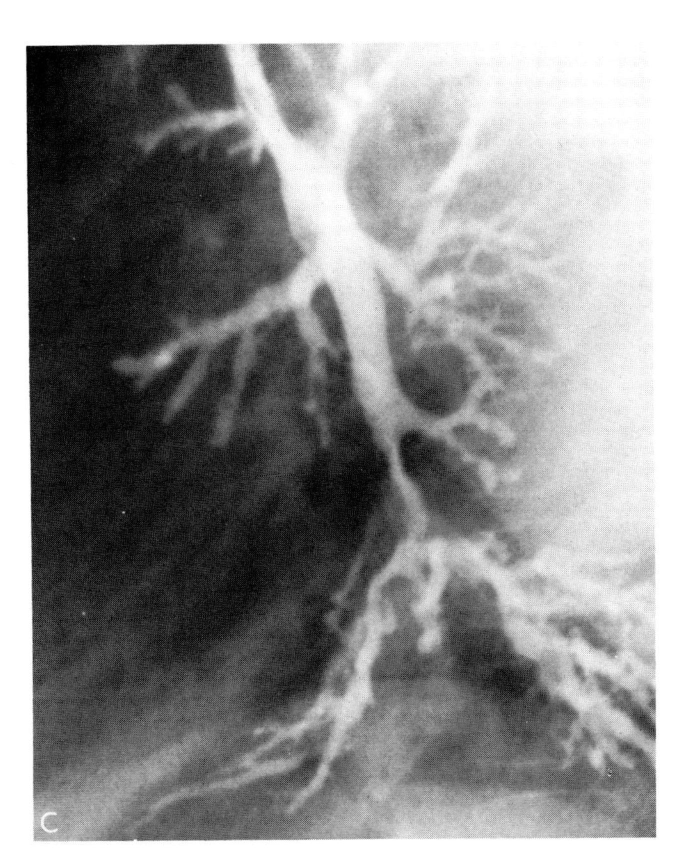

Figure 7–1 Continued. C. Lateral spot film during bronchography reveals nonfilling of the right middle lobe. Mild cylindrical bronchiectasis is demonstrated in the right lower lobe. Bronchoscopy revealed a tiny right middle lobe orifice. Subsequent surgery was performed, with resection of the right middle lobe. The lobar bronchus was compressed and narrowed by adjacent large lymph nodes.

dren in the first decade of life, as well as in older children who are not cooperative. General anesthesia properly administered carries a negligible risk, and the examination can be completed as fast or faster than with topical anesthesia. Many patients undergo bronchoscopy immediately prior to bronchography, and this has not been found to interfere with the procedure. The two procedures are usually performed in combination in the radiology department, where the use of fluoroscopy greatly expedites the performance of the bronchogram and improves the quality of the radiographs obtained. With image intensification the room can be kept well-lighted, allowing satisfactory observation of and easy access to the patient.

The type of premedication administered should routinely include a parasympathetic blocking agent, such as atropine, in order to reduce bronchial secretions and produce better mucosal coating by the contrast medium. The dose of atropine in children is 0.02 mg./kg.—minimum 0.15 mg., maximum 0.60 mg.[12]

The catheter is inserted through the endotracheal tube and is positioned under fluoroscopic control. A curved connector between the ventilating bag and the endotracheal tube is used, with a side opening for insertion of the catheter (Fig. 7–4). A rubber sleeve with a small central orifice is placed over this opening. This prevents air leakage during the examination and therefore promotes dispersion of contrast medium into peripheral bronchi and aids in preventing segmental pulmonary collapse. A straight polyethylene or polyurethane angiographic catheter is employed, the diameter determined by the size of the endotracheal tube and tracheobronchial tree. Angiographic catheters offer moderate rigidity, which facilitates catheter passage and manipulation. The use of curved catheters is not necessary to obtain satisfactory studies.

The problem of segmental or lobar pulmonary volume loss during pediatric bronchography deserves special attention, since it is a potential complication of performing the study under general anesthesia. A re-

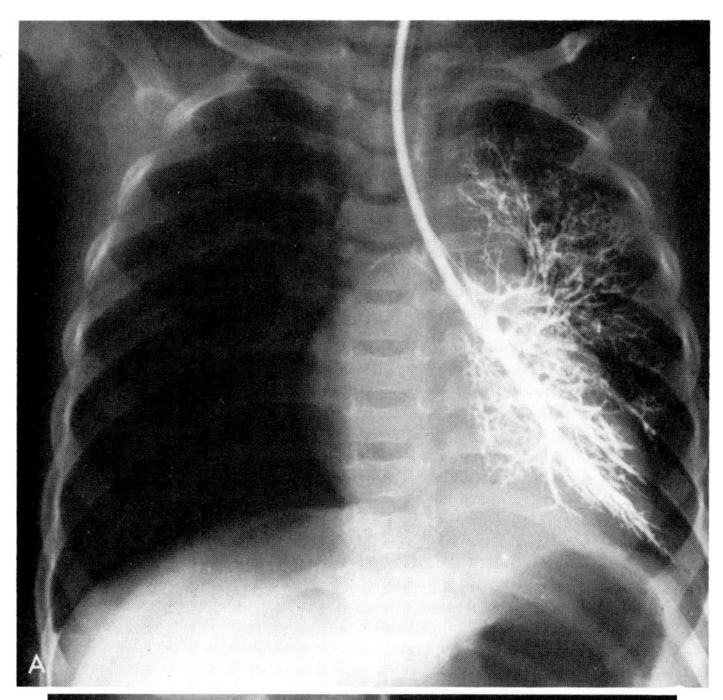

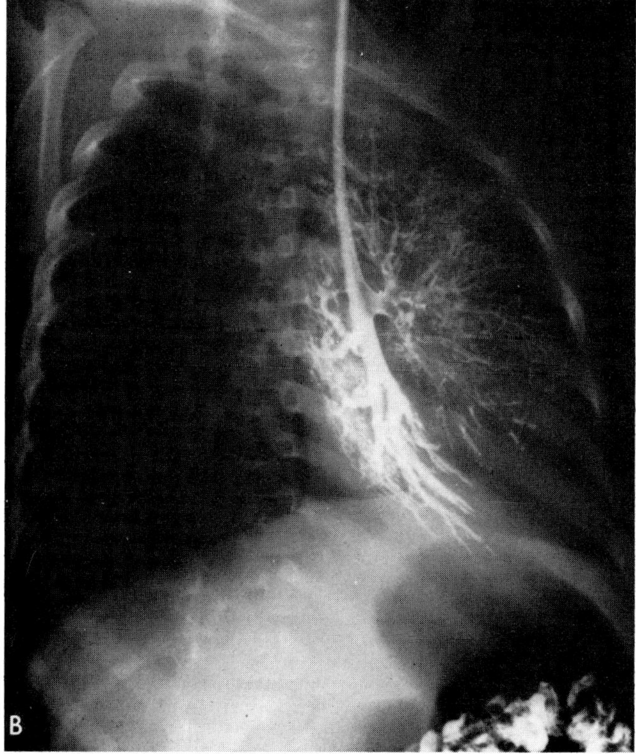

Figure 7–2. Extralobar pulmonary sequestration. *A* and *B*. Frontal and left posterior oblique roentgenograms during bronchography in a 15 month old boy. The peripheral bronchi in the left lower lobe are filled and outline a wedge-shaped extrapulmonary mass in the posteromedial portion of the left hemithorax.

Legend continued on the opposite page

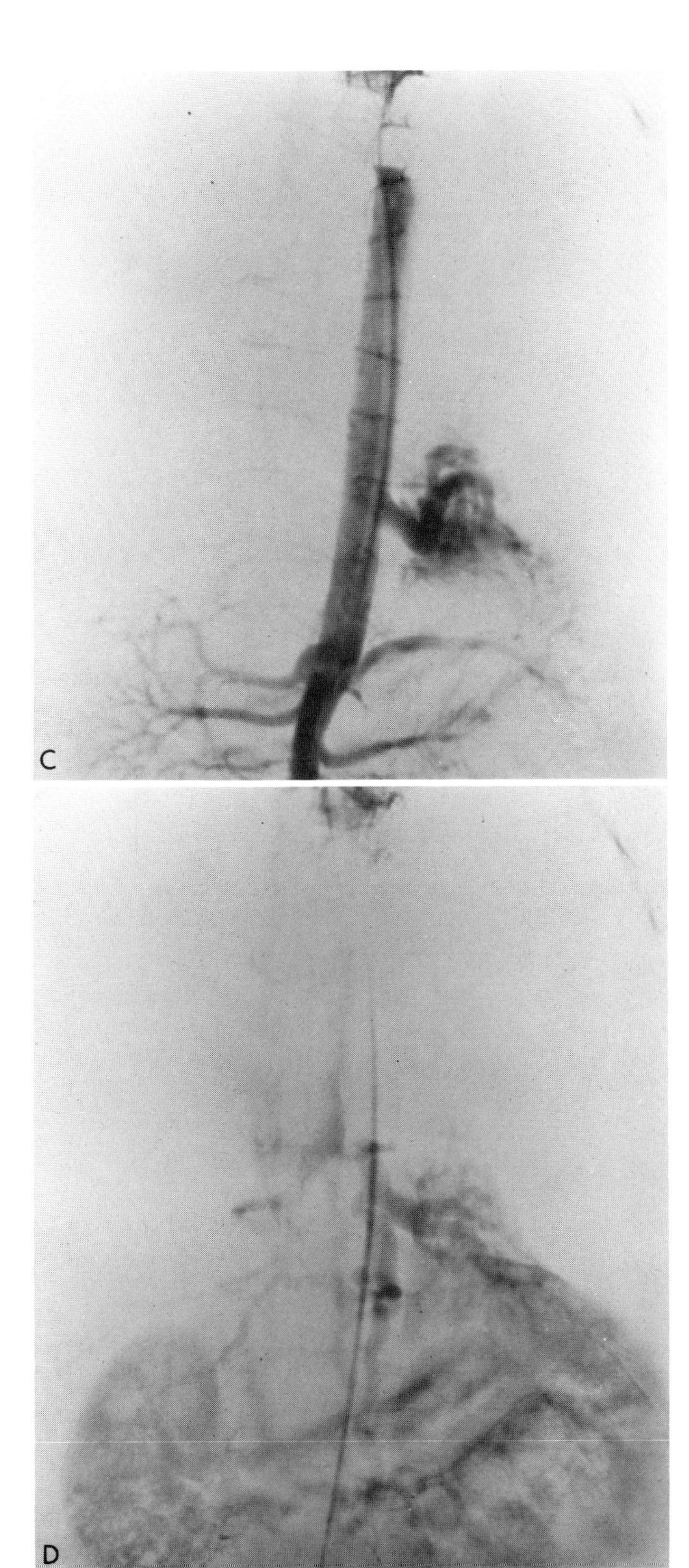

Figure 7–2 Continued. *C* and *D*. Arterial and venous phases of a thoracic aortogram. A large artery supplying the sequestration originates from the lower thoracic aorta, with venous drainage into the hemiazygos system.

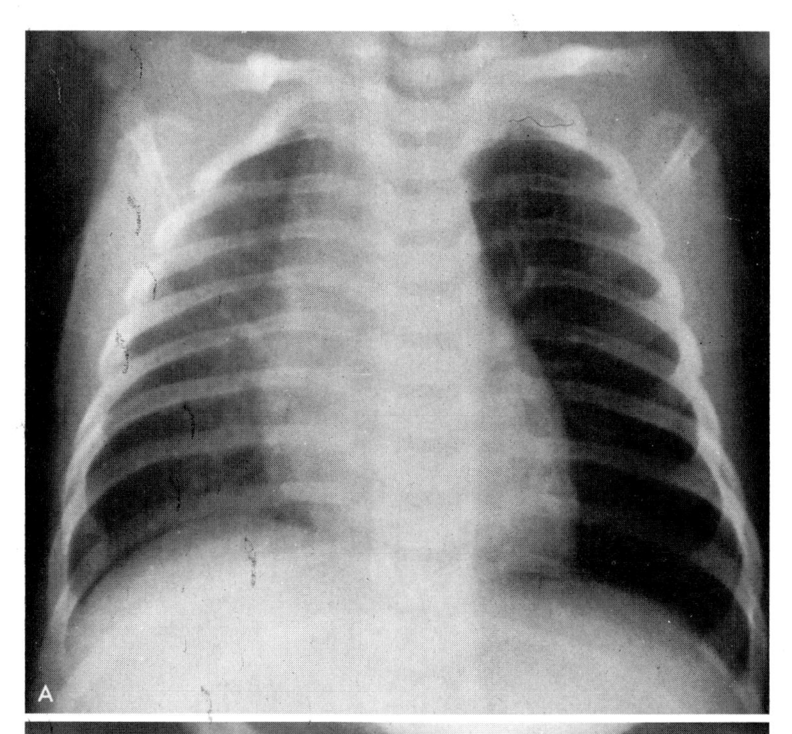

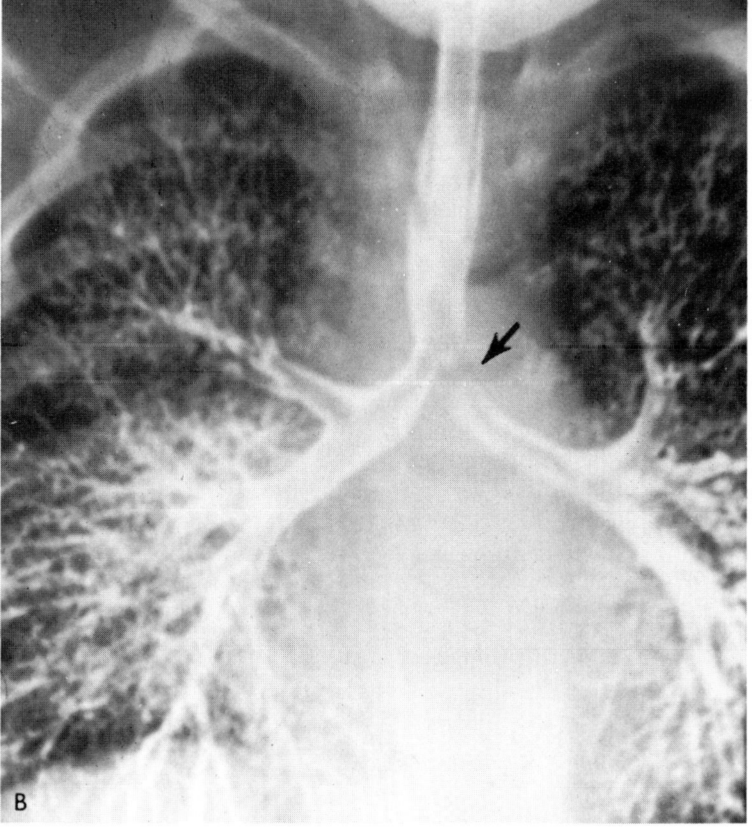

Figure 7–3. Pulmonary artery sling producing obstructive emphysema of the left lung. *A.* Frontal chest roentgenogram in a 3 month old boy shows hyperlucency of the left lung. *B.* Bronchography reveals narrowing of both mainstem bronchi due to compression by the aberrant left pulmonary artery. The narrowing is more severe on the left (arrow), accounting for the obstructive emphysema of the left lung.

Legend continued on the opposite page

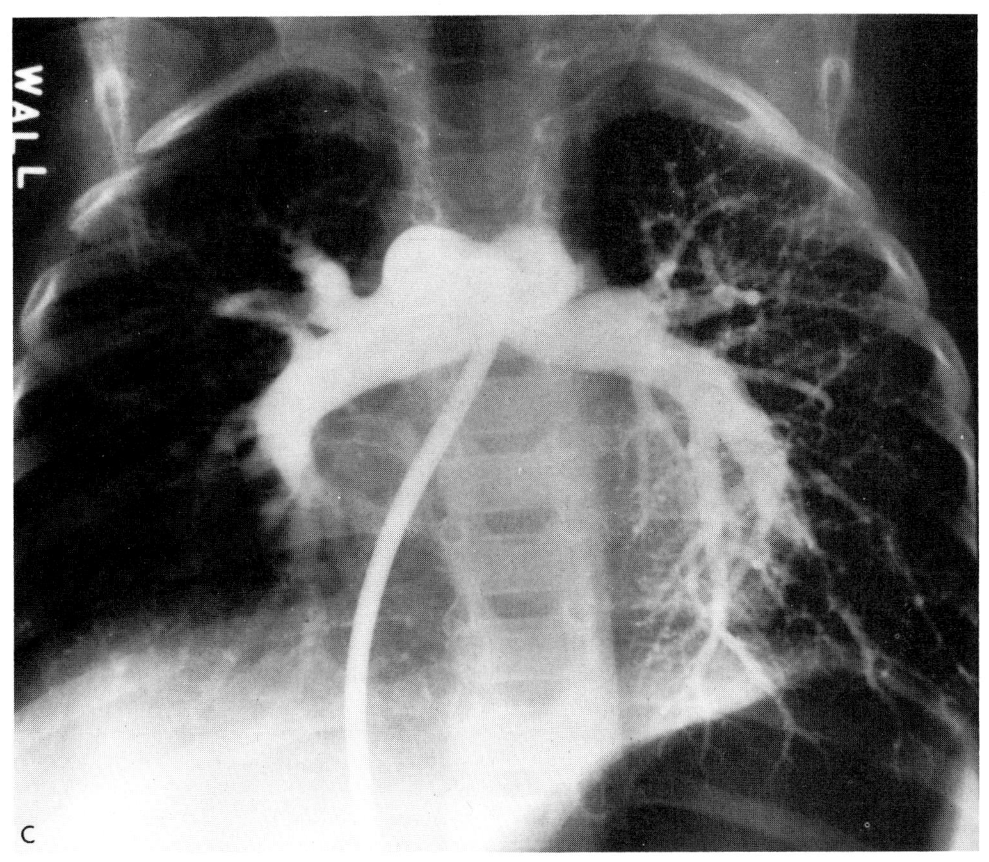

Figure 7–3 Continued. *C*. Pulmonary arteriogram reveals origin of the left pulmonary artery from the right pulmonary artery.

trospective review found volume loss in 45 per cent of 165 pediatric bronchograms performed under general anesthesia.[14] Factors related to collapse, but not necessarily causative, included the use of halothane anesthesia and aqueous contrast agents, and a history of asthma or other allergic states. In addition, volume loss correlated with the use of readily diffusible ventilating gas mixtures. The latter may be the crucial factor in the development of collapse, and support for this thesis was gained from an experimental study in dogs by the same authors.[15] The use of a highly diffusible gas such as 100 per cent oxygen results in absorption of the gas distal to the partially obstructing contrast agent faster than it can be replaced, thus leading to collapse. Because of these data, a less diffusible ventilating mixture, usually 50 per cent oxygen and 50 per cent nitrous oxide, is preferred. This practice, as well as the employment of the rubber sleeve over the opening in the connector through which the catheter is inserted, has greatly reduced the occurrence of segmental volume loss during pediatric bronchography.

As with the adult, oily Dionosil is utilized, with half of the layer of oil decanted prior to shaking the bottle to mix the contents. This practice increases the viscosity of the contrast medium and prevents excessive peripheral filling ("alveolarization").

At the end of the examination, as much of the contrast agent as possible should be removed by suction. Fluoroscopy can facilitate positioning of the suction catheter. This is of utmost importance in children undergoing bronchography under general anesthesia, as transient hypoventilation and depressed cough reflex predispose to atelectasis. Periodic postural drainage is performed until the contrast medium has been nearly completely eliminated.

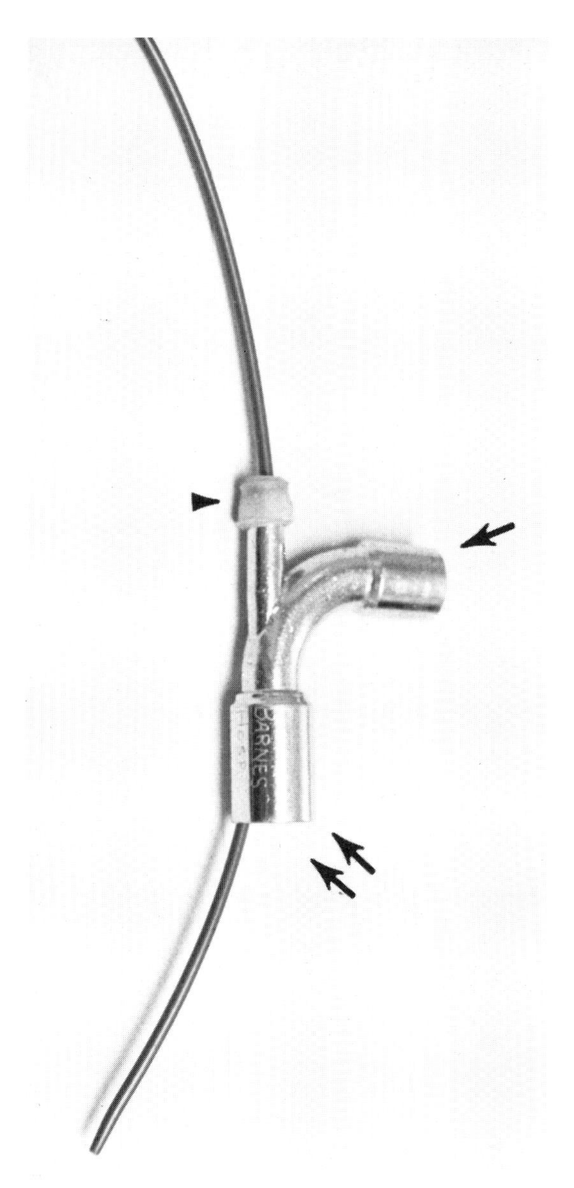

Figure 7–4. Connector device for bronchography under general anesthesia. The inflating bag is attached to the proximal orifice (single arrow). The bronchogram catheter passes through a side opening over which a rubber sleeve is placed to prevent air leak (arrowhead). The connector is attached to the endotracheal tube at the distal orifice (double arrows).

CONTRAINDICATIONS. Pediatric bronchography should not be performed in children with acute pulmonary disease or significant respiratory compromise. The latter contraindication is purposely loosely stated. Each case should be individualized in considering a patient for bronchography. The contrast medium is a partially obstructing substance, and bronchography may be very hazardous in a child with pre-existing airway compromise. Bilateral bronchography can be performed safely during the same examination in most patients, but this should be contingent upon satisfactory clinical status after examination of the first side is completed.

TRACHEOBRONCHIAL WASHOUT FOR ATELECTASIS IN INFANTS AND CHILDREN

A technique for tracheobronchial catheterizaton and lavage in newborn infants with atelectasis has recently been described.[18] While this procedure was initially performed in infants with atelectasis complicating hyaline membrane disease, it can also be utilized in neonates with other underlying lung disease as well as in older children with postoperative atelectasis or mucus impaction secondary to cystic fibrosis.[11] Its use should be restricted to cases in which the atelectasis cannot be alleviated by blind catheter passage and suctioning in the intensive care unit or on the ward (Fig. 7–5). A bedside technique for tracheobronchial washout utilizing pre-curved angiographic catheters has apparently increased the frequency of successful re-expansion on the ward.[9] However, the advantage of fluoroscopically monitored positioning of the catheter directly in the occluded bronchus makes this technique the preferred alternative in instances in which other measures have failed to produce re-expansion.

A properly planned and meticulously performed procedure can be carried out with only minor stress, even in infants with severe respiratory distress. A warmed environment is provided on the fluoroscopic table. An angiographic catheter with a Luer-Lok attachment and a mild "J" curve at the distal end is employed routinely. Catheters with different curves may be used as needed. The catheter is introduced through a previously inserted endotracheal tube and is positioned in the occluded bronchus under direct fluoroscopic control; 0.5 ml. of normal saline is instilled, and manual suction with a syringe is applied. Multiple lavages and suctions may be per-

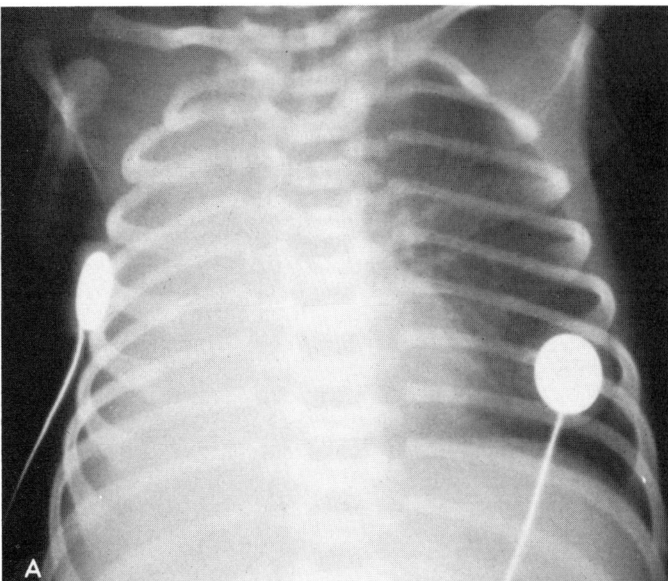

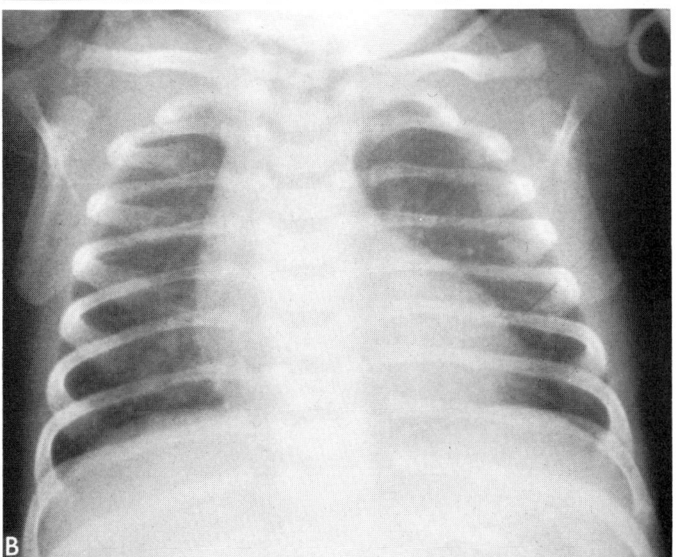

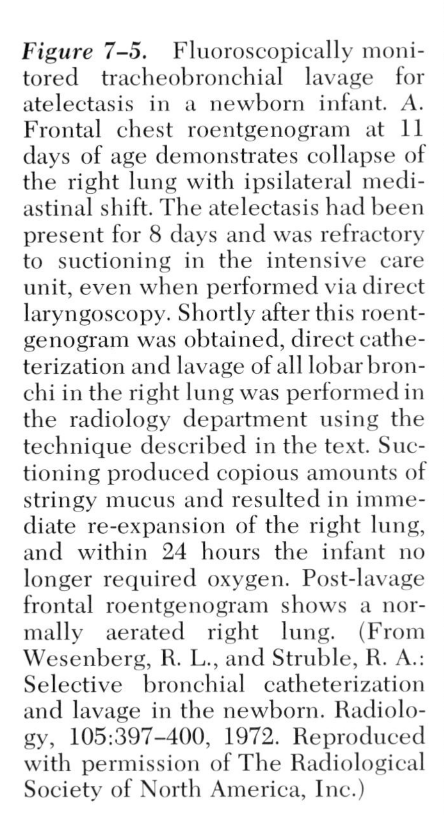
Figure 7–5. Fluoroscopically monitored tracheobronchial lavage for atelectasis in a newborn infant. *A.* Frontal chest roentgenogram at 11 days of age demonstrates collapse of the right lung with ipsilateral mediastinal shift. The atelectasis had been present for 8 days and was refractory to suctioning in the intensive care unit, even when performed via direct laryngoscopy. Shortly after this roentgenogram was obtained, direct catheterization and lavage of all lobar bronchi in the right lung was performed in the radiology department using the technique described in the text. Suctioning produced copious amounts of stringy mucus and resulted in immediate re-expansion of the right lung, and within 24 hours the infant no longer required oxygen. Post-lavage frontal roentgenogram shows a normally aerated right lung. (From Wesenberg, R. L., and Struble, R. A.: Selective bronchial catheterization and lavage in the newborn. Radiology, 105:397–400, 1972. Reproduced with permission of The Radiological Society of North America, Inc.)

formed as needed, with oxygen administered during the intervals.

PULMONARY AND THORACIC ARTERIOGRAPHY

The most common indication for pulmonary arteriography in children is the study of suspected congenital malformations of the lungs or pulmonary vessels.[10] Anomalies of the thoracic aorta or its branches constitute the major indication for thoracic aortography.

Many of these anomalies have respiratory signs and symptoms as their primary clinical manifestation. Vascular rings, tracheal indentation by an anomalous innominate or left common carotid artery, and pulmonary artery sling may produce stridor. The latter condition may also produce regional hyper- or hypo-aeration of either lung[6] (Fig. 7–3). Pulmonary arteriography has also been found to be safe and diagnostic in other conditions producing unequal aeration of the lungs in children, including absent or hypoplastic pulmonary artery and lung, scimitar syndrome, and hyperlucent lung or lobe.[8] Other conditions with primary pulmonary manifestations which can be diagnosed by pulmonary arteriography include total anomalous pulmonary venous return with obstruction to venous return, and pulmonary arteriovenous fistula.

The safety of pulmonary arteriography in the small infant constitutes one of the chief advantages of this procedure and makes it preferable to bronchography in many instances. This is particularly true in children with significant underlying pulmonary disease or partial airway obstruction, in whom the partially obstructing bronchographic contrast medium may further compromise the airway. In addition, thoracic and pulmonary angiography permit definitive diagnosis of those conditions with vascular anomalies, such as sequestration (Fig. 7–2) or pulmonary artery sling (Fig. 7–3).

The examination is performed with the child under sedation. There is no need for general anesthesia. Percutaneous entry into the femoral artery or vein is the preferred method of catheter insertion.[16] With practice the necessary skill can be acquired, and the study can be completed in a shorter period of time and with less trauma to the vessel than with the cut-down approach.

TOMOGRAPHY

Tomography has limited applicability and utility in pediatric chest disease, especially in very young children. Technical problems created by a necessarily long exposure in a patient who cannot remain apneic throughout its duration often render an image of poor quality. High quality plain roentgenograms, fluoroscopy, and spot filming usually provide satisfactory information with less radiation dosage to the patient than with tomography. High kilovoltage radiography has proved to be particularly valuable in the delineation of the central tracheobronchial tree and has further lessened the need for tomography—and even tracheobronchography—in the evaluation of these structures.

Nevertheless, there are occasional instances in which tomography in young children can provide diagnostically useful information, as in evaluating masses for presence of calcification, in distinguishing enlarged hilar lymph nodes from vessels, in demonstrating feeding arteries and draining veins in sequestrations and arteriovenous malformations, and in outlining the central tracheobronchial tree in cases in which plain roentgenograms have not successfully done so.

Tomography is most readily accomplished with the child in the supine position and securely immobilized. It is impossible to obtain exposure times short enough to abolish all respiratory motion in patients too young to cooperate, but by increasing the thickness of the section the exposure time can be decreased somewhat, resulting in more acceptable clarity. The number of exposures should be strictly limited to those which are absolutely necessary, since the radiation dose is considerably greater than with plain roentgenograms.[3]

DIRECT MAGNIFICATION TECHNIQUE

Direct magnification chest radiography is a technique which is not widely used in newborn infants, primarily because of the lack of necessary equipment. Most radiologists are conversant with the essentials of direct magnification radiography, which include a small effective focal spot, air-gap between patient and film, and, usually, no grid. Technical factors for a newborn chest examination producing a magnification factor of 2.5× include 114–125 kVp (3 phase), 3 mA, focus-to film distance 57 in., focus-to-midchest distance 23 in., approximately 0.3 mm. effective focal spot size, par-speed screen, and Kodak Blue Brand film.[1] For use with 90-second processing, a Kodak X-OMATIC Regular Intensifying Screen with X-OMATIC G film can be used, with identical technical factors.

Advantages of the direct magnification technique are that it can demonstrate small structures or densities not visible or poorly seen on conventional roentgenograms, such as faint granularity of early hyaline membrane disease, and that it facilitates the differentiation of parenchymal lung densities from vessels (Fig. 7–6). A major

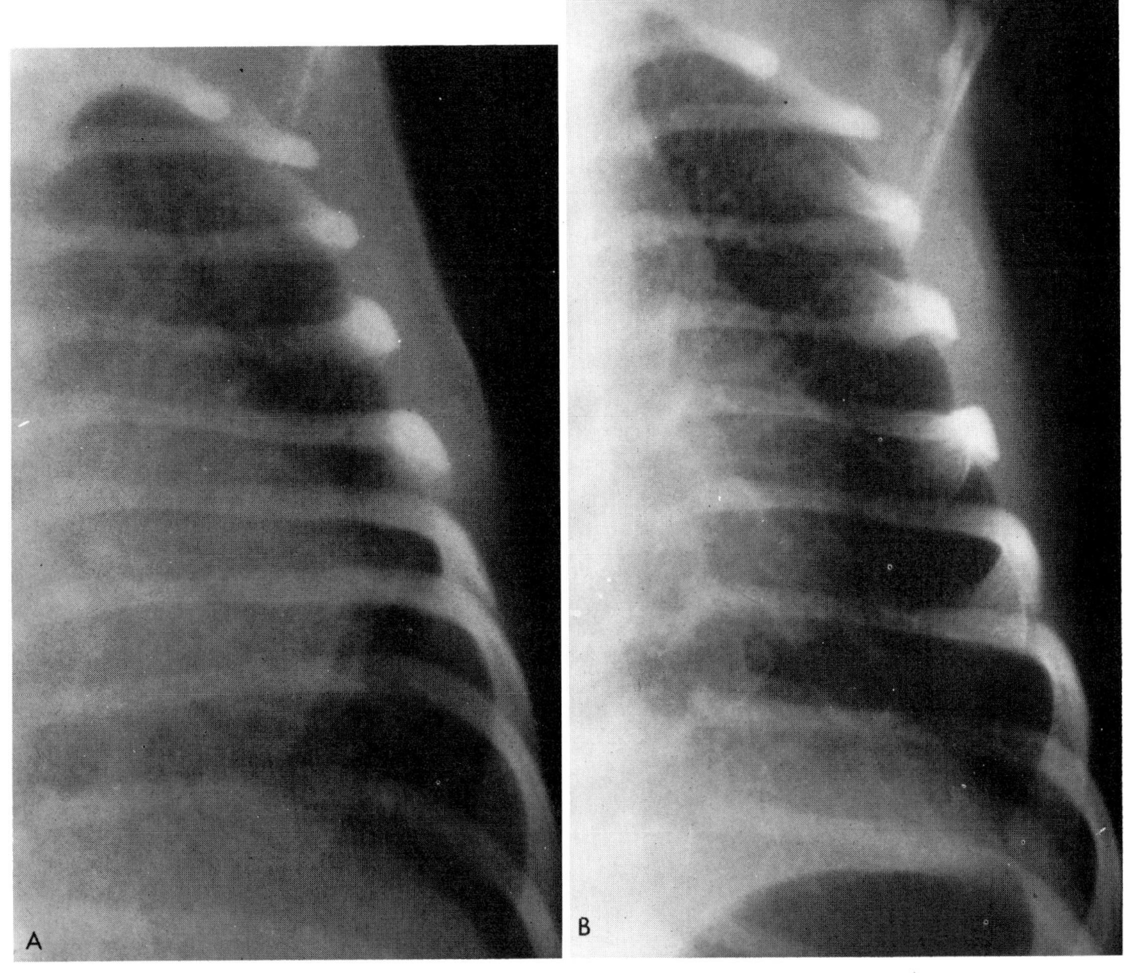

Figure 7–6. Magnification chest roentgenography. *A.* Left lung, anteroposterior roentgenogram, standard technique with 1 mm. focal spot. *B.* Left lung, anteroposterior roentgenogram, direct roentgenographic magnification technique utilizing 0.3 mm. focal spot. Note increased, sharper detail.

disadvantage, however, is a considerable increase in radiation dose to the patient, which is approximately seven times greater than with conventional radiography.[1]

In view of the noted advantages and disadvantages, magnification roentgenograms are generally obtained only when conventional radiographs are inconclusive.

BIBLIOGRAPHY

1. Ablow, R. C., Greenspan, R. H., and Gluck, L.: The advantages of direct magnification technique in the newborn chest. Radiology, 92:745–750, 1969.
2. Avery, M. E.: Bronchography: Outmoded procedure? Pediatrics, *46*:333–334, 1970.
3. Bernard, J., Sauvegrain, J., and Nahum, H.: Tomography of the lungs in infancy and childhood: Techniques, indications and results. Progr. Pediat. Radiol., *1*:59–90, 1967.
4. Brünner, S.: Tracheography and bronchography: Techniques and indications during infancy and childhood. Progr. Pediat. Radiol., *1*:45–58, 1967.
5. Caffey, J.: Pediatric X-Ray Diagnosis, Sixth Edition. Chicago, Year Book Medical Publishers, 1972, p. 1533.
6. Capitanio, M. A., Ramos, R., and Kirkpatrick, J. A.: Pulmonary sling. Roentgen observations.
7. Dees, S. C., and Spock, A.: Right middle lobe syndrome in children. JAMA, *197*:78–84, 1966.
8. Franken, E. A., Jr., Hurwitz, R. A., and Battersby,

J. S.: Unequal aeration of the lungs in children. The use of pulmonary angiography. Radiology, *109*:401–408, 1973.

9. Galvis, A. G., White, J. J., and Oh, K. S.: A bedside washout technqiue for atelectasis in infants. Amer. J. Dis. Child., *127*:824–827, 1974.
10. Gooding, C. A.: Pulmonary angiography. *In* Gyepes, M. T., editor: Angiography in Infants and Children New York, Grune and Stratton, Inc., 1974, pp. 99–138.
11. Heller, R. M., Galvis, A. G., and Oh, K. S.: Angiographic catheters for tracheobronchial procedures in infants and children. Radiology, *106*:702–703, 1973.
12. Nelson, W. E.: Textbook of Pediatrics, Ninth Edition. Philadelphia, W. B. Saunders Co., 1969, p. 314.
13. Robinson, A. E., and Campbell, J. B.: Bronchography in childhood asthma. Amer. J. Roentgen., *116*:559–566, 1972.
14. Robinson, A. E., Hall, K. D., Yokoyama, K. N., and Capp, M. P.: Pediatric bronchography: The problem of segmental pulmonary loss of volume. I.A. Retrospective study of 165 pediatric bronchograms. Invest. Radiol., *6*:89–94, 1971.
15. Robinson, A. E., Hall, K. D., Yokoyama, K. N., and Capp, M. P.: Pediatric bronchography: The problem of segmental pulmonary loss of volume. II. An experimental investigation of the mechanism and prevention of pulmonary collapse during bronchography under general anesthesia. Invest. Radiol., *6*:95–100, 1971.
16. Takahashi, M.: Percutaneous catheterization in infants and children. *In* Gyepes, M. T., editor: Angiography in Infants and Children. New York, Grune and Stratton, Inc., 1974, pp. 29–48.
17. Takahashi, M., Ohno, M., Mihara, K., Matsuura, K., and Sumiyoshi, A.: Intralobar pulmonary sequestration. With special emphasis on bronchial communication. Radiology, *114*: 543–549, 1975.
18. Wesenberg, R. L., and Struble, R. A.: Selective bronchial catheterization and lavage in the newborn. A new therapeutic procedure for diagnostic radiology. Radiology, *105*:397–400, 1972.

INDEX

Page numbers in *italics* indicate illustrations.